EDUCATING HEALTH PROFESSIONALS: BECOMI

PRACTICE, EDUCATION, WORK AND SOCIETY
Volume 8

Other books in this Series:

1. Higgs, J., Horsfall, D., & Grace, S. (2009). *Writing qualitative research on practice*. Rotterdam, The Netherlands: Sense Publishers.

2. Higgs, J., Cherry, N., Macklin, R., & Ajjawi, R. (Eds.) (2010). *Researching practice: A discourse on qualitative methodologies*. Rotterdam, The Netherlands: Sense Publishers.

3. Higgs, J., Fish, D., Goulter, I., Loftus, S., Reid, J., & Trede, F. (Eds.) (2010). *Education for future practice*. Rotterdam, The Netherlands: Sense Publishers.

4. McAllister, L., Paterson, M., Higgs, J., & Bithell, C. (Eds.) (2010). *Innovations in allied health fieldwork education: A critical appraisal*. Rotterdam, The Netherlands: Sense Publishers.

5. Higgs, J., Titchen, A., Horsfall, D., & Bridges, D. (Eds.) (2011). *Creative spaces for qualitative researching: Living research*. Rotterdam, The Netherlands: Sense Publishers.

6. Higgs, J., Barnett, R., Billett, S., Hutchings, M., & Trede, F. (Eds.) (2012). *Practice-based education: Perspectives and strategies.* Rotterdam, The Netherlands: Sense Publishers.

7. Higgs, J., Letts, W., Sheehan, D., Baldry Currens, J., & Jensen, G. (Eds.) (2013). *Realising exemplary practice-based education*. Rotterdam, The Netherlands: Sense Publishers

Educating Health Professionals: Becoming a University Teacher

Edited by

Stephen Loftus
The Education For Practice Institute
Charles Sturt University, Australia

Tania Gerzina
Faculty of Dentistry
The University of Sydney, Australia

Joy Higgs
The Education For Practice Institute
Charles Sturt University, Australia

Megan Smith
Faculty of Science
Charles Sturt University, Australia

and

Elaine Duffy
School of Nursing and Midwifery
Griffith University, Australia

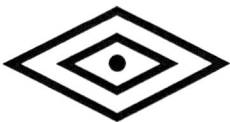

SENSE PUBLISHERS
ROTTERDAM / BOSTON / TAIPEI

A C.I.P. record for this book is available from the Library of Congress.

ISBN 978-94-6209-351-5 (paperback)
ISBN 978-94-6209-352-2 (hardback)
ISBN 978-94-6209-353-9 (e-book)

Published by: Sense Publishers,
P.O. Box 21858, 3001 AW Rotterdam, The Netherlands
https://www.sensepublishers.com/

Printed on acid-free paper

TABLE OF CONTENTS

Section 3: Teaching and Research

Section 4: Case Studies

Section 5: Future Directions

JOY HIGGS

SERIES INTRODUCTION

Practice, Education, Work and Society

This series examines research, theory and practice in the context of university education, professional practice, work and society. The series explores places where two or more of these arenas come together. Themes that are explored in the series include: university education of professions, society expectations of professional practice, professional practice workplaces and strategies for investigating each of these areas. There are many challenges facing researchers, educators, practitioners and students in today's practice worlds. The authors in this series bring a wealth of practice wisdom and experience to examine these issues, share their practice knowledge, report research into strategies that address these challenges, share approaches to working and learning and raise yet more questions.

The conversations conducted in the series will contribute to expanding the discourse around the way people encounter and experience practice, education, work and society.

Joy Higgs, Charles Sturt University, Australia

FOREWORD

This book is intended for academics and for health professionals in workplace settings who are involved in educating health professionals. Some of these educators are scientists from outside the health professions, some have taken an academic path soon after graduating from the health professions and bring both a (sometimes distant) professional background as well as academic qualifications and experience to their role, some are practitioners newly entering academia and some are practitioners who take on the role of workplace educators for health professional students.

For each group there are many issues to deal with. These issues range from learning about teaching and learning strategies, learning to do research (often for the first time), managing workplace learning or interprofessional learning, learning to deal with assessment, engaging with issues of educational internationalisation, coping with the demands of standards and accreditation, to becoming involved in curriculum review and design. These issues cannot be dealt with superficially and they will seriously engage the attention of health professional educators. These are issues that are complex and have no easy answers but which are at the heart of higher education in general and health professional education, in particular.

There is a growing volume of literature on the education of health professionals. Many publications can be seen as 'survival guides' helping newcomers to survive their first few weeks in a university environment. This book is different. While there is much sound, practical advice in this book that can be applied quickly, its main intention is more long term, i.e. to introduce newcomers to the conversations and issues that will occupy a great deal of their time and attention as educators. We have endeavoured to provide an introduction to the major concerns that will confront health professional educators so that they will be informed and able to engage with the complexities that make up university and workplace teaching and learning in the health professions, today and for years to come.

There are several sections to this book:

1. **Introduction**: This section looks at what it means to be a health professional who is also an educator.

2. **Health professional education in context**: This section explores issues such as the personal and professional development of educators as well as the expectations that society has of our graduates.

3. **Teaching and research**: This section opens up a range of issues such as curriculum, standards, the student experience and interprofessional education among others.

4. **Case studies**: In this section we take a close look at examples that include internationalisation, blended learning, workplace learning and the teaching of clinical reasoning.

5. **Future directions**: The final section takes a critical look at current trends and discusses how the future of health professional education could develop.

Stephen Loftus

SECTION 1: INTRODUCTION

STEPHEN LOFTUS AND TANIA GERZINA

1. BEING A HEALTH PROFESSIONAL EDUCATOR

Understanding the Context

The core purpose of health professional education is to prepare practitioners who can cope with the many demands of working in a range of health settings, not only as these settings exist today but also as they might exist tomorrow. This can include traditional clinical roles in metropolitan and regional hospitals, suburban and rural clinics, specialist centres and the many varieties of community care.

Many health professionals will become involved in other responsibilities besides the purely clinical, such as management, research and education. This complex mixture of demands means that the education we provide must equip our new graduates with the knowledge, the skills and the resources of character that will enable them to cope with the uncertainty that arises out of such complexity.

However, we want our graduates to do more than just cope. We want them to flourish and thrive as health professionals who are not only competent technically, but who understand and embody the underlying values of their chosen profession. We want them to be health professionals who relate to patients/clients as human beings and who can integrate new knowledge and insights into their practice as these become available in the course of their careers. Preparing people for the health professions of the 21st century is therefore a formidable task and not to be taken lightly.

THE PROFESSIONAL PRACTICE OF HIGHER EDUCATION

Educating new practitioners for the health professions can be, and should be, a rewarding and interesting experience. For many practitioners a career in higher education offers the chance to combine an interest in their professional practice with the opportunity to prepare new practitioners who will themselves go on to be enthusiastic, well-prepared, and capable of carrying on the profession to high standards. Some might describe such a teaching career as a vocation rather than just a career, as it requires real commitment from those who undertake it.

There are challenges in becoming a professional teacher and academic which are not to be underestimated. Most prominent of these challenges is the state of seemingly never-ending change imposed by a range of parties and communities. Professional practice itself may be steadily changing in many ways, but our understanding of what university education is, and how to conduct it, is also undergoing rapid change and is likely to do so into the foreseeable future. New and prospective academics need to be fully aware of these challenges and ready and

S. Loftus et al. (Eds.), Educating Health Professionals:
Becoming a University Teacher, 3–14.
© *2013 Sense Publishers. All rights reserved.*

willing to deal with them if they are ever to be successful university teachers. Perhaps the journey is best taken by those willing and prepared to cope with change as normal and expected.

Living in a World of Change

It is almost a cliché to say that we live in a world of change, but this is certainly true of academic life in the early 21st century. Change comes from many different directions, from educational technology, from new understandings of what professional education should entail, from educational policy change that might, for example, affect the balance between service, research and teaching activity.

Society's expectations of higher education are also changing, with more people being encouraged and expected to complete tertiary education. This means that higher education is no longer seen as a privilege reserved for an intellectual elite who are strongly motivated and need little support. The increased participation rate in higher education brings with it the requirement to provide greater support so that people from a wide variety of backgrounds can engage with tertiary education and graduate at the level required for professional practice.

To highlight the first example of change in higher education, the emergence and continued development of educational technology now allows us to provide much richer learning experiences for our students – but only if applied wisely. Educational technology allows us to offer open-source and mobile options including sophisticated simulations through which students can try out many scenarios and develop different kinds of expertise and, above all, make mistakes where patients will not be harmed if things go wrong. There is further discussion of educational technology and blended learning in Chapter 21. Mastering educational technology is just one aspect of the modern practice of higher education.

Research and Scholarship of Higher Education

One of the most exciting aspects of being involved in higher education today is that it has been and continues to be the subject of sustained and rigorous research and scholarship. This scholarly activity has raised our awareness of many issues and produced insights that are of real and practical use for university teachers seeking to offer a high-quality education. Some insights seem obvious. For example, the notion of constructive alignment in the curriculum is now widely accepted and consciously implemented.

In the past there have been many examples of courses that espoused noble aims, such as developing critical thinking in their students. Yet close examination of the enacted curricula often revealed that in many cases these lofty goals were rarely or poorly taught and might not even have been assessed. Research demonstrates that, for students, assessment drives what they learn and the choices they make in their learning habits. (For an introduction to this work see Biggs & Tang, 2011.) Therefore, careful attention to assessment and ensuring that it aligns with what we aspire to teach and what we actually teach (i.e. constructive alignment) is more

4

likely to bring about a course that achieves its aims. This may seem obvious, but it is remarkable how often it is still not realised in many courses. Chapter 20 provides further exploration of assessment. Assessment can also be linked to the ideas of self-assessment and metacognition. This creates yet another challenge for university teachers to address, in shared responsibility with students, students' capacity for and commitment to lifelong learning.

There is now a renewed awareness of the importance of thinking about curriculum issues more deeply, beyond constructive alignment (refer to the discussion of curriculum theory in Chapter 11). For now, we simply note that simplistic understandings of what constitutes learning and teaching have led to unnecessary suffering for students in the past, because some university teachers in the past have thought of students as blank slates (*tabula rasa*) to be filled in and have followed a strategy of cramming as much material into a course as possible. We now realise that this led to superficial or surface learning, where students were required simply to memorise material in order to reproduce it in an exam, but without having the chance to truly understand what it was they were learning or how it might apply to practice. Students often struggled with such over-burdened courses. Poor learning outcomes were blamed on students rather than on courses deeply in need of "decompression".

MODELS OF EDUCATION

There are reports going back to the mid-19th century (see General Medical Council, 1993) claiming that medical courses were too full, but because the underlying belief was that students had to be "filled up" with knowledge, the practice of cramming courses continued, and arguably became worse. As medical science advanced there was competition between different disciplines, with each believing that its disciplinary knowledge was crucial and had to be included in the educational program.

Another problem, for the education of doctors in particular, was that medical schools were able to point out that the doctors they graduated did, on the whole, become proficient practitioners. What was ignored was the fact that medical students tend to be bright and highly motivated, and that medical students were graduating from medical school and becoming good doctors not because of the educational experience provided but in spite of it.

Fortunately, this situation began changing in the latter half of the 20th century when newer models of education, such as those utilising problem-based learning, began to emerge. Instead of expecting students to simply know everything, there was recognition that it was possible to focus on a "core" body of knowledge and how it was to be used in practice. It began to be accepted that professional practitioners could never know everything upon graduation, or at any time in their careers, and they would need to become lifelong learners.

In light of such an approach, discovering an area of ignorance is now generally regarded as a prompt to go and find out, rather than as a fault that needs to be punished. Newer educational models make a conscious and explicit attempt to foster lifelong learning. On a critical note, however, the question of whether the newer courses will truly encourage students to become lifelong learners is still contentious (Newman, 2003).

More recently, courses that are oriented around whole-of-course frameworks as opposed to collections of subjects have been widely adopted across health professional programs. A typical example of a whole-of-course framework, now widely accepted, is that of problem-based learning (PBL). In PBL the curriculum is founded on a series of clinical cases, based on real patients. In designing the cases, the curriculum team makes a conscious effort to integrate as many relevant subjects as possible. So, for example, a patient with heart disease will prompt students to study the anatomy, physiology and biochemistry of the heart and how they are relevant to the present case. The same case could be used to integrate the social sciences if it turns out that smoking, lack of exercise and poor diet have been contributing factors. Further subjects, such as ethics and medical economics, can be integrated into the case by creating a "patient" who is elderly, incapable of living alone, and occupying a bed in an acute ward that is desperately needed for other patients. The strength of the PBL approach is that the different subjects can be related to each other and to real-world practice in a relatively seamless manner.

In these courses, academics need to adopt a new mind-set in their teaching. In such courses, academics who are used to more old-fashioned pedagogy will need to exercise restraint and resist the temptation to impart as much information as possible, as quickly as possible, to their students. Becoming a facilitator of other people's learning rather than a lecturer who simply dispenses knowledge is just one of the challenges to be met by anyone who aspires to be a professional and a university educator today. Beginning teachers need to educate themselves about the range of new educational models; problem-based learning just happens to be one of the most popular. How successful, or otherwise, teachers are in engaging with new educational models has not been widely investigated. The predominant focus of research is often on students rather than on teachers. There is much scope for research into how academics can become successful university teachers.

For university teachers in the health professions, the knowledge that needs to be learned includes what is relevant both to the professional practice of healthcare and the professional practice of university teaching. About the same time as the newer educational models began to emerge, education of other health professions began moving into universities and, unburdened with a long tradition of university education, these professions were willing to question and critique prevailing models of medical and dental education and to rethink how health professionals should be prepared for the world of professional practice.

Nursing, for example, largely adopted a model of patient care. There was a conscious attempt to put an emphasis on the care of patients as human beings rather than as biological organisms that had pathology to be treated (Meerabeau, 2004). This was nursing care that, while informed by biomedical science, was quite different from the treatment of pathology that seemed to dominate the curricula of the older health professions that had participated in university education for many decades.

6

The emergence of higher education for other health professions highlighted the need to examine other aspects of healthcare besides the biomedical sciences, such as sociocultural aspects. The growing literature on clinical reasoning can be seen as an attempt to integrate all these aspects (Higgs, Jones, Loftus, & Christensen, 2008). This need for integration highlights another quality required by the professional who is also a teacher and an academic, which is the ability to access, interpret, value, apply and contribute to research and evidence-based practice, often of both their professional knowledge and their teaching. One response to this call has been research-based teaching.

Fish and Coles (2005) wrote of research-based teaching as one of three models that can be used to categorise the majority of courses provided to health professionals. The oldest model they called the *product model*, in which education was seen as a product to be passed on as efficiently as possible from teacher to student. This has been by far the most common model used in the education of health professionals. Some of the weaknesses of this model have been mentioned earlier, but can be summarised as assuming that the transmission of knowledge is simple and unproblematic. It is now clear that this is a simplistic view, even though there will be occasions where it is appropriate to use a transmission model. Many of the newer courses fit within what Fish and Coles described as a *process model*; case-based approaches such as problem-based learning fit within this model. Here, teachers are seen as facilitators, encouraging students to manage their own learning.

However, teachers are still very much in control of the process and provide strong direction as to what students should learn. Fish and Coles promoted a third model, which they called the *research model*. Here, the ideal is that students and teachers learn together and students use academics more as supervisors of their developing understanding than as learning facilitators. One particular version of the research model is research-led teaching, about which we say more below.

The emphasis in the research model of education is on the development of a critical understanding of knowledge, and especially a critical understanding of the underlying principles of professional practice that can contextualise knowledge in any setting. The implication is that in settings where practitioners do not hold all the necessary knowledge to deal with new professional problems they can still base their actions on underlying principles and make professional judgements that are considered and justifiable. Underpinning all this, there is an emphasis on professional values.

Fish and Coles (2005) claimed that when designing or reviewing a curriculum it is important to begin by articulating the professional values that would underpin the course and characterise the graduates who go out into the workplace. These values, such as being professional, being reflective, being critical or being ethical, must explicitly inform the course, and conscious attention should be given to making them explicit to staff and students, with the express intention that the students should come to accept and embody these values for themselves.

This raises the question of how we can teach these aspects of professional practice. The answer is that we must provide role models and we, the teachers, must be those role models. Professional practitioners who are also university teachers must embody these qualities in their own practice so that students can see the qualities being enacted. Students have to see that *we* behave professionally, reflectively, critically and ethically.

A well-designed curriculum is likely to produce many occasions when these values can be enacted, and at key points a perceptive practitioner/teacher can point out to students how and when these values are playing an important role. It is also important to encourage students to engage with these values and become familiar with discussing them. This explicit engagement with values can bring a degree of authenticity to education. It is said that students have a strong resonance with education and careers that support their plans for an authentic quality to their lives; this is a dimension to be considered when a practitioner is a role model (Osipow, 1990). For example, many cases in a problem-based learning course can be designed to raise ethical and social issues for staff and students to explore together.

RESEARCH-ENHANCED LEARNING AND TEACHING

Among the central goals of any university is the continued development of its intellectual environment. Research-enhanced learning and teaching attempts to capture this goal by describing teaching that is directly informed by research conducted or interpreted by the teacher and sometimes by the student as well. The term "research-enhanced learning and teaching" is also referred to in the literature and other knowledge avenues as "research-led learning and teaching" but "enhanced" may be more fitting to the concept for discussion here.

Research-enhanced learning and teaching include the integration of disciplinary research findings into courses and curricula such that students are both an audience for research and are engaged in research activity. Equally important is the provision of opportunities for students to experience and conduct research, learn about research throughout their courses, develop the skills of research and inquiry and contribute to the university's research effort.

A further matter of interest is research on learning and teaching itself as opposed to research into basic medical sciences or clinical practice, which is what most students and practitioners think of when they consider research. Research on learning and teaching itself might be better thought of in terms of the scholarship of learning and teaching. This is because "scholarship" is a wider term that includes other activities besides what is conventionally seen as pure research. Scholarship can include the critique and integration of existing knowledge from disparate sources. When both teachers and students engage in scholarship and/or research on learning and teaching it is argued that there is great promise of improving education (Boyer, 1990). This is because there is considerable motivation to students to engage with an activity that directly concerns them and can enrich their experience of education. Research-enhanced learning and teaching can also encourage students to see teachers as colleagues and collaborators in a joint enterprise rather than merely as the transmitters of knowledge.

An important aim of research-enhanced teaching and learning, therefore, is to engage students in the discovery, engagement and elaboration of new knowledge in collaboration with academics. To start, the objective is to make teachers' research interests transparent to students. The curriculum captures this endeavour in student–teacher learning activities and in assessments that are clearly valued and linked to such research. The world of research, often a realm exclusive to researchers and postgraduate students, is opened to both teachers and undergraduate students and thus expands students' horizons. This may be the real purpose of research-enhanced teaching and learning.

How well such teaching and learning achieves deep learning and its objectives is contested. Debate continues about the objective of effectively combining the strands of research and teaching into a cohesive educational experience (Brew, 2003; Jenkins, Healey, & Zetter, 2007). Positions range from a positive view that teaching and research fit naturally together (e.g. Sullivan, 1996) to a negative view that such a combination is a waste of an academic's time and resources (e.g. Ramsden & Moses, 1992). It may be that the divergence of opinion reflects perceptions of what research-led teaching is understood to be. It can be as simple as presenting research to students, or as complex as engaging students in conducting their own research.

Whether academics believe that research can or cannot be integrated with undergraduate teaching seems to be related to how one understands knowledge and its relation to research (Robertson & Bond, 2001, 2005). It can be argued that students are most likely to gain the greatest depth of learning from research when they are actually engaged in doing some research. However, there has been little evaluation of students' experiences of learning from research and how they develop research-related understanding and skills. The few studies that have focused on students' experiences and perceptions of the relevance of academic research to their learning are mixed (e.g. Volkwein & Carbone, 1994).

PRACTICE-BASED EDUCATION

Higher education, along with professional practice, faces the challenge of establishing richer vocabularies and discourses to conceptualise what we do. There is, for example, a growing body of literature on practice-based education that is changing the way we visualise much of what we now do in higher education. The two authors of this chapter happen to be dentists. We can both testify that dentistry education has been practice-based for decades. There have also been dental simulations for many years, although these were for many decades admittedly "low-tech". The bulk of a dental course takes place in clinics with students treating real patients, doing exactly what they will do in practice after graduation.

What has changed is that we now have a new vocabulary and discourse that allows us to articulate and conceptualise professional practice and its education in ways that can deepen our understanding of what it is our students learn and how it is learned (Higgs, Loftus, & Trede, 2010). Also emerging from this new vocabulary and discourse is the growth of new approaches to educational practices that exist outside the classroom. Two such pedagogies are research-enhanced learning and teaching and work-integrated learning, both of which have particular significance in health professional education and are part of practice-based education.

Courses that emphasise the role of regular and frequent practice can help students bring theory and its application together. There is now a growing realisation of the importance of practice-based education. This is a whole-of-curriculum approach that emphasises the importance of integrating theory with practice throughout a course (Higgs et al., 2010). Such integration occurs through work-integrated learning (WIL) which is a common aspect of courses that are practice-based. Problem-based learning is another example of practice-based education, which makes an explicit effort to regularly and consciously integrate theory into practice, as well as integrating different subjects as described above. For instance, a medical student with a previous degree in biomedical sciences had this to say about his experience of a course founded on problem-based learning.

> I've gone through my old notes and progressively thrown them out as I've rewritten them into a different format ... now I approach learning the diseases in the same way that I would ... a patient. (Loftus, 2009, p. 100)

In other words, the scientific knowledge this student already had was being reformatted to make it applicable to his emerging experience of professional practice. It can be argued that the student was reformatting his knowledge into the narratives that comprise the case-based knowledge so important to medical practice as opposed to the straightforward factual knowledge of medical science.

Critical and Narrative Thinking

As our understanding of what constitutes professional education develops there are now moves to borrow ideas from other disciplines such as those of the humanities and social sciences (Loftus, 2011). The example referred to just above is one instance where *narrative knowing*, a construct from the humanities, is utilised to understand how health professionals formulate their practice knowledge. There is a growing and informative literature around the importance of narrative in the health professions (Charon, 2006; Frank, 2004; Loftus & Greenhalgh, 2010).

Other ideas borrowed from the humanities include the importance of critical thinking. Sullivan and Rosin (2008) claimed that integrating insights and skills (such as critical thinking) from the humanities into professional education could foster what they called "practical reasoning". This is reasoning aimed at working out what is to be done in a particular situation, in other words, contextualised thinking for this particular patient, in this particular time and setting with all its limitations. They contrasted this with theoretical reasoning or scientific thinking which is aimed at working out knowledge that is context-free and true in all times and places. Professional reasoning is primarily the former, practical reasoning, although it is informed by the latter, scientific knowledge. A key aspect of such practical reasoning is criticality.

Real-world Experience

It has long been assumed, ever since the Flexner Report (1910), that the education of most health professionals needs to occur in tertiary teaching hospitals in large metropolitan centres where there is a concentration of specialties and extreme cases in need of specialised treatment. This means that the practitioners who provide the role models for students, in these early and impressionable years, are the specialists in such tertiary centres.

Most graduates, not surprisingly, want to continue working in such metropolitan centres and are reluctant to work in rural environments that are very different from the environments that have formed them as early career professionals. Because of this, many countries which have a sharp division between rural and metropolitan living, Australia and Canada in particular, have long experienced significant shortages of health professionals, particularly doctors, willing to work in rural settings. In recent years there have been attempts to move some portion of education into remote and rural settings. However, attempts to move most of the education into remote and rural clinics have generally met with fiscal and cultural resistance.

Despite this resistance there are now examples where medical schools have made a deliberate attempt to provide the bulk of their education in rural clinics. Some such schools make a point of being predominantly rural. In these rural settings, the role models who provide the examples of what it is to *be* a health professional are the practitioners in the rural clinics who take on the teaching and supervision of such students. The result is that many of the graduates from these institutions are happy to pursue careers in rural settings and are just as capable and competent as their peers schooled in the cities (Tesson, Hudson, Strasser, & Hunt, 2009). Some graduates drift back to seeking city practice, perhaps seeking a different quality of life, while strongly valuing their rural experience. A key aspect of education in both rural and metropolitan settings is the direct experience of actual professional practice.

For too long, many university courses assumed that (scientific) theory comes first and that practice, as applied scientific theory, will simply follow on naturally. This naivety resulted in generations of newly graduated practitioners who struggled to cope with real-world practice, knowing that they had learned relevant scientific knowledge but being unsure as to how to use it with real patients.

This problem can range from simply trying to apply textbook knowledge of diabetes to the individual patient to trying to integrate that same textbook knowledge with the complex sociocultural issues that many patients bring to the clinical encounter. For example, how closely can a well-educated medical graduate raised in a comfortable middle-class environment understand the complexities of the situation faced by an Indigenous patient, living in poverty, who may, for a large number of reasons, have difficulty complying with a medical plan? We now realise that direct involvement in supervised practice is probably the most important learning experience of all. As Davey (2006, p. 245) wrote:

What makes a practice a practice rather than a method is precisely the fact that it is based upon acquired and accumulated experience. The acquisition of discernment, judgment, and insight is based not so much upon what comes to us in a given experience but what comes upon us by involvement and participation in a whole number of experiences.

Work-Integrated Learning (WIL)

WIL describes educational programs that integrate classroom learning and workplace experience. Other terms are also in common use, such as workplace learning, and this subject is dealt with in more detail elsewhere in this book. WIL is now a serious topic of interest in academic circles (e.g. Atchison, Pollock, Reeders, & Rizzetti, 1999) and has become a distinctive pedagogy (Boud, Solomon, & Symes, 2001). Boud (2001, pp. 44-58) has outlined the characteristics of work-based learning programs as those that:

- are established in a partnership between an organisation and an educational institution
- are where learners enrolled on the program work in the partner-organisation
- are developed out of the needs of the workplace and of the learner
- have a starting point that often involves accreditation of prior learning or work experience
- have learning projects that are undertaken in the workplace
- assess learning outcomes and awards academic credits.

WIL promotes authentic student learning outcomes. Moreover, it captures the dimension of situated learning, with workplace culture, values and understandings, thus providing the four conditions for effective learning: a knowledge base, a motivational context, learning activity and interaction (Biggs & Tang, 2011).

CONCLUSION

The world of higher education is experiencing change and has been changing significantly for decades. The future seems to promise yet more change to come. This change offers both opportunities and challenges for those who seek to become university teachers of future health professionals. Challenges range from the provision of support to the broader range of students participating in higher education to curriculum reform that endeavours to integrate practice-based education, research, professional values and other demands into a coherent whole. The opportunities for newcomers to university teaching are to become involved in, and to contribute to, all these activities in a manner that not only enriches the education of our students but also enriches their own professional and personal engagement.

REFERENCES

Atchison, M., Pollock, S., Reeders, E., & Rizzetti, J. (1999). *Guide to WIL*. Melbourne: RMIT.

Biggs, J., & Tang, C. (2011). *Teaching for quality learning at university: What the student does* (4th ed.). Maidenhead, UK: Open University Press.

Boud, D. (2001). Creating a work based curriculum. In D. Boud & N. Solomon (Eds.), *Work-based learning: A new higher education?* (pp. 44-58). Buckingham, UK: Open University Press & Society for Research into Higher Education.

Boud, D., Solomon, N., & Symes, C. (2001). New practices for new times. In D. Boud & N. Solomon (Eds.), *Work-based learning: A new higher education?* (pp. 18-33). Buckingham, UK: Open University Press & Society for Research into Higher Education.

Boyer, E. (1990). *Scholarship reconsidered: Priorities of the professoriate*. Princeton, NJ: Carnegie Foundation for the Advancement of Teaching.

Brew, A. (2003). Teaching and research: New relationships and their implications for inquiry-based teaching and learning in higher education. *Higher Education Research & Development, 22*(1), 3-18. doi:10.1080/0729436032000056571

Charon, R. (2006). *Narrative medicine: Honoring the stories of illness*. Oxford: Oxford University Press.

Davey, N. (2006). *Unquiet understanding: Gadamer's philosophical hermeneutics*. Albany, NY: State University of New York Press.

Fish, D., & Coles, C. (2005). *Medical education: Developing a curriculum for practice*. Maidenhead: Open University Press.

Flexner, A. (1910). *Medical education in the United States and Canada: A report to the Carnegie Foundation for the Advancement of Teaching*. Bulletin No. 4. Retrieved from http://www.carnegiefoundation.org/sites/default/files/elibrary/Carnegie_Flexner_Report.pdf

Frank, A. W. (2004). *The renewal of generosity: Illness, medicine and how to live*. Chicago: University of Chicago Press.

General Medical Council UK. (1993). *Tomorrow's doctors*. Education Committee of UK General Medical Council.

Higgs, J., Jones, M. A., Loftus, S., & Christensen, N. (2008). *Clinical reasoning in the health profession*s (3rd ed.). Oxford: Butterworth-Heinemann.

Higgs, J., Loftus, S., & Trede, F. (2010). Education for future practice. In J. Higgs, D. Fish, I. Goulter, S. Loftus, J-A Reid & F. Trede (Eds.), *Education for future practic*e (pp. 3-13). Rotterdam: Sense.

Jenkins, A., Healey, M., & Zetter, R. (2007). *Linking teaching and research in disciplines and departments*. York, UK: The Higher Education Academy.

Loftus, S. (2009). *Language in clinical reasoning: Towards a new understanding*. Saarbrücken: VDM Verlag.

Loftus, S. (2011). Pain and its metaphors: A dialogical approach. *Journal of Medical Humanities, 32*(3), 213-230.

Loftus, S., & Greenhalgh, T. (2010). Towards a narrative mode of practice. In J. Higgs, D. Fish, I. Goulter, S. Loftus, J.-A. Reid & F. Trede (Eds.), *Education for future practice* (pp. 85-94). Rotterdam: Sense.

Meerabeau, E. (2004). Be good, sweet maid, and let who can be clever: A counter reformation in English nursing education? *International Journal of Nursing Studies, 41*, 285-292.

Newman, M. (2003). *A pilot systematic review and meta-analysis on the effectiveness of problem based learning*. ISBN 0 7017 0158 7. London: Report from the Learning and Teaching Support Network.

Osipow, S. H. (1990). Convergence in theories of career choice and development: Review and prospect. *Journal of Vocational Behavior, 36*, 122-131.

Ramsden, P., & Moses, I. (1992). Associations between research and teaching in Australian higher education. *Higher Education, 23*(3), 273-295.

Robertson, J., & Bond, C. (2001). Experiences of the relation between teaching and research: What do academics value? *Higher Education Research & Development, 20*(1), 5-19.

13

Robertson, J., & Bond. C. (2005). Being in the university. In R. Barnett (Ed.), *Reshaping the university: New relationships between research, scholarship and teaching* (pp. 79-91). New York: Society for Research into Higher Education.

Sullivan, A. V. S. (1996). Teaching norms and publication productivity. *New Directions for Institutional Research, 90*, 15-21.

Sullivan, W. M., & Rosin, M. S. (2008). *A new agenda for higher education: Shaping a life of the mind for practice*. San Francisco, CA: Jossey-Bass.

Tesson, G., Hudson, G., Strasser, R., & Hunt, D. (2009). *The making of the Northern Ontario School of Medicine: A case study in the history of medical education*. Montreal: McGill-Queen's University Press.

Volkwein, J. F., & Carbone, D. A. (1994). The impact of departmental research and teaching climates on undergraduate growth and satisfaction. *Journal of Higher Education, 65*, 147-167.

Stephen Loftus PhD
The Education For Practice Institute
Charles Sturt University, Australia

Tania Gerzina PhD
Faculty of Dentistry
The University of Sydney, Australia

MEGAN SMITH AND JOY HIGGS

2. HEALTH PROFESSIONALS BECOMING UNIVERSITY TEACHERS

This chapter provides a context for understanding the characteristics and motivations of health professionals who become university teachers and explores the nature of their experiences. Health professionals who become university teachers may do so motivated by varied individual factors. These factors could include an interest in teaching, a positive experience of teaching students in a clinical setting, a strong desire to educate new practitioners in their field, lifestyle choices or an interest in a career direction as an academic. Being a university teacher may involve teaching students on a part-time or casual basis while maintaining some clinical work or a complete change to full-time employment in a university setting. Although health professionals can be involved in teaching in clinical settings or providing occasional specialist lectures, we have limited the scope of the discussion to teaching in university settings.

Becoming a university teacher in contemporary higher education clearly involves teaching, but teaching is only one element of a full academic appointment. Being an academic comes with expectations of teaching as well as involvement in research and university administration. As we discuss in this chapter the experience of becoming a university teacher is shaped by these broader responsibilities and expectations of academia. Therefore in using the term "university teacher" in this chapter we are including the wider elements associated with becoming an academic in a university context. Health professionals who become university teachers often follow a pathway to academia that has involved a considerable period in clinical practice. Smith and Boyd (2012) observed that the pathway to becoming teachers for health professionals differs to the experience for other academic posts. For example in the sciences the pathway typically involves doctoral study linked to disciplinary research. In contrast health professionals often consider teaching once they are well-established in their profession. Data collected in a survey of nursing, midwifery and allied health academic staff supports the view that becoming a university teacher is frequently regarded as a mid-career decision for health professionals (Smith & Boyd, 2012). For example, this study of academics with between one and five years' experience in higher education, found that 32% of the respondents to the survey, were aged 30-39 years and 53% were aged 40-49 years.

The experience of becoming a university teacher involves identifying and securing a teaching or academic position, beginning work and then developing skills as a teacher. We will explore each of these phases to pursue an understanding of the particular experiences and challenges for the individuals involved. In the subsequent section we explore proposed strategies to support health professionals in their journey to becoming university teachers.

S. Loftus et al. (Eds.), Educating Health Professionals:
Becoming a University Teacher, 15–22.
© 2013 Sense Publishers. All rights reserved.

THE EXPERIENCE OF BECOMING A UNIVERSITY TEACHER

Applying for and Securing a Position as a University Teacher

The experience and knowledge of practice that health professionals bring to teaching is highly regarded and valued. However, there are a number of particular challenges for health professionals who apply for positions as university teachers. One of the most significant challenges is that experience as a health professional is often only one of the selection criteria for university positions. Although health professionals may have experience of teaching in clinical settings they may have limited experience of teaching in contemporary higher education settings, limited experience in the administration involved in university education and may not have attained formal qualifications (such as teaching qualifications or higher degree qualifications) in their field. Health professionals may also have very limited backgrounds in research and established research track records. These factors can make the initial entry into academia difficult, particularly in a competitive employment environment. If this is the case then experienced practitioners may be offered junior academic appointments at reduced salaries compared to their clinical appointments. This is a problem for institutions in attracting skilled practitioners and for the practitioners whose clinical expertise is seemingly valued but not rewarded in academic status and salary. These new university teachers can experience tension between the value placed on their professional expertise and the capacity for gaining acceptable positions and remuneration.

Increasingly those seeking to enter academia from the health professions are recognising the value of pursuing postgraduate research studies prior to entering university employment or during their early academic years. Both pathways into academia (experienced clinicians and practitioners who engage in postgraduate studies earlier in their careers) reflect the link between levels of academic appointments and varied practice, teaching and research capabilities and achievements. Mid to higher level academic appointments typically require the appointee to hold a doctoral qualification. In some circumstances there is a significant financial disincentive for health professionals to become university teachers. The implication of these challenges point to the need for new university teachers to consider carefully their move into academia and their motivations. Becoming a university teacher may be best regarded as a career change or "new profession" and therefore may require further training and entrance at a lower level rather than a career progression from expert status as a health professional. However, it is also important for universities to recognise that professional knowledge is not only acquired from research but also from practice and that the expertise of academics needs to cover both spheres for the advancement of the knowledge base of the profession and for the education of new graduates.

Beginning Work as a University Teacher

Once a teaching position has been secured, either on a permanent basis or a casual basis, the literature has identified a number of common experiences shared by new teachers. These are reflected in health professional academics and compare with the experiences of other professionals such as school teachers. Smith and Boyd (2012) summarised these challenges as relating to the practice of being a teacher and the development of an identity as a teacher in a new professional role. New university teachers become very quickly immersed into the responsibility for teaching and supporting students requiring a rapid adaptation to their new role (Boyd, 2010). Health professionals who become university teachers bring high levels of content knowledge related to their professional practice field to their new jobs. In contrast they may have limited knowledge of teaching beyond clinical education.

Teaching in a university context requires knowledge of how to promote learning and skills in teaching. Some of the differences between clinical education practice and teaching practices experienced by new university teachers are teaching larger numbers of students, different assessment and marking strategies, using new teaching technologies, involvement in curriculum design, and interpreting and applying university regulation and policy and supporting students (see McArthur-Rouse, 2008; Smith & Boyd, 2012).

In addition to developing core skills in teaching, new university teachers need to develop what Shulman (1987) referred to as pedagogical content knowledge. This is the knowledge of how university teachers use their content knowledge from practice and transform it for students; to be able to present and explain concepts in multiple ways and to be able to diagnose and resolve student errors in understanding. These skills differ from those used in clinical teaching which often involves smaller groups of students in practice contexts. New teachers entering academia from professional practice may experience challenges in transferring knowledge of teaching learnt in the practice context to their new role (Trowler & Knight, 2000). However, they have the advantage of a deeper knowledge and experience of practice (in comparison to academics in physiology and sociology) that serves them very well in relation to their capacity to be practice role models for their students and sharing with students real life experiences of professional practice and the practice world.

In university settings new academic staff describe an expectation of independence and autonomy in the conduct of their work that they may not have experienced in a practice context (Trowler & Knight, 2000). Trowler and Knight have represented university settings as having local cultures, practices, languages and ways of working that new teachers need to come to understand.

Traditionally university academics have experienced autonomy and independence. In professional practice the concept of professional autonomy exists but the reality of health professional settings typically involves large numbers of people working in close relationships and through teamwork with a higher degree of job clarity, line management, supervision and scrutiny of work. Thus universities have often been experienced as less structured than healthcare settings in terms of tasks and routines.

For new university teachers their roles can be associated with a lack of clarity, broad job descriptions and lack of task specificity in traditional academic settings which allow new academics to "find their own feet". McArthur-Rouse (2008), for instance, found that new nursing academics felt a lack of clarity in their role and had difficulty judging their effectiveness in their new role, particularly when they came into environments where established staff were already functioning and the skills required were taken for granted. For example timetables are flexible, teachers are given relative freedom to plan their work days and teaching activities and there are long periods of the year when students are off-campus. The cycles of workload in universities can vary from periods of high teaching and assessment load to other periods when there is time for planning, curriculum development and research. The new teacher may be inexperienced in how to manage the new workload to meet new targets and deadlines or to fill unstructured time. Universities are also characterised by distributed leadership where there are much flatter organisational structures and there is less direct supervision of work. Some health professionals may be unfamiliar with this and find themselves feeling alienated and lacking support and guidance and being unaware of where to find information and appropriate communication channels in the organisation (McArthur-Rouse, 2008; Trowler & Knight, 2000). McArthur-Rouse (2008) identified that although health professionals joining academia may have skills in management and organisational knowledge these were not readily transferable to working in an academic context.

It is interesting to note that in recent decades the shift of universities to be education providers within a higher education market has emphasised the commodification of higher education and external accountability. In this context the level of academic autonomy has diminished with a greater degree of role specificity and performance targets - another adaptation context for new and experienced academics alike.

The process of becoming a university teacher is most frequently represented in the literature as a transition (Hurst, 2010) and there is a tendency to explore the transition in terms of stages. Although a staged view of transition can be critiqued on the basis that using stages simplifies a complex individual process of adaptation to new roles, individual choices and pathways plus an ongoing connection to previous roles and identities, the concept of using stages to understand becoming a teacher as requiring a process and period of change is useful. Health professionals joining academia have been reported as experiencing feelings of anxiety, uncertainty, lack of confidence but also more positive feelings of excitement, stimulation and exhilaration that aligned to expectations in their new role (Hurst, 2010; Smith & Boyd, 2012). In the initial period of becoming a teacher the health professional typically retains strong feelings of identity as a health professional in a new context, such that academics describe themselves in terms of their health profession, for example as a nurse or physiotherapist (Boyd, 2010). New teachers draw on their feelings of expertise in their profession to validate and add credibility to their role as a teacher (Hurst, 2010).

A second phase in the transition to becoming a university teacher is a period when health professionals experience feelings of being novices in their new profession. New academic staff may experience a perceived loss of status when they join a university when they are no longer regarded as an expert among other experts (Boyd, 2010). The notion of identity has been frequently applied to make sense of the experience of new academics (Clegg, 2008; Trowler & Knight, 2000).

The experiences of health professionals as they become university teachers involves a process of socialisation that provides changes and challenges to re-shape individuals' sense of their identity as they become involved in the work and social practices in their university department (Trowler & Knight, 2000). The socialisation process involves the development of an identity where health professionals see themselves as teachers, not as clinicians who are teaching their craft, but as teachers embracing the profession of teaching and the skills and expectations of this role (Boyd, 2010). There exists a complex, dynamic set of demands upon the new academic related to identity formation which emerges from tensions and their resolution (Smith and Boyd). Trowler and Knight (2000, p. 34) proposed that new university teachers need to do identity "work" as they establish themselves in their new environment and cultures and need to "make and re-make their identities".

A further phase of development can be experienced when individuals redefine their identity as, for example a "nurse lecturer", in which they integrate their identity as a professional but also their new career identity as an academic. New academics who are unable to redefine themselves as having a new identity may experience discomfort in their new role and may choose not to continue in academia and return to clinical practice (McArthur-Rouse, 2008).

Health professionals who become new university teachers often experience considerable pressure, as well as a desire, to maintain currency or identity within their profession. Clegg (2008) proposed that for academics there are porous boundaries between the university and the professional practice world. New university teachers may feel pressure as they face expectations to learn new knowledge for teaching while maintaining existing knowledge to sustain their identity as a credible practitioner (Smith & Boyd, 2012). For example, Hurst identified that physiotherapists felt the need to retain competency and remain professionally up-to-date, and their established identities as clinical experts. It has been our experience that a number of health professionals often transition into academia and university teaching in a staged way where they prefer to commence with part-time positions, retaining some clinical work or seeking opportunities either in or outside of their academic roles to continue clinical work. This may be related to factors such as their desire to maintain currency and credibility but also to experience comfort in a familiar environment where their identity is well-established and they reaffirm their (professional) self-worth.

As we noted above, the new university teacher may be drawn to an academic role by their motivation to teach resulting in the primacy of teaching in their perception of their role (Smith & Boyd, 2012). Smith and Boyd identified in their 2008 survey of health professionals becoming university teachers that few health professionals entered academia with doctoral qualifications (4%). Most new academics in the study reported the considerable stress they experienced as they faced expectations that they would conduct research and publish.

SUPPORTING HEALTH PROFESSIONALS TO BECOME UNIVERSITY TEACHERS

The nature of the challenges that new academics face are significant and understanding these challenges is important for new university teachers and their employers. McArthur-Rouse (2008) identified that it is an important issue for universities to effectively recruit but also retain health professionals in the academic workforce to ensure the quality of teaching. From the work described above this implies ensuring that health professionals who become university teachers are supported to develop strong academic identities and to develop the skills required for university teaching.

There have been a number of factors identified and proposed in the literature which contribute to health professionals being supported in the transition to becoming university teachers. Health professionals considering becoming university teachers conceptualise the process as a career change, requiring support through the transition process and realistic expectations of the transferability of their existing skills to the university context. It would appear to be perilous for individuals to hold to a view that expertise as a clinician will transfer directly to recognition, status and expertise as a university teacher. There needs to be expectations that taking on this role will require learning new abilities and knowledge, participation in training and learning how to cope with changing identity and roles. This means that good information about the role and expectations of academics needs to be part of recruitment and induction and that ongoing support is required. Such support could take the form of decreased workload in the first year of employment, having an assigned mentor, clear specification of and performance targets, online staff development modules, workshops and drawing early career academics into new tasks like designing curricula, publishing and grant writing.

Smith and Boyd (2012) identified from their participants' feedback that there was value in ensuring new university teachers had access to others at the same peer level. Trowler and Knight (2000) argue, in a theorisation of universities as activity systems and communities of practice, that understanding how new staff become socialised and have access to learning the systems are important to their successful induction. The authors proposed that induction activities are needed for the support of new university teachers, such as providing them with access to discussions with existing staff about their daily activities and experiences of working in their department, giving them opportunities to shadow and work collaboratively with other staff and providing leadership which supports socialisation and positive cultures. Trowler and Knight draw on the recognised value of local informal cultures to promote learning and development of university teachers, to propose that "the most important way to improve induction of new university teachers is to concentrate on the normal quality of communication and relations in teams and departments" (p. 33). Smith and Boyd (2012) suggested new university teachers learnt more from less experienced peers; they found more experienced teachers less accessible and less helpful.

The discussion above also indicates the importance for induction into university teaching for health professionals to pay attention to the unique experiences of health professionals, with their later entry into academia and the support required for identify formation. Such processes could include discussions about expectations and role clarity, awareness of what new staff are likely to experience, familiarity with the culture and acknowledgement of the changes in structure to established routines. Supervision may also need to be structured to provide feedback on effectiveness of performance initially until individuals are able to draw on intrinsic feedback within their role. There is also a need to explore the tensions around maintaining currency of practice with expectations from the university and also the individuals desires to maintain their credibility. Further, specific attention is needed to support new academics to develop an identity as a researcher, particularly if they bring to the role only expectations about teaching with limited ideas about how they will engage in research.

Becoming a university teacher is a personal journey of career change. In this chapter we have described the motivations and challenges that are experienced by those undertaking this journey. To conclude we offer a reprise as our reflection of the unexpected, testing and rewarding journey to a career in academia.

REPRISE

In my profession I was a senior clinician.
For fifteen years - I had built my expertise
expanded my practice knowledge
my patients told me I was good,
so did my students I enjoyed being a practitioner –
I was part of a community and a workplace
I had a good sense of who I was
what my role was
and where my career was going

I was a senior staff member
I had status
I had earned respect

I enjoyed clinical teaching
which led me to consider
becoming a university teacher.

So I applied for a job at university
But a university job is so much more than teaching

First – my pay went backwards – signficantly
Next – I became a junior all over again
Then – I lost my sense of professional self
Who was I?
Did my practice expertise matter any more?
My head was in a spin
Every day I went to work
it was to an unknown world
to some new unexpected challenge
to something else
I was not prepared for

A really big deal
was "the wall"

RESEARCH

"you have to do research"
"you have to do a PhD"
I don't know how this will look for me

I started out at this part-time
I kept my feet grounded in my practice world
Sometime in the next two years
I'll find out if this is really the place for me.

For now I love teaching
And there is such satisfaction in seeing students learn and share my passion for my
practice world.

REFERENCES

Boyd, P. (2010). Academic induction for professional educators: Supporting the workplace learning of newly appointed lecturers in teacher and nurse education. *International Journal for Academic Development, 15*(2), 155-165.

Clegg, S. (2008). Academic identities under threat? *British Educational Research Journal, 34*(3), 329-345. doi:10.1080/01411920701532269

Hurst, K. M. (2010). Experiences of new physiotherapy lecturers making the shift from clinical practice into academia. *Physiotherapy, 96*(3), 240-247.

McArthur-Rouse, F. J. (2008). From expert to novice: An exploration of the experiences of new academic staff to a department of adult nursing studies. *Nurse Education Today, 28*, 401-408.

Shulman, L. S. (1987). Knowledge and teaching: Foundations of the new reform. *Harvard Educational Review, 57*(1), 1-23.

Smith, C., & Boyd, P. (2012). Becoming an academic: The reconstruction of identity by recently appointed lecturers in nursing, midwifery and the allied health professions. *Innovations in Education and Teaching International, 49*(1), 63-72.

Trowler, P., & Knight, P. T. (2000). Coming to know in higher education: Theorising faculty entry to new work contexts. *Higher Education Research & Development, 19*(1), 27-42. Retrieved from http://chelt.anu.edu.au/sites/default/files/Trowler%20and%20Knight.pdf

Megan Smith PhD
School of Community Health, Faculty of Science
Charles Sturt University, Australia

Joy Higgs PhD
The Education For Practice Institute
Research Institute For Professional Practice, Learning & Education
Charles Sturt University, Australia

TANIA GERZINA AND KIRSTY FOSTER

3. BEING A UNIVERSITY TEACHER

Teaching in Professions

There is a common view that becoming and being a university teacher is a relatively straightforward process, and there are popular websites that provide what appear to be simple steps to achieve this (e.g. http://www.wikihow.com/Become-a-College-Professor). We argue, however, that becoming a university teacher is a complex process and not to be taken lightly.

Identity and Recognition

University teachers are a heterogeneous group, reflective of the society from which they are drawn, but can be considered in three loose groupings. One group is made up of people who are primarily educators and who hold educational qualifications in support of their academic roles. Another group hold qualifications in a health profession such as nursing and forego their professional practice in order to become full-time university teachers. Many such teachers have no formal education credentials and find themselves in a teaching role simply because of expertise in their professional field. A third group are those who decide to contribute to their professional community in a teaching role while continuing regular professional work. Universities often employ the latter teachers on a casual, infrequent basis despite the valuable contribution they can make to teaching. Indeed, the existence of all three groups of teachers provides rich variety in university teaching as a discipline. In particular, the knowledge and practical experience they bring from the "real" world of work is crucial within a learning institution where the focus is on the need for graduates who are able to perform in the workplace. One further note of interest is that, although a teaching qualification is optional, research training is essential to progress in an academic career. This clear inequity is reflected in the perceived value of research over teaching which still exists in the tertiary sector, despite the growing realisation that education is just as important as research. On closer inspection, therefore, the process of developing an identity as a university teacher is rather more complex than it seems at first.

Moving from a workplace environment where one was a health professional into the academic space of a university requires a shift in professional identity. Coming as they do from many different backgrounds, it is not surprising that university teachers forge their new identities in diverse ways. Skelton (2012) differentiated three types of teachers: those who are "specialists in teaching" and spend much time in face-to-face teaching activity; "blended" professionals who regard both teaching and research as

S. Loftus et al. (Eds.), Educating Health Professionals:
Becoming a University Teacher, 23–32.

contributing to learning; and "researchers who teach". Teaching specialists see their educational role as encompassing a broader professional responsibility than simply lecturing or taking tutorials. They tend to take a holistic view of teaching and are aware of the need to spend time supporting students in their learning beyond the mere transmission of information characteristic of recognised teaching activities such as lecturing. In contrast, for those who consider themselves researchers who teach, teaching is often an activity secondary to research. This impoverished view of teaching seems to be still widely held in many academic institutions and needs to change if high-quality teaching and learning within universities is to flourish. Those who Skelton dubbed "blended professionals" approach the issue from a different perspective. For them, learning is the primary activity of a university, and they consider that everyone, be they staff member or student, is a learner. Blended learners tend to regard both teaching and research as learning activities and therefore can more comfortably combine the two aspects of their work.

Not everyone can successfully blend teaching and research identities. Skelton (2012) captured the tension that can arise for individuals as they seek to establish a new identity as a university teacher. He referred to the "identity struggles" that occur when people try to integrate a teacher identity alongside a researcher identity. This is because it is hard to meet teaching responsibilities as well as attend to the research activities expected of academics in tertiary institutions. New academics can feel overwhelmed by these demands. These professionals can find themselves working with two quite separate groups of people, a research community and a teaching community, but feel they are not being embraced by either. A further challenge for academics who identify themselves as teachers is the strong sense of duty they feel towards their students (Calvert, Lewis, & Spindler, 2011). Tension also exists for teachers in the dynamic environment of universities where the breadth of scholarly activity extends to high calibre and well-qualified professional staff who work alongside academics and where traditional academic boundaries in work allocation are blurred (Whitchurch, 2012). This blurring has resulted in expanding the range and heterogeneity of academic identities. In addition to all this, university teachers are under extra pressure as financial constraints on higher education and higher student numbers have an impact on what they are expected to do. As the tertiary education sector adopts more business-oriented processes in response to this pressure, academics must take on new roles and identities that are becoming increasingly fragmented (Clegg, 2008; Gale, 2011). An idea that allows us to conceptualise teaching identities in more depth is the community of practice (Wenger, 1998).

The Teaching Community of Practice

The website *How to Become a College Professor* suggests that one of the steps you can take to become a university teacher is:

> when searching for a full-fledged professor position, apply everywhere. Start by looking at universities that are looking to expand the department you are interested in becoming a part of.

The advice is clearly to look broadly for a community of practice in which you would fit. The higher education literature focuses not only on teacher approaches and tips for teaching but also on conceptions of learning and how to engage students and teachers in a learning community. This can be seen as an attempt by university teachers to form an open and collegial *community of practice* (Lave & Wenger, 1991) dedicated to improving their contribution to the university. This is much more than just a *community of interest* where participation is reduced to little more than a passing interest in a topic. A community of practice is distinguished by structural characteristics that Wenger, McDermott, and Snyder (2002) described as a "domain of knowledge; … a community of people; … and … shared practice" (p. 27). The emphasis is particularly on the shared practice of the community. The community grows and develops a shared understanding of the value of the knowledge and practice of its members by exchanging information, expressing opinion, and providing support. The underlying motivation is that members of a community of practice need to share knowledge to constantly improve their practice both as individuals and as a community.

There is strong motivation to join a community of practice when knowledge is valued in this way. The strength of the motivation can overcome potential barriers to forming a community such as time poverty or geographic separation (Ardichvilli, Page, & Wentling, 2003). The engagement of teachers within a community of practice can encourage the exchange of practice stories, for example, that will enhance their ability to do their job as teachers. A good community of practice, therefore, deliberately sets out to foster strong social engagement and collaboration where participants can continue to negotiate the meaning of their knowledge and their practice and develop a sense of identity. In this way participants can develop a sense of the professionalism needed in being a university teacher. This raises the issue of what teachers need to know in order to teach.

Imparting Discipline-specific Knowledge Versus Deep or Lifelong Agentic Learning

We might ask, what do university teachers need to know in order to teach? Several authors have addressed this question in the context of higher education. A common conclusion is that teachers need to possess a range of skills, attitudes, knowledge and values in both discipline-specific and pedagogical areas. Discipline-specific knowledge is essential knowledge, described by Ramsden (1999, p. 25) as involving

> an understanding of the main issues in a subject, an appreciation of the nature of appropriate arguments in it, an awareness of what counts as relevant evidence, and the wisdom to think critically and admit one's deficiencies in knowledge.

There is clearly much more involved than simply imparting textbook information. For example, in the health professions, teachers who are also practitioners provide a unique dimension with their experiential understanding of professional practice. The value to students is that their teacher's experiential understanding is important in supporting students to develop their own notions of the realities of professional practice from an "insider" perspective. In other words, teachers can convey the realities of the profession to students and the meaning of professionalism. This is why teaching in the clinical environment presents a challenging and complex task, a task many clinicians often assume without adequate preparation or orientation. Harden and Crosby (2000), in the medical profession, described six major roles that the clinical teacher takes on: information provider, role model, facilitator, assessor, curriculum and course planner, and resource material creator. All these roles must be co-ordinated and used to help students become members of the community of practice that is their profession.

Billett (2009) calls university-based discipline knowledge "canonical", adding that these concepts need to be augmented by learning experiences of authentic professional practice where that knowledge can be applied in ways that can allow students to develop a deeper understanding of what professional practice entails. Discipline-specific knowledge is also constrained by complex institutional requirements and the demands of accreditation bodies that validate and certify courses. This means that professional practitioners who are also teachers must carefully integrate their experiential practice knowledge and skills with the knowledge and competencies that are formally stated within the curriculum. It is now clear that discipline-specific experiential knowledge is essential but not sufficient to become an effective teacher. An important implication of this is that a great deal of interpretation is needed when deciding what to teach and how to teach it (i.e. pedagogy).

Pedagogical knowledge, or ways of knowing, is knowledge of instructional strategies, curriculum resources and tools that are effective in supporting students' learning. We now realise that successful pedagogy requires engagement with the prior conceptions and experiences that students bring to their learning. Therefore, professional development of teachers in pedagogical knowledge is increasingly focused on helping teachers to understand and engage with student thinking. But just as discipline-based experiential knowledge is essential but not sufficient for effective teaching, understanding of student thinking addresses only part of the challenge. The challenge of effective teaching is to combine these different aspects of education. We must make the complex knowledge, from both the curriculum and our own practice knowledge, accessible to students in a manner that relates to their abilities to understand. This means that teachers need to able to use a range of instructional strategies and techniques and know when and how to use them. All this activity must be constructively aligned with the aims of the course and with the way learning is assessed. Moreover, we should be encouraging students to become autonomous learners who have the intrinsic motivation to manage their own learning (i.e. self-directed learning). Students need to be *agentic*.

Billett (2009) described agentic learners as those who are "pro-active and engaged in making meaning and developing capacities in ways that are intentional, effortful and actively critical in constructing their knowledge" (p. 5). It is remarkable, though not unexpected, how closely this definition matches that provided by patients when asked what expectations they have of the health professional who provides their care (Gerzina, unpublished). It is not surprising that there is alignment between the qualities patients expect to see in their healthcare providers and the objectives of health professional education in universities. However, university teachers should also think of themselves as agentic and active learners.

Teacher Approaches to Teaching

McLaughlin and Zarrow (2001) claimed that teachers should consider themselves active learners in both the evolution of their understanding of discipline knowledge and their abilities as teachers. There is a need to be engaged in ongoing development of teaching, assessment, observation and reflection. Ongoing development as a teacher should be seen as a professional commitment, part of the professionalism of being a teacher. Both successes and failures may occur, reflected in teaching evaluations by students, peers, supervisors and institutions, but ongoing development as a teacher can be sustained by the accumulated wisdom of experience over time (Dadds, 2001). It must be remembered, however, that individual development as a teacher takes place in a social context that is always changing. Higher education in the Western world has been characterised by constant and regular change in response to pressures from a wide range of organisations and governments. The demands and expectations of institutions seem always to be undergoing reform and renewal. University teachers are expected to keep abreast of such change and adapt to it. For example, it is now accepted that student ratings of teacher effectiveness are a normal part of being a university teacher because these evaluations are seen as valid metrics of teacher effectiveness (Cohen, 1981). Such evaluations are now a reality that many university teachers must come to terms with, no matter what reservations they may privately hold about the claims to accurately measure effectiveness. One reservation is that these measures take no account of a teacher's approaches to teaching and learning. For example, what attitude do teachers have towards issues such as student-centred learning?

Student-Centred Learning

Åkerlind (2003), reviewing studies that examined university teachers' conceptions of and approaches to teaching, considered two issues. The first is a perception of teaching as a transmission of information to students vs. the development of conceptual understanding in students; the second is teachers and their teaching strategies vs. students and their learning and development. The first issue emphasises the importance of encouraging students to undertake higher order thinking about what they learn by providing structured learning activities that require substantial engagement in decision-making and critical thinking. The second issue concerns the teacher-student axis and the need to find a fine balance between what the teacher does and what the student does in order to achieve the learning goals. Ramsden (1999) adds that students should undergo a gradual change in their perceptions of a subject, from a simplistic view of knowledge and learning towards a more relational view where they become aware of the sophisticated relations and connections between different bodies of knowledge. This means that the balance between academic teaching and student learning is dynamic and changing. These concerns have led to a growing interest in student-centred learning.

For many years, a growing number of scholars have argued for a form of education that puts students rather than teachers at the centre of educational activity (e.g. Vygotsky, 1978). Student-centred learning contrasts with teacher-centred learning in the balance of power, the function of content, the role of the teacher, the responsibility for learning, and the purpose and processes of evaluation (Weimer, 2002). The term *student-centred learning* was articulated by the psychologist Carl Rogers (1951), and it is often considered to be synonymous with other terms like active learning and participatory learning. Rogers asked:

> If the creation of an atmosphere of acceptance, understanding, and respect is the most effective basis for facilitating the learning which is called therapy, then might it not be the basis for the learning which is called education? (p. 384)

There is a clear link between student-centred learning and adult education. Knowles (1970) argued that adult learners consider themselves to be independent, bringing experience to their learning and having a problem-centred or problem-solving approach. The problem-solving approach also links with patient-centred teaching, with the complex relationship between teacher, student and patient playing an important role in the education of health professionals. The aim of patient-centred teaching and learning is to provide authentic education. Further complexity is added by the involvement of other stakeholders, adding further tensions to teaching.

Tensions in the Teaching Environment

Many tensions exist in the teaching environment of the university. Sources of tension include heavy workload expectations vs. the quality of life balance for teachers, the tension between teaching and research, the requirement to constantly master the pedagogical implications of new technologies and media, and the shifting view of tenure with a growing trend towards casualisation and short-term contracts. It is important for new academics to be aware of all these tensions so that they can engage with these issues, which are likely to be with us for many years to come. One particular tension at the present time is the issue of workload.

Teaching workload typically includes all time spent on instructional and scholarly activities face-to-face with students, and the preparation of those activities. This is an issue because there is a widespread sense that workload demands are steadily increasing with rising student numbers but often without a concomitant rise in staff and resources. Many academics feel that they are being asked to do more with less. This is complicated by the casualisation of many teaching roles and the uncertainty this can bring.

The uncertainty brought about by casualisation and short-term contracts means that it can be difficult for an academic department to establish continuity in research, scholarship and teaching. Percy and Beaumont (2008) argued that there are significant risks to teaching if casualisation merely reduces the costs of providing education. This situation is not helped by the growing number of staff who are required to generate grant funding to help pay their own salary, although this relates more to those with a research commitment. On top of all this is the demand for all academics to generate more publications in order to be seen to be productive.

The teaching environment for practitioner teachers is further complicated by additional elements at play, each with distinct challenges. The teaching environment may consist of inpatient, hospital outpatient and community settings, all with different practice cultures and ways of doing things. All these settings need to be understood by the teacher so that students can be successfully introduced to them. What students learn in practice settings takes on particular relevance for them, as they can see that it relates directly to what they will do as autonomous practitioners (Spencer, 2003). In these settings a university teacher also needs to balance patient care with the requirement to teach and supervise students as they practise their emerging skills, apply their knowledge, communicate with patients and do so in a professional manner. It is one of the duties of a practitioner teacher in these settings to provide a role model, embodying and demonstrating the values and attitudes of the profession. Yet until recent years very little preparation has been provided for prospective university teachers to take on these roles.

For many practitioner teachers the only preparation for teaching is their own experience of learning or being taught. This is problematic for a number of reasons. The tendency is to emulate one's teachers, regardless of whether the experience was good or bad. In some of the health professions, particularly medicine, there has often been a tradition of intimidation and humiliation in clinical teaching (Knight & Bligh, 2006), which is now recognised as counterproductive for students and can have detrimental consequences for the teaching practice of new medical teachers if it is allowed to continue. One response to this situation is to provide formal preparation in higher education for new university teachers.

Preparation for Teaching at Tertiary Level

Formal courses to orient newcomers to the teaching environment of the university and to impart knowledge about theories of education and methods of instruction have been shown to improve understanding and skills of teaching (Foster & Laurent, 2013; Gibbs & Coffey, 2004). This alone is not sufficient. Research shows that interaction with and support from colleagues within the community are essential experiences in the process of identity development as a university teacher (Trowler & Knight, 2000). New university teachers most value work-related discussion with more experienced colleagues, but in general find that opportunities for talking about teaching are rare (Remmick, Karm, Haamer, & Lepp, 2011). This experience can be isolating, and such loneliness saps the self-confidence essential to be an effective teacher. It is increasingly recognised that successful professional socialisation and preparation for teaching require collegial support for novice teachers as they become familiar with the culture and practice of their new environment (Boyd & Harris, 2010; Remmick et al., 2011) and gain confidence in teaching. In other words, besides formal preparation to teach it is important to be a member of a community of practice of teachers who can provide regular support for each other.

Remmick et al. (2011) showed that when new teachers have the opportunity to observe teaching colleagues at work they tend to adopt the norms and values of the particular department or institution. Support and guidance from more experienced teachers is as important for novice teachers as instruction in teaching methods. The warmth of interpersonal relationships within a community of practice can be the foundation to successful integration into the university teaching community. New university teachers need to adopt a critical and questioning attitude to existing educational practices and values that they encounter. This is another reason for new teachers to take advantage of any formal preparation offered to become an educator. A well-designed course will encourage teachers to be critical and questioning of educational and professional practice and to encourage this in their students. No community of practice is perfect; new members of the community of university teachers need to accept responsibility for reforming and gradually improving the practice of educating health professionals.

Conclusion

We have attempted here to describe the stresses, large and small, that confront those who choose the vocation of university teacher. The community of practice of health professional educators is complex, though reflective of society at large with all its expectations and tensions. Such teachers are required to bring a deep understanding of a *profession* to their teaching while bringing a degree of *professionalism* to the teaching as they fathom their emerging identity as a teacher. Having deep and thorough discipline-specific knowledge on its own does not equip someone to be a university teacher. Teachers are responsible for student engagement with this knowledge and are obliged to support the construction of a professional reality for their students, who are, after all, junior colleagues of the teacher. Teaching approaches should place the student in the centre of the endeavour, and encourage student-centred learning. There is a great range of issues to consider when setting out to become a university teacher. A final tip comes from our opening website, *How to Become a College Professor*:

Remain humble. Don't succumb to "professor's disease". Just because you spend your days in front of students who, by definition, have a lot to learn, doesn't mean you are omniscient or have an exalted place in the universe.

REFERENCES

Ardichvilli, A., Page, V., & Wentling, T. (2003). Motivation and barriers to participation in virtual knowledge sharing in communities of practice. *Journal of Knowledge Management, 7*(1), 64-77.
Åkerlind, G. S. (2003). Growing and developing as a university teacher: Variation in meaning. *Studies in Higher Education, 28*(4), 375-390.

Billett, E. (2009). *Developing agentic professionals through practice-based pedagogies.* Final report for the Australian Learning and Teaching Council Associate Fellowship. Retrieved from http://www.olt.gov.au/search/apachesolr_search/Billett

Boyd, P., & Harris, K. (2010). Becoming a university lecturer in teacher education: Expert school teachers reconstructing their pedagogy and identity. *Professional Development in Education, 36*(1-2), 9-24.

Calvert, M., Lewis, T., & Spindler, J. (2011). Negotiating professional identities in higher education: Dilemmas and priorities of academic staff. *Research in Education, 86*(1), 25-38.

Clegg, S. (2008). Academic identities under threat? *British Educational Research Journal, 34*(3), 329-345. doi:10.1080/01411920701532269

Cohen, P. A. (1981). Student ratings of instruction and student achievement: A meta-analysis of multisection validity studies. *Review of Educational Research, 51*, 281-309.

Dadds, M. (2001). Continuing professional development nurturing the expert within. In J. Soleer, A. Craft and H. Burgess (Eds.), *Teacher development: Exploring our own practice* (pp. 23-34). London: Paul Chapman Publishing & the Open University.

Foster, K., & Laurent, R. (2013). How we make good doctors into good teachers: A short course to support busy clinicians to improve their teaching skills. *Medical Teacher, 35*(1), 4-7. doi:10.3109/0142159X.2012.731098

Gale, H. (2011). The reluctant academic: Early career academics in a teaching-orientated university. *International Journal for Academic Development, 16*(3), 215-227.

Gibbs, G., & Coffey, M., (2004). The impact of training of university lecturers on their teaching skills, their approach to teaching and the approach to learning of their students. *Active Learning in Higher Education, 5*(1), 87-100.

Harden, R. M., & Crosby, J. R. (2000). AMEE Guide No 20. The good teacher is more than a lecturer: The twelve roles of the teacher. *Med Teach, 22*, 334–347.

Knight, L. V., & Bligh, J. (2006). Physicians' perceptions of clinical teaching: A qualitative analysis in the context of change. *Advances in Health Sciences Education, 11*(3), 221-234.

Knowles, M. S. (1970). *The modern practice of adult education. Andragogy versus pedagogy.* Chicago: Association Press.

Lave, J., & Wenger, E. (1991). *Situated learning: Legitimate peripheral participation.* Cambridge: Cambridge University Press.

McLaughlin, M. W., & Zarrow, J. (2001). Teachers engage in evidence-based reform: Trajectories of teachers' inquiry, analysis and action. In A. Lieberman & L. Miller (Eds.), *Teachers caught in the action: Professional development that matters.* New York: Teachers College Press. Retrieved from http://www.dest.gov.au/archive/highered/eippubs/eip00_5/fullcopy.pdf

Percy, A., & Beaumont, R. (2008). The casualisation of teaching and the subject at risk. *Studies in Continuing Education. 30*(2), 145-157.

Ramsden, P. (1999). *Learning to teach in higher education.* London: Routledge.

Remmick, M., Karm, M., Haamer, A., & Lepp, L. (2011). Early career academics' learning in academic communities. *International Journal for Academic Development, 16*(3), 187-199. Retrieved from http://www.tandfonline.com/doi/pdf/10.1080/1360144X.2011.596702

Rogers, C. R. (1951). *Client-centered therapy.* Boston: Houghton Mifflin.

Skelton, A. (2012). Teacher identities in a research-led institution: In the ascendancy or in the retreat? *British Educational Research Journal, 38*(1), 23-39.

Spencer J. (2003). Learning and teaching in the clinical environment. *British Medical Journal, 326*, 591-594.

Trowler, P., & Knight, P. T. (2000). Coming to know in higher education: Theorising faculty entry to new work contexts. *Higher Education Research and Development, 19*(1), 27-42. Retrieved from http://chelt.anu.edu.au/sites/default/files/Trowler%20and%20Knight.pdf

Vygotsky, L. S. (1978). *Mind in society: The development of the higher psychological processes.* Cambridge, MA: MIT Press.

Weimer, M. (2002). *Learner-centered teaching: Five key changes to practice.* San Francisco: Jossey-Bass.

Wenger, E. (1998). *Communities of practice: Learning meaning and identity.* Cambridge, MA: Cambridge University Press.

Wenger, E., McDermott, R., & Snyder, W. M. (2002). *Cultivating communities of practice: A guide to managing knowledge.* Cambridge MA: Harvard Business Press.

Whitchurch, C. (2012). Expanding the parameters of academia. *Higher Education, 64*, 99-117.

Tania Gerzina PhD
Faculty of Dentistry
The University of Sydney, Australia

Kirsty Foster PhD
Sydney Medical School
The University of Sydney, Australia

SECTION 2: HEALTH PROFESSIONAL EDUCATION

IN CONTEXT

GARY D. ROGERS AND DAWN FORMAN

4. THE CONTEXT OF HEALTH PROFESSIONAL EDUCATION TODAY

There is no doubt that graduates entering the health professions in the second and third decades of the twenty-first century will face an environment that is different in a range of important ways from that which most of their teachers encountered at the same point in their own professional careers. It is vital that we, as health professional educators, help our students to develop the perspectives and skills that will enable them to thrive and develop further in this changed context. We argue that foremost among these is a critical posture, where they are encouraged from the beginning to question the assumptions and culturally received knowledge that they will encounter in clinical and educational spaces. The fact that many of our students come to us after training in positivist scientific paradigms, at school or undergraduate levels, makes this a particular challenge

In this chapter we first survey the sociopolitical context of current health professional practice and education. Then we consider recent changes in the system of healthcare delivery with which our students will have to grapple, before examining recent trends in educational practice that will impact on us as health professional educators. We also reflect on how the world view of current healthcare students may differ from our own and the influences that these differences may have on the process of learning. Finally, we offer some suggestions for how we might best equip our students to become effective health practitioners at this point in history.

SOCIOPOLITICAL CONTEXT

Currently, hardly a day passes without the news media featuring some "crisis" in relation to healthcare (Sweet, 2010), leaving the average health professional student or educator in developed countries with an uneasy sense that something is deeply wrong with our health system, but no sense at all of what exactly that something is, or how it might be addressed. In this section we attempt to describe the sociopolitical currents that bear on the current state of healthcare delivery in the developed world.

Individualism, the Neoliberal Agenda and the Commodification of Health

Neoliberalism is a political philosophy that emphasises individual liberty and responsibility over community responsibility and the role of the state in improving human welfare. Coming to prominence during the 1980s under Ronald Reagan in

S. Loftus et al. (Eds.), Educating Health Professionals:
Becoming a University Teacher, 35–48.

the United States (US), Margaret Thatcher in the United Kingdom (UK) and the Hawke-Keating governments in Australia, it remains the dominant paradigm underpinning health policy in most developed countries (McGregor, 2001).

Neoliberalism as an historical movement represented a resurgence of the "free markets" principle first proposed by Adam Smith in the Eighteenth Century. Pellegrino (1999, p. 245) summarised Smith's central tenet very succinctly as "if … everyone pursues his or her own interests, the interests of all will be served". Smith argued in *The Wealth of Nations* (1776, 1976, p. 356) that in the operation of an economy:

> every individual … intends only his own gain, and he is in this … *led by an invisible hand* to promote an end which was no part of his intention. … By pursuing his own interest he frequently promotes that of the society more effectually than when he really intends to promote it. (emphasis added)

This "invisible hand" of self-interest, re-worked and re-stated by many other thinkers, including Friedrich Hayek and Milton Freidman, forms the basis for a set of beliefs about the ability of unfettered economic activity – buying and selling in markets that are as free as possible from "interference" by governments – to solve all the problems of humankind. McGregor (2001, p. 84) described the basic elements of Neoliberalism as:

> (a) the necessity of [a] free market (in which we work and consume); (b) individualism; and (c) the pursuit of narrow self-interest rather than mutual interest, with the assumption that these three tenets will lead to social good.

In relation to health, pursuit of the free market philosophy by Western governments in the last three decades has led to a range of policy outcomes. First among these has been a focus on individual responsibility in the prevention of ill-health. This view is exemplified by the "just say no" drug use prevention campaign in the US (Elliott, 1993) and the pronouncements of former Australian health minister Tony Abbott on issues as diverse as obesity (2006) and blood borne virus infection (2003). It posits that all that is needed to reduce the incidence of diseases linked to personal behaviours such as smoking, unprotected sex with multiple partners, overeating or inadequate exercise is for informed individuals simply to decide to change their behaviour. In this view, state institutions have no role beyond simply informing citizens of the causal associations between the behaviours and the health outcomes. What individuals do with such information is considered entirely a matter for them. Such a view has been stringently criticised, since it ignores what is known about the complex causation of health and health-related behaviours (Krieger, 2001), including the deliberate efforts of the manufacturers of unhealthy products to influence behaviour through marketing.

A second outcome of the Neoliberal agenda in relation to health is the trend towards privatisation and corporatisation of healthcare delivery. The compulsory transfer of funds from one individual to another by governmental action, such as through taxation of the healthy to fund care for the chronically ill, is seen in the

Neoliberal model to be transgressive of the free market principle and "a type of discrimination for those who do not get to benefit" (McGregor, 2001, p. 85). Thus, the Neoliberal approach emphasises the responsibility of individuals to make personal provision for the possibility of accident or illness through savings or private insurance.

Related to this is the notion that, because of the absence of a profit motive, the delivery of services by state institutions inherently "lacks efficiency, while private markets are more cost-effective and consumer friendly" (Horton, 2007, p. 2). As a result, governments motivated by the Neoliberal agenda will seek to move responsibility for the provision of healthcare services from public institutions to private companies.

Pellegrino (1999) has argued that these processes amount to a "commodification of health care"; that is, treating healthcare as if it were a commodity like iron ore or coffee beans, with the intention that "quality" will be assured "through the usual mechanisms of competition"(p. 243). However, as Pellegrino further demonstrated, healthcare does not, in fact, have the fundamental characteristics of a commodity. It is not "fungible"; that is, instances of it cannot be mutually substituted. Rather, each episode of healthcare is, or at least should be, a unique and particular human interaction between provider and patient or client that is inherently different from any other. Nor is healthcare "proprietary", meaning that it is the property of the vendor. As Pellegrino argued, the knowledge and skills of health providers do not wholly belong to them, since they are based on the collective historical wisdom of their professions and the heritage of health research, much of which has been supported by the resources of the community. In this view, professionals are seen as "stewards" rather than proprietary owners of the wherewithal to provide healthcare (p. 251).

Additionally, as Kaveny (1999) pointed out, commodities are distributed within a market "to each according to their willingness (and ability) to pay" (p. 211), but there are ethical imperatives for healthcare to be provided according to other principles such as "to each according to need" or "to each according to the degree that his or her receipt of the good is likely to improve the general health status of the population" (p. 216).

Callahan (1999, p. 229) suggested that market-based approaches to healthcare will fail to benefit humankind because of "a fundamental, intrinsic conflict between market values and traditional medical values". He argued that healthcare is "explicitly altruistic in its formal goals, aiming for health" and thus fundamentally at odds with the market, which is "explicitly oriented to the maximization of choice and efficiency, aiming at satisfying individual self-interest." In attempting to answer the question of why, in the light of this conflict, many policymakers persist in attempts to use commodity principles to organise healthcare, Callahan further noted that "it is a matter of indifference to many market proponents that health care does not lend itself well to a … market model". He concluded that "the reasons for this appear as much ideological as efficiency oriented" (p. 229).

On the other hand, while Timmermans and Almeling (2009, pp. 24-25) agreed that the imposition of market mechanisms in health had a range of negative outcomes, they pointed out that it is possible that the commodification of some aspects of healthcare could have beneficial consequences for patients and clients, such as "bringing new products to market" or "raising awareness of treatment options".

Either way, it appears likely that, along with the predominance of Neoliberal ideals more generally in the developed world, market-oriented approaches to healthcare provision will continue to dominate for the foreseeable future. Thus it will be important for the health professionals of the future to have the understanding and skills needed to optimise outcomes for their patients, clients and communities in the face of the challenges they provide, while simultaneously applying a critical perspective to the Neoliberal model and its consequences.

Empowerment of Patients and Clients – Health Consumerism

Although, as has been discussed, the characterisation of healthcare provision as a commercial transaction between vendor and customer can have a range of negative consequences, one idea borrowed from the commercial sphere, that of the empowered consumer, has considerable potential to benefit the health of individuals. As Herrmann (1970) documented, consumer movements probably began in the 1880s with community mobilisation that ultimately led to "pure food" legislation in the US and, as early as 1938, following the death of more than a hundred recipients of a new preparation of sulphanilamide, healthcare issues have been among their foci.

As Hibbard and Weeks (1987, p. 1020) observed, the role of the empowered consumer for a recipient of healthcare "is in stark contrast to the traditional patient role". Under this model, they argued, a patient or client is "questioning, willing to make independent judgments on whether to accept [healthcare provider] advice, and seeks out alternative sources of information", rather than being "compliant, trusting, and uncomplaining". This shift in role has occurred in parallel with the organisational changes in healthcare already discussed. Kizer argued in 2001 that the shift had been driven by a range of socio-historical factors, namely:

> the aging of the "baby boomers" and greater prevalence of chronic conditions, the explosion of biomedical scientific knowledge and technology, changes in the prevailing method of health care financing, a recent prolonged period of economic prosperity, widespread community concerns about patient safety, return of disproportionate health care cost increases, and the democratization of medical knowledge consequent to widespread use of the Internet. (p. 1213)

The organised consumer movement in relation to healthcare has also been actively supported by governments in several countries, such as New Labour's reforming of the National Health Service in Britain around the turn of the current century (Newman & Vidler, 2006) or the establishment of the Consumers Health Forum of

Australia by the Hawke-Keating government in 1987, and its subsequent funding from government revenue since that time (Consumers Health Forum of Australia, 2012).

There is little doubt that the empowerment of consumers has led to an improvement in the quality of relationships between health practitioners and their patients or clients (Ouschan, Sweeney, & Johnson, 2006) and there is some evidence of associated improvements in health outcomes (Segal, 1998). Social researchers such as Lupton (1997) have pointed to complexity in real provider-recipient relationships, however, where health service users "may pursue both the ideal-type 'consumerist' and the 'passive patient' subject position simultaneously and variously, depending on the context" (p. 373).

Breen (2001, p. 21) emphasised the importance of reforms to health professional education so that graduates in the traditionally more directive professions such as medicine, in particular, are "better equipped" for these changed healthcare relationships. He pointed out that all medical schools in Australia have adjusted their programs to "emphasize the development of communications skills and appropriate professional attitudes" with these issues in mind. Improving educational programs to optimise acquisition of these critical skills may be more challenging, however, in less well-resourced health professional programs, with larger learning group sizes.

Patient Safety

Another major recent development that bears on health professional education is the "patient safety" discourse, which arguably began with the publication of the report *To Err is Human: Building a Safer Health System* by the Institute of Medicine of the (US) National Academy of Sciences in 1999 (Kohn, Corrigan, & Donaldson, 2000). The report estimated that more people died as a result of healthcare error in the US each year, at the time of its writing, than from motor vehicle accidents, breast cancer or AIDS. The patient safety agenda has focused on analysis of the systemic causes for healthcare error, in recognition of the extreme complexity of contemporary healthcare delivery, and the failure of a legalistic, blame-oriented, approach to prevent adverse outcomes.

A particular area of attention with the patient safety movement has been the importance of effective collaboration between healthcare workers from different professions in the safe provision of care to patients and clients. Interprofessional practice was defined by Freeth and colleagues (2005) as "two or more professions working together as a team with a common purpose, commitment and mutual respect". Enquiries into healthcare misadventure in multiple developed world settings (Bristol Royal Infirmary Inquiry, 2001; Garling, 2008) have highlighted the importance of high-quality interprofessional practice in the assurance of patient safety. Recently, the World Health Organization (2010), supported by a series of international conferences under the moniker of *All Together Better Health*, has sought to advance the approach as a solution to problems with healthcare delivery in both developed and developing countries. As a consequence there has been considerable work on how best to equip health professional graduates to become effective members of interprofessional teams (see Interprofessional Education below and Chapter 16).

Changes in the Media

The advent of television stations dedicated to the continuous provision of news, which began in the 1980s, as well as the increasing use of the Internet to access information, especially on portable devices, has fundamentally changed the rhythm of information gathering by individuals across the world (Croteau, Hoynes, & Milan, 2012). Whereas formerly, information about current events was assimilated on a daily basis through reading a newspaper, or later through an evening television news bulletin, now "cable news, websites, and other sources of news are constantly updated throughout the day" (p. 301). Individuals seek to access new information on a continuous basis, but with little opportunity for analysis or reflection.

Similarly, gaining an understanding of the cause of health symptoms formerly required either a trip to the local library or, more commonly, consultation with a trusted practitioner. Now, more adults (59%) reported having accessed health-related information on the Internet in the preceding year than having consulted a medical practitioner (55%) according to Elkin (2008). In another study, 51% of adult respondents reported using the Internet to access health-related information "typically weekly" and 11% reported that they had discontinued prescribed treatment on the basis of information obtained online (Weaver, Thompson, Weaver, & Hopkins, 2009, p. 1376).

The impact of the "24-hour news cycle" on the quality of public discourse and behaviour of political leaders has also been the subject of considerable concern (Tanner, 2011), not least in relation to health policy (CBS News, 2009; Sammut, 2012). As a result of these developments, it is clear that health practitioners now have to work with patients and clients who are more informed, but not necessarily better informed, than those of their predecessors. Health practitioners will need to help patients and clients to be critical of the information they access. This is yet another important reason for practitioners themselves to have well-developed critical skills.

Alternative and Complementary Therapies

Another important trend in the sociopolitical context of healthcare practice in recent times is the increasing interest, on the part of citizens in the developed world, in understandings of health and disease that are outside of the Western scientific paradigm (Kessler et al., 2001). In a recent population survey of Australians aged 50 or more, Morgan et al. (2012) found that 46% of respondents had used a non-conventional medicinal product in the 24-hour period that was the subject of the study. Among the respondents, 87% had also used a conventional medicine within the same period, supporting the contention that non-Western interventions are not only very widely used but are now commonly seen by patients and clients as "complementary to" rather than "alternative to" conventional healthcare. Comparison to earlier studies suggests that engagement with complementary health traditions continues to increase (Thompson & Feder, 2005) and there is little doubt that it will be a major feature of future healthcare practice.

Increased Scrutiny of Healthcare Practice

The shift towards a consumerist stance for patients and clients, as well as the changes in media usage, both discussed above, have also had a major impact on the degree of scrutiny to which healthcare practice is now subject. Widely publicised examples of criminal behaviour on the part of healthcare workers have also had a profound negative effect on public trust in the caring professions. Examples include Harold Shipman, the British general practitioner who is thought to have murdered 250 patients (Baker & Hurwitz, 2009), Charles Cullen, the US nurse convicted of murdering 29 clients (Associated Press, 2006) and surgeon Jayant Patel in Australia, who was found guilty and gaoled for three counts of manslaughter and one of grievous bodily harm in relation to injudicious and incompetent surgery (Burton, 2010), but was, at the time of writing, awaiting re-trial following a High Court challenge.

These influences have changed forever an environment where the healthcare worker can expect to be trusted implicitly, and it is important that we prepare our students for a world where they will be subject to continuous scrutiny and need always to be prepared to defend their clinical decisions and actions.

CHANGES IN HEALTHCARE PRACTICE

The changing demographics and consequent changes in the healthcare needs of people in developed countries (Crisp, 2010) have demanded significant reassessment of the ways in which healthcare is delivered. Recent reviews of health systems in Australia (Health Workforce Australia, 2012) and internationally (World Health Organization, 2010) point to the need for new models of healthcare delivery. Many aspects of healthcare have been called into question, including service inequalities, sociocultural issues with regard to refugees, geographical and regional aspects, aged care, a perceived need for greater efficiency, integration of primary and tertiary care, integration of private and public healthcare initiatives, clarity of communication systems, the impact of information technology, skill mix and new roles of health assistants. It is also interesting to compare the approach to these issues in developed countries with the innovations being implemented in developing countries (World Health Organization, 2010). Given that healthcare in any country is expensive, it is high on any government agenda to ensure efficient and effective use of the resources while maintaining quality.

Research comparing healthcare expenditure with outcomes is an ongoing enterprise in developed countries. Davis, Schoen, and Stremikis (2010) compared health expenditure with measures of healthcare quality and accessibility in a number of countries for the same year. They found that the United Kingdom had the second highest quality ranking overall (after the Netherlands), with perhaps some further need to focus on patient-centred care, despite much lower per capita health expenditure than the US or Canada, which were ranked 7th and 6th respectively.

Perhaps it is unsurprising, therefore, that a British White Paper on the National Health Service (NHS) published in the same year (Department of Health, 2010) emphasised the need to:

- put patients at the heart of everything the NHS does
- focus on continuously improving those things that really matter to patients – the outcome of their healthcare
- empower and liberate clinicians to innovate, with the freedom to focus on improving healthcare services.

This emphasis on quality can be traced through white papers in the UK over the eight years from 2004 to 2012. Initially it was couched in the language of "key performance indicators", but in 2008 there was a shift to include more of the views of the staff working in the NHS – a result, many believe, of the influence of the then Parliamentary Under Secretary of State for the Department of Health, Lord Darzi. He researched health service provision in London and published *Health Care for London: A Framework for Action* (2008). The document was based on five main principles:

- Services focused on individual needs and choices
- Localise where possible; centralise where necessary
- Truly integrated care and partnership working, maximising the contribution of the entire workforce
- Prevention is better than cure
- A focus on health inequalities and diversity.

Inevitably, as these changes are implemented, health professional educators will need to adjust their curricula and pedagogies accordingly.

CHANGES IN EDUCATIONAL PRACTICE

Operationalising Workforce Reform

Internationally, developed countries have been reviewing health and education policy to ensure that they have a workforce ready for changing healthcare needs and an aging population (Crisp, 2010). Health Workforce Australia (HWA) has recently undertaken a review of that country's health professional workforce requirements with the intention of "preparing for 2025" (HWA, 2012).

To address the healthcare practice changes alluded to in the previous section, HWA contends that higher education institutions and health professional educators may need to:

- adjust the skill mix of practitioners being developed in higher education. For example, are sufficient support workers being educated? Are new types of health professionals needed?
- ensure that health professionals can work to their full, or even an expanded scope of practice and have an appropriate balance of specialism and generalism
- ensure that graduates are able to examine the current roles of each health profession and respond creatively to any identified need for role adjustments
- enable health professional graduates to work collaboratively in new and changing service models
- ensure that graduates are ready to work with emerging technologies, including e-health and tele-health.

The process of workforce reform has also led to a renewed focus on accurate delineation of the capabilities required by health professionals in particular settings. There has been increasing pressure from government agencies to define these in very precise terms, according to the approach developed by the "competency movement" in vocational education (Reeve, Fox, & Hodges, 2009, p. 451). Considerable controversy has surrounded this development, in relation to both the definition of the word "competency", as applied to healthcare, and the risk that complex, higher-level cognitive and human elements of healthcare practice will be ignored or undervalued because they cannot be easily reduced to short competency statements (Australian Medical Council, 2010).

Learning-Centred Pedagogies

The last three decades have seen significant advances in learning theory, as well as recognition of the critical importance of lifelong learning for health practitioners, in the face of continually developing human knowledge. This has led to a major shift in the orientation of educational practice from a focus on the transmission of information by teachers to a concentration on student-regulated learning and acquisition of the capacity to continue to learn throughout professional careers.

This change of approach has been manifest through a range of educational innovations such as problem-based learning (see Chapter 11) and simulation (see Chapter 22), as well as learning approaches that blend face-to-face and computer-based strategies (see Chapter 21).

Interprofessional Education

The importance to patient safety of collaborative interprofessional practice has been emphasised above. Interprofessional education (IPE) is defined by the World Health Organization (2010, p. 13) as occurring:

when students from two or more professions learn about, from and with each other to enable effective collaboration and improve health outcomes.

Participation in IPE is generally agreed to be critical to the development of the skills, understandings and attitudes needed for interprofessional practice. A global movement, supported by the World Health Organization (2010), aims to ensure the inclusion of IPE opportunities in all health professional training programs.

Australia has recently undertaken a national review of IPE efforts and is in the process of developing a national curriculum framework to guide the implementation of the approach by educational institutions. The framework will utilise a four-dimensional model for health professional curriculum development developed by Lee, Steketee, Rogers, and Moran (2013). The methodology recognises the real potential for organisational and logistic barriers to impede the implementation of IPE, and provides the impetus for overcoming these problems by reconnection with the high-level societal purpose for change. IPE is explored more fully in Chapter 16.

CHANGES IN HEALTH PROFESSIONAL STUDENTS

Many of the societal changes discussed earlier in this chapter have had an impact not only on patients, clients and the public, but also specifically on the young (and often not so young) people who are our students. The learners of today are different in a wide range of ways that are explored more fully in Chapter 13. One aspect that many higher education practitioners talk about, in our experience, is the difference in the place of work and study in the complex lives of contemporary students compared with their forebears. Billett (2010) encapsulated this well when he suggested that:

> more than being time poor many of today's higher education students are actually time jealous. That is, they jealously guard and manage their time, including that allocated to their ... studies. The difference between being time poor (i.e., not having enough time) and being time jealous is quite distinct. The latter means that students are more likely to actively and critically evaluate demands upon their time made by their university studies, and then respond according to those activities they view as being worthy of the investment of their time.

Billett's (2010) suggestion that "managing time jealous students' learning may become a key challenge" for contemporary higher education practitioners is particularly relevant in health professional education, where concepts are difficult, repetitive practice of skills essential and the welfare of the community depends on the outcome.

We may have to encourage our students to adopt a critical stance to their own education. Through this approach they might come to appreciate that the demands of a course are, in fact, worth the investment of their time and effort, because of the potential impact on their future patients and clients.

PREPARING OUR GRADUATES FOR PRACTICE

So how might we approach preparing our graduates for practice and further training in the complex and fluid environment that we have outlined in this chapter? Our collective experience suggests that among the most important tools that we can provide is a capacity for deliberation and reflection. We emphasise again that it is also vital to ensure that learners adopt a critical posture, through which they can, at all times, question the assumptions and culturally received knowledge that they encounter in clinical environments.

We find that early, examined, clinical exposure can be very useful for this purpose. Being able to observe healthcare delivery cultures with the "innocent eyes" of a neophyte, especially when accompanied by facilitated critical reflection, allows students to see the dehumanisation that is evident in many clinical settings but which becomes hidden from senior students and practitioners who are deeply acculturated in existing practices. We see this process as rather akin to "immunising" our students to the effects of acculturation to which they will subsequently be exposed as they progress in clinical training, with the aim of maintaining a patient/client-centred orientation in the face of the rigours of professional life.

An illustration from popular culture that one of us has found useful and engaging for contemporary students is the "red-pill/blue-pill" scene from the Australian/US movie *The Matrix* (Wachowski & Wachowski, 1999). In the scene, Keanu Reeves' character, Neo, is invited by Laurence Fishburne's Morpheus to make a choice between taking the blue pill and returning to the unquestioning but safe monotony of ordinary life or taking the red pill, which will lead to finding out how things really are and where "nothing will ever be the same again". If we liken the adoption of a critical posture to "taking the red pill", our students can come to understand that only if they are continuously vigilant, question all assumptions and think deeply about their clinical lives will they be able to have the greatest positive effect on the welfare of their patients and clients. It is also likely to result in a much more rewarding professional life.

REFERENCES

Abbott, T. (2003). Cited in Hopwood M. (2007). Globalisation, healthism and harm reduction: Responsibility, blame and cultures of care. *Polare, 74*(4). Retrieved from http://www.gendercentre.org.au/74article4.htm

Abbott, T. (2006, May 10). Plan to win the battle of the bulge. *Sydney Morning Herald*. Retrieved from http://www.smh.com.au/news/opinion/a-plan-to-win-the-battle-of-the-bulge/2006/05/09/1146940545446.html

Associated Press. (2006, March 2). Nurse who killed 29 sentenced to 11 life terms. *NBCNews.com*. Retrieved from http://www.msnbc.msn.com/id/11636992/ns/us_news-crime_and_courts/t/nurse-who-killed-sentenced-life-terms/#.UDXnpOG7Oco

Australian Medical Council. (2010). *Competence-based medical education*. Consultation paper. Retrieved from http://www.amc.org.au/images/publications/CBEWG_20110822.pdf

Baker, R., & Hurwitz, B. (2009). Intentionally harmful violations and patient safety: The example of Harold Shipman. *Journal of the Royal Society of Medicine, 102*(6), 223-227.

Billett, S. (2010). From time poor to time jealous. *Campus Review*, July 5. Woolloomooloo, Australia: APN Educational Media. Retrieved from http://www.campusreview.com.au/blog/analysis/from-time-poor-to-time-jealous/

Breen, K. J. (2001). The patient-doctor relationship in the new millennium: Adjusting positively to commercialism and consumerism. *Clinics in Dermatology, 19*(1), 19-22.

Bristol Royal Infirmary Inquiry. (2001). *Learning from Bristol: The report of the public inquiry into children's heart surgery at the Bristol Royal Infirmary 1984-1995*. London: Stationery Office. Retrieved from http://www.bristol-inquiry.org.uk/final_report/index.htm

Burton, B. (2010). Surgeon sentenced to seven years in jail for patient deaths. *British Medical Journal, 341*. doi:10.1136/bmj.c3646 Retrieved from http://www.bmj.com/content/341/bmj.c3646.full

Callahan, D. (1999). Medicine and the market: A research agenda. *Journal of Medicine and Philosophy 24*(3), 224-242.

CBSNews. (2009). *Obama: 24-hour news cycle feeding anger*. Retrieved from http://www.cbsnews.com/2100-3460_162-5324017.html

Consumers Health Forum of Australia. (2012). *CHF's history*. Retrieved from https://www.chf.org.au/history.php

Crisp, N. (2010). Global health capacity and workforce development: Turning the world upside down. *Infectious Disease Clinics of North America, 25*(2), 359-367.

Croteau, D., Hoynes, W., & Milan, S. (2012). *Media society: Industries, images and audiences* (4th ed.). Thousand Oaks, CA: Sage.

Darzi, A. (2008). *Health care for London: A framework for action*. London: National Health Service. Retrieved from http://www.nhshistory.net/darzilondon.pdf

Davis, K., Schoen, C., & Stremikis, K. (2010). *Mirror mirror on the wall: How the performance of the U.S. health care system compares internationally*. The Commonwealth Fund. Retrieved from http://www.commonwealthfund.org/Publications/Fund-Reports/2010/Jun/Mirror-Mirror-Update.aspx?page=all

Department of Health. (2010). *NHS white paper – Equity and excellence: Liberating the NHS*. The Stationery Office: London. ISBN: 9780101788120.

Elkin, N. (2008). *How America searches: Health and wellness*. Scottsdale, AZ: iCrossing. Retrieved from http://www.icrossing.com/research/how-america-searches-health-and-wellness.php

Elliott J. (1993, May). Just say nonsense – Nancy Reagan's drug education programs. *Washington Monthly*, 18-21. Retrieved from http://www.unz.org/Pub/WashingtonMonthly-1993may-00018

Freeth, D., Hammick, M., Reeves, S., Koppel, I., & Barr, H. (2005). *Effective interprofessional education: Development, delivery and evaluation*. Oxford: Blackwell with CAIPE.

Garling, P. (2008). *Final report of the special commission of inquiry: Acute care in NSW public hospitals*. Retrieved from http://www.dpc.nsw.gov.au/__data/assets/pdf_file/0003/34194/Overview_-_Special_Commission_Of_Inquiry_Into_Acute_Care_Services_In_New_South_Wales_Public_Hospitals.pdf

Health Workforce Australia. (2012). *Health workforce 2025: Doctors, nurses and midwives*. Adelaide, Australia: Health Workforce Australia. Retrieved from http://www.hwa.gov.au/publications

Herrmann, R. O. (1970). Consumerism: Its goals, organizations and future. *Journal of Marketing, 34*(4), 55-60.

Hibbard, J. H., & Weeks, E. C. (1987). Consumerism in health care. *Medical Care, 25*(11), 1019-1032.

Horton, E. (2007). Neoliberalism and the Australian healthcare system (factory). In *Creativity, enterprise, policy: New directions in education. Proceedings of the 2007 conference of the Philosophy of Education Society of Australasia*. Wellington, New Zealand. Retrieved from http://eprints.qut.edu.au/14444/1/14444.pdf

Kaveny, M. C. (1999). Commodifying the polyvalent good of health care. *Journal of Medicine and Philosophy, 24*(3), 207-223.

Kessler, R. C., Davis, R. B., Foster, D. F., Van Rompay, M. I., Walters, E. E., Wilkey, S. A. et al. (2001). Long-term trends in the use of complementary and alternative medical therapies in the United States. *Annals of Internal Medicine, 135*(4), 262-268.

Kizer, K. W. (2001). Establishing health care performance standards in an era of consumerism. *JAMA, 286*(10), 1213-1217.

Kohn, L. T., Corrigan, J. M., & Donaldson, M. S. (Eds.). (2000). *To err is human: Building a safer health system.* Washington, DC: National Academy Press. Retrieved from http://www.nap.edu/openbook.php?isbn=0309068371

Krieger, N. (2001). Theories for social epidemiology in the 21st century: An ecosocial perspective. *International Journal of Epidemiology, 30*(4), 668-677.

Lee, A., Steketee, C., Rogers, G. D., & Moran, M. (2013). Towards a theoretical framework for curriculum development within and between health professions. *Focus on Health Professional Education, 14*(3).

Lupton, D. (1997). Consumerism, reflexivity and the medical encounter. *Social Science & Medicine, 45*(3), 373-381.

McGregor, S. (2001). Neoliberalism and health care. *International Journal of Consumer Studies, 25*(2), 82-89.

Morgan, T. K., Williamson, M., Pirotta, M., Stewart, K., Myers, S. P., & Barnes, J. (2012). A national census of medicines use: A 24-hour snapshot of Australians aged 50 years and older. *Medical Journal of Australia, 196*(1), 50-53.

Newman, J., & Vidler, E. (2006). Discriminating customers, responsible patients, empowered users: Consumerism and the modernisation of health care. *Journal of Social Policy, 35*(2), 193-209.

Ouschan, R., Sweeney, J., & Johnson, L. (2006). Customer empowerment and relationships outcomes in healthcare consultations. *European Journal of Marketing, 40*(9), 1068-1086.

Pellegrino, E. D. (1999). The commodification of medical and health care: The moral consequences of a paradigm shift from a professional to a market ethic. *Journal of Medicine and Philosophy, 24*(3), 243-266.

Reeve, S., Fox, A., & Hodges, B. D. (2009). The competency movement in the health professions: Ensuring consistent standards or reproducing conventional domains of practice? *Advances in Health Sciences Education, 14*(4), 451-453.

Sammut, J. (2012). NSW health history shows Carr's feet of clay. *The Drum Opinion.* Sydney: Australian Broadcasting Corporation. Retrieved from http://www.abc.net.au/unleashed/3920084.html

Segal, L. (1998). The importance of patient empowerment in health system reform. *Health Policy, 44*(1), 31-44.

Smith, A. (1776, 1976). The Glasgow edition of the works and correspondence of Adam Smith, Vol. 2a *The Wealth of Nations* (eds. R.H. Cambell & A.S. Skinner). Oxford: Clarendon Press.

Sweet, M. (2010). *Problems with media coverage of health policy ... and some suggested solutions.* Retrieved from http://blogs.crikey.com.au/croakey/2010/06/29/problems-with-media-coverage-of-health-policy-and-some-suggested-solutions/

Tanner, L. (2011). *Sideshow: Dumbing down democracy.* Brunswick, VIC: Scribe Publications.

Thompson, T., & Feder, G. (2005). Complementary therapies and the NHS. *British Medical Journal, 331,* 856-857.

Timmermans, S., & Almeling, R. (2009). Objectification, standardization, and commodification in health care: A conceptual readjustment. *Social Science & Medicine, 69*(1), 21-27.

Wachowski, L., & Wachowski, A. (Writers and Directors). (1999). *The matrix.* Melbourne, VIC: Village Roadshow Pictures.

Weaver, J. B., Thompson, N. J., Weaver, S. S., & Hopkins, G. L. (2009). Healthcare non-adherence decisions and Internet health information. *Computers in Human Behavior, 25,* 1373-1380.

World Health Organization. (2010). *Framework for action on interprofessional education and collaborative practice.* Geneva, Switzerland: World Health Organization. Retrieved from http://www.who.int/hrh/resources/framework_action/en/index.html

Gary D. Rogers MBBS, MGPPsych, PhD
School of Medicine and Health Institute for the Development of Education and
Scholarship (Health IDEAS)
Griffith University, Australia

Dawn Forman PhD MBA PG Dip Research PG Dip Executive Coaching MDCR
TDCR
Curtin Health Innovation Research Institute
Faculty of Health Sciences
Curtin University, Australia

OLANREWAJU SORINOLA, TANIA GERZINA AND
JILL THISTLETHWAITE

5. HEALTH PROFESSIONAL EDUCATION PROGRAMS

How the Teacher Develops

Health professionals who teach may be salaried health sector employees who are directly engaged by a higher education institution in adjunct or conjoint academic appointments. Many teaching health professionals also provide learning activities through good will and altruism. Another group consists of academics with health professional degrees for whom academia is the primary employment; these professionals may engage in professional clinical practice in only a limited capacity.

Many assume that practising health professionals will be adequate educators: that as clinical (content or discipline) experts, they should naturally also be competent teachers. We know, however, that there may be little correlation between clinical proficiency, seniority and teaching excellence. Thus there is a need for health professional *educators* to be provided with the opportunities to develop skills in educating. The provision of teaching development in this area has expanded over the last few decades. Many universities now offer degree programs such as certificates and masters level degrees so that health professionals can gain formal education qualifications, thus legitimising their teaching in a professional context.

Such legitimisation is also increasingly viewed as important by national health systems and services and/or learners (at both pre- and post-qualification levels). Moreover, as the cost of health professional training continues to rise, students as consumers of education are beginning to expect their educators to be formally qualified to teach, facilitate and supervise. This chapter presents an overview of these developmental initiatives, referred to as education development (also known as faculty development) and analyses evidence that shows what works and why. The ultimate aim of this development is to improve teaching practices, the quality of graduates and ultimately patient care, but the evidence for this sort of impact remains weak (Steinert et al., 2006). We include as educators health professionals teaching in any of the following environments: tutorial rooms in academic centres, clinical settings (primary, secondary and tertiary), simulation centres and lecture theatres.

Development of the Health Professional as a Teacher

Only from the second half of the 20th century has teaching in medical schools been acknowledged as a skill independent of content expertise. The theories underpinning student learning have played a major role in this shift in emphasis. In some higher education institutions, attendance of educators at sessions to develop or enhance

S. Loftus et al. (Eds.), Educating Health Professionals:
Becoming a University Teacher, 49–60.

teaching skills is mandatory. Goody's (2007) review confirms that nearly 75% of Australian universities now offer teaching preparation activities with requirements for staff participation. Course material in such teaching preparation activity programs includes the theory of adult learning and principles of learning and teaching, curriculum design, evaluation and assessment for a general audience about to start teaching, in addition to specifically addressing needs of health professional educators. The World Federation for Medical Education (WFME) has recommended that medical teachers professionalise their practice through teaching qualifications, in conjunction with a medical school policy to include teacher training, development, appraisal and reward (WFME, 2000). However, the status of such development varies greatly within different national contexts: from established programs in the USA and Canada, to a developmental framework in the UK and compulsory engagement in Scandinavia, to absence of activities in France (Saroyan & Frenay, 2010).

National regulatory bodies for health professional education and training, such as the national professional councils, are also taking an increasingly prominent role in defining standards and scopes of practice for quality in health professional education at undergraduate and postgraduate levels. During the last few years, the Australian Medical Council (AMC) has outlined requirements for the accreditation and re-accreditation of specialty training programs. Increasingly there is a requirement for medical colleges providing specialty training and continuing professional development to acquire greater expertise in areas such as curriculum development, assessment methodology and program evaluation. Some health professional industrial awards that list the salary rates for hospital-employed workers, such as nursing, have particular classifications for educators. These classifications require specialist qualifications in education for health professionals. A factor that may drive more development in health professional education in the Australian environment is the national (Australian) Health Practitioner Regulation Agency (AHPRA) that administers professional registration and will inevitably influence policy in professional education as analysis drawn from the combined logistical data generated is published.

Health professional education development programs aim to improve performance in teaching, research and administration (Sheets & Schwenk, 1990). A comprehensive development program may therefore include several components (Box 5.1).

- Orientation to the institution and to faculty member roles
- Educational theory – particularly adult learning principles
- Educational/teaching improvement and mentoring
- Leadership development
- Organisational development such as an understanding of policies and procedures
- Research and governance

Box 5.1. Suggested components of generic faculty development
(adapted from Wilkerson & Irby, 1998)

The Heath Professional Education Development Literature

A significant amount of the published literature is informed by medical education research, with three main categories comprising context, content/process and evaluation (Box 5.2). The main interest to health professional educators lies in the articles on content/process and evaluation.

In the next sections we consider both content/process and evaluation.

- Context: articles discussing the historical development, evolution, background, implementation, drivers and barriers affecting health professional education
- Content: articles primarily focused on describing a health professional educator intervention or program on teaching, which they may also have a small section on evaluation
- Evaluation: articles with detailed descriptions of health professional educator program evaluation

Box 5.2. Themes of health professional educator articles from medical education

Content and Process of Health Professional Education Initiatives

The learning processes most frequently used in health professional educator development are based on the theory of adult learning (McLaughlin, 2005), with active learning (Frohna, Hamstra, Mullan, & Gruppen, 2006), self-directed, experiential/reflective learning (Amin, Hoon Eng, Gwee, & Chay Hoon, 2006) and conceptual change theory (Hewson, 2000) also prominent. The last is a process in which educators are helped to develop or change their existing educational ideas into more elaborate concepts of teaching, such as from a teacher-centred to a learner-centred conception (Pratt, 1992; Hewson, 2000; Light & Calkins, 2008).

Educator development tends to be delivered mainly as *ad hoc* short courses, workshops, seminars or accredited university awards. More innovative approaches include longitudinal programs, where faculty members commit a proportion of their time on a regular basis over 1–2 years to develop their knowledge and skills leading to certification, advanced degrees or fellowships (Steinert, Nasmith, McLeod, & Conochie, 2003; Steinert & McLeod, 2006), or hybrid programs, that is, a combination of workshops or seminars and web-based or online learning (Fidler, Khakoo, & Miller, 2007).

Mentorship is an under-utilised method. Mathias (2005) indicated that the use of mentors, that is, staff with expertise in education, can establish a genuine collegial partnership between participants' departments and the program providers, as mentors can support the development of participants' teaching roles, both generically and within the context of the subject-discipline. Clark et al. (2002) also suggested that mentors can support participants by encouraging new staff to discuss teaching with colleagues and can address issues related to translating the generic learning acquired on programs into specific teaching contexts: moving from theory to practice. Mentorship is also an important way of ensuring that staff have an appreciation of their role and the organisation in which they are working.

The literature reveals little consistency in the way programs are offered; the skills and experience acquired by participating staff differ from program to program and there is no uniformity as to whether attendance is mandated. In the UK, faculty development or similar programs are important for probationary purposes but this is less common in other parts of the world (Clark et al., 2002). Dearn, Fraser, and Ryan (2002) and Gibbs and Coffey (2000) suggested that a disparity in approaches exists between the USA, where training focuses on teaching practices, and the UK, where reflective practice is emphasised. Some programs have only medical school participants whereas others are multidisciplinary, involving health sciences departments, nursing, pharmacy, physical and occupational therapy and communication sciences (Steinert & McLeod, 2006; Fidler et al., 2007). There are also interventions that are university-wide across different disciplines (Steinert et al., 2010).

Formal development interventions range from one hour to 3 years in duration. Most programs use a multimodal approach, involving methods such as small group discussions, workshops, interactive exercises, role-play, simulations, videotaped teaching review, real-time video critique, case-based workshops, peer coaching, web-based learning and mentoring (Lang, Everett, McGowen, & Bennard, 2000; Newland, Newland, Steele, Lough, & McCurdy, 2003; Boucher et al., 2006).

Evaluation of Non-Award Programs

So far we have shown that there are major differences among programs. The reasons for these differences are not always clear but are likely to be pragmatic and dependent on resources. While this may not in itself be problematic it does make comparisons difficult. Hence there is little comparative research on which components of faculty development are most useful or whether one method, such as a workshop, is more effective than another, such as a longitudinal course (Steinert et al., 2006). With the current emphasis on evidence-based practice and the need to justify time and resources within higher education, it is important that we explore impact and what works for whom, and why. Workshops and short courses, the most common interventions, have in most studies been evaluated mainly by participants' satisfaction, most often at the end of the activity rather than in the long term. The impact of the training upon actual teaching is not usually assessed, and the duration for which this effect is sustained is seldom measured (Gall, Weathersby, & Dunning, 1971; Bland, 1980; Foley & Smilansky, 1980; Mahler & Benor, 1984). In the only systematic review of faculty development activities, Steinert et al. (2006) concluded that such activities appear to be highly valued by participants, leading to changes in learning and behaviour, but that subsequent changes in organisational practice or in student learning were not frequently reported. The review summarised the characteristics of effective educational development as using multiple instructional methods, an experiential learning approach, peer/collegial support and adherence to principles of teaching and learning. Although some authors (Barlett & Rappaport, 2009) have suggested that it is the experience of education development rather than the particulars of length, content, or delivery that have lasting importance, at present no conclusions can be drawn as to the most effective development activity or the optimal time for reinforcement.

Health Professional Education Degrees

The academic rationale for a postgraduate degree in health professional education arises from changing expectations in health professional education and reflects the wider changes that are occurring locally and globally within the higher and continuing professional education sectors. These include changes in healthcare delivery systems and their implications for learning and teaching, public and professional demand for more relevance in educational programs for the health professions, demands from funding bodies and government for accountability and quality education and training, and new pedagogies of curriculum design and delivery. Such degrees are also important for health professionals who want to pursue an academic career, though some may choose to focus more on their discipline area or on research rather than education. Curricula for these degrees reflect workforce changes, the political environment, and societal expectations of quality of care in health support, by strategically addressing increased demand for professional education and formal teaching qualifications (McLean et al., 2008).

As with all disciplines, the education literature is expansive, growing and difficult to keep up-to-date with, particularly as many health professional educators must provide evidence of continuing development in profession-specific areas as well maintaining professional registration. Examples of current "hot topics" are: the consideration of learning theories in developing and aligning curriculum elements; a focus on learners as a proactive participants in constructing their own learning; the use of innovative methods, such as high-fidelity simulation and e-learning; engagement of students in interprofessional learning; early involvement of undergraduate students in clinical settings; professionalism; work-based assessment; the development of a community of practice in learning; and a focus on developing clinical reasoning skills. Work-integrated learning has also developed its own pedagogy.

Programs Offered

Globally, qualifications in health professional education are offered at many universities, demonstrating the market that exists for such initiatives. In Australia there are eight health professional education programs; Table 5.1 is presented as an example of offerings. There are 20 in the UK and many more in North America and Asia. Of note is that, building on strong advances in medical education, an increasing number of these courses are adapted for all the health professions rather than just for medical education. For some academic health professionals there is also the opportunity to pursue a PhD in medical or health professional education, reflecting a requirement for career progression in the university system.

Programs vary widely in basic logistic characteristics, such as the award obtained, length of candidature, type of enrolment (full- or part-time), credit points, mode of educational delivery and aspects of clinical placement. A comparison of these characteristics is given in Table 5.2.

Table 5.1. Summary of health professional education courses in Australia, as an example

Institute	Competitive offering	Website
The University of Sydney	Certificate, Diploma, Master of Education (Health Professional Education)	http://sydney.edu.au/education_social_work /future_students/postgraduate/med/health_ professional_education.shtml
Charles Sturt University	Graduate Certificate in Clinical Education	http://www.csu.edu.au/courses/postgraduate /clinical_education/course-overview
Flinders University	Graduate Certificate, Graduate Diploma, Master of Clinical Education	http://www.flinders.edu.au/courses/ postgrad /ce/
Griffith University	Graduate Certificate in Clinical Education	http://www148.griffith.edu.au/programs-courses/Program/OverviewAndFees? ProgramCode=3221
Macquarie University	Master of Higher Education (Medical Education)	http://staff.mq.edu.au/teaching/workshops_ programs/postgrad_program/faq_ postgradprogram/
Monash University	Graduate Certificate, Masters in Health Professional Education. Graduate Certificate in Clinical Simulation	http://www.monash.edu.au/study/ coursefinder/course/3860/
University of Queensland	Graduate Certificate in Health Sciences – Clinical Education stream	http://www.uq.edu.au/study/program.html? acad_prog=5431
University of Western Australia	Master of Health Professional Education	http://www.meddent.uwa.edu.au/courses/ postgraduate/coursework/mast-health-prof-ed

Table 5.2. Summary of characteristics of health professional education courses

Award	– MHPE, MMEd, MMedSci, MScClinEd. – Diplomas, Graduate Certificates
Length of candidature	– 3-4 years part-time – 1 year full-time (for masters level)
Admission	– Undergraduate degree in health discipline with or without required professional teaching experience
Intake	– Clinical teachers in the health professions, administrative officers, clinical educators and health program co-ordinators, junior academics with university appointments
Organisation/ administration	– Often committee of health discipline academics
Type of enrolment	– Part- or full-time
Educational delivery	– Face-to-face, distance and online or blended – 3-4 core units plus electives coursework, group work or discussion
Curriculum	– Health education related to educational theory – Curriculum design and evaluation in the health sciences – Teaching and instructional methods – Research design and methods in health education – Measurement, assessment and psychometrics – Learning and cognition
Assessment	– Practical, focused, project-based application of principles to students' own work-integrated or clinical settings. Includes e-portfolio, peer feedback, assignments, and examinations, thesis or dissertation or portfolio
Clinical placement	– Mandatory, immersion in coursework
Further careers for graduates	– Academic, clinical educator/supervisor, clinical academic, academic in health school
Student outcomes	– Enhanced skills in curriculum development, implementation and evaluation, and student assessment – Proactive approach to continuous quality improvement in teaching and learning – Deeper understanding of principles and practices which underpin teaching and learning in health – Attitude to health education informed by best evidence and aligned to learner-centredness
Additional notes	– Graduate Certificate credit toward masters enrolment. – May impact on working conditions and promotion for health service employed graduates

Curricula of Health Professional Education Programs

Most programs emphasise core educational principles and practices relevant across the health professions and to students from a wide range of health professional backgrounds. They particularly target those wishing to enhance their teaching skills at undergraduate and postgraduate level; curriculum developers; those involved in assessment and evaluation; and individuals given new teaching responsibilities. Students from across the health professions (including health sciences, medicine, nursing, dentistry, pharmacy and allied health) enrol in the programs. Some courses are aimed at particular professional groups (e.g. Masters of Medical Education), and although students may be from different health professions, the aims are mainly related to the teaching of a specific profession.

The interprofessional nature of some educational programs, as students learn with, from, and about each other, may model interprofessional practice itself (refer to the Centre for Advancement of Interprofessional Education (CAIPE, http://www.caipe.org.uk) and the Australasian Interprofessional Practice and Education Network (AIPPEN, http://www.aippen.net) for a comprehensive list of publications on the topic, including the *Journal of Interprofessional Care*). Academics develop and deliver the courses, modelling the cooperative and collaborative interdisciplinary aspirations often articulated in university strategic learning and teaching plans. An example of an interprofessional program is the Master of Education (Health Professional Education) program at The University of Sydney, Australia.

It is a collaboration between four faculties (Education and Social Work, Health Sciences, Medicine, and Nursing and Midwifery) and is designed to maximise economies of scale and eliminate the duplication that occurred in disciplinary programs. Teaching is shared, and units of study are cross-listed among the four faculties. Current offerings are two units of study from the Faculty of Health Sciences, one unit from the Faculty of Nursing, two units from Sydney Medical School, and up to three choices from the Faculty of Education and Social Work. The university's Faculty of Education and Social Work maintains administrative oversight of the program and administers the degree enrolments, progression and graduations. Each of the collaborating faculties utilises existing staff to provide teaching in its own units of study and each faculty undertakes the marketing of the degree to its own constituencies, professional bodies and colleges. All aspects of curriculum oversight are undertaken by a multidisciplinary steering committee consisting of the collaborating faculties. Although administered by four faculties, enrolment is open and encouraged from professionals in all health professions.

Graduate Attributes in Health Professional Education

Programs aim to equip health professional educators with knowledge, skills and attitudes relevant to undergraduate, postgraduate and continuing education. Students are expected to emerge with a deeper understanding of contemporary, internationally recognised educational pedagogies and practices that underpin teaching and learning in the health professions. The learning outcomes of the programs reflect this aim and focus on the application of evidence-based educational practice to the education and supervision of health profession students in clinical environments. Universities also expect inclusion of the development of capacity in research, information literacy, personal and intellectual autonomy, ethical, social and professional understanding and communication.

Curriculum Framework

Participants in education development programs include clinical nurses, nurse educators, medical staff specialists, surgeons, physiotherapists, medical diagnostic radiography course co-ordinators and health lecturers. The practicalities of the often complex teaching commitments of these (usually part-time) students require the curriculum to be delivered in blended modes that include face-to-face, online, elective and group learning. Face-to-face delivery varies markedly, from one session a week per semester to a week-long interactive workshop. Some courses allow students to study and participate solely online, with interaction occurring through discussion boards. This method enables students from different countries to undertake the same program, with concomitant cultural challenges for course developers and facilitators.

The Impact of Faculty Development

As mentioned earlier there is little published evidence of the impact of education development programs on individuals, their learners or their organisations. This is an area ripe for further evaluation and research. In our experience of working within this area (and the ongoing doctoral work of one of the chapter's authors), there are a number of benefits from undertaking such study. Firstly, participants enhance their understanding of the education process and are usually able to apply their learning in their own clinical environments. We have seen participants begin to define learning outcomes for their students and enhance the feedback they deliver. Secondly, participants value the community of practice (Wenger, 1998) involved in such courses and the opportunity to discuss their work and challenges with other educators, as discussed in Chapter 1. Thirdly, many participants are motivated to pursue careers in academia or educational leadership as their confidence improves; for some this may involve undertaking doctoral studies.

Another significant impact of these programs has been to contribute to the advance of research and pedagogy in health professional education. There are a number of networks and associations whose members focus on such research and scholarship. In Australia and New Zealand, for example, the Australian & New Zealand Association for Health Professional Educators (ANZAHPE) is the largest group of this nature and "promotes supports and advances education in the health care professions. It aims to recognise, facilitate and disseminate high-quality educational research in health professions education". The evolution of medical education to widen engagement with other health professions is exemplified in the history of ANZAHPE (http://anzahpe.org/), which began in 1972 as ANZAME (the Australasian and New Zealand Association for Medical Education). ANZAHPE provides an annual conference, bulletins, grants and a journal for its membership of health education professionals.

In the USA, the Alliance for Continuing Education in the Health Professions (ACEHP, http://www.acehp.org) was founded in 1975 as the Alliance for Continuing Medical Education (AHCME) in support of certified medical education for physicians. In 2010 it expanded in scope to include healthcare-related education and continuing professional development. Membership is now open to all healthcare professionals involved in continuing education and professional development. The Canadian Association of Medical Education (http://www.came-acem.ca) is similar to the UK's Association for the Study of Medical Education (http://www.asme.org) which publishes the journals *Medical Education* and *The Clinical Teacher;* and in Europe (but truly global) the Association for Medical Education in Europe (http://www.amee.org) which publishes *Medical Teacher.* Despite the "medical" in their titles, these associations attract a wide range of health professional educators. The Asian Medical Education Association (http://www.med.hku.hk/amea) is an institution-based association of the Asian medical schools and was established in 2001 to strengthen and promote good pedagogy and research on medical education.

The Future for Faculty Development Programs

Further research in this area should help to identify the optimal methods for delivering such education, with more flexible programs being tailored for individual needs. More in-depth realistic evaluation should lead to greater understanding of what works best, for whom, and in what circumstances (Pawson & Tilley, 1997). We do have to consider that there is a finite market for such programs and only those that provide what participants value will survive; programs need to be profitable and thus have a minimum number of students. Students as consumers will push for quality courses and expect value for money. Program deliverers will need to review and refresh programs to ensure that they are up-to-date and fit for purpose.

Education development is under threat. There is a diminishing academic pool of teachers willing and able to contribute to teaching in the health professions rather than practise in a full-time capacity in their fields. The academic promotion of educationally-qualified health professionals through the ranks to professor continues to be slow; attractive only to the totally committed. Funding for health professional educational research, although gaining some traction in public health sectors, trails behind that for educational research in other fields, both in money, diversity of sources and timelines. Research outcomes in areas that support and inform health professional education programs are often set in long time-frames that do not meet funding agencies' expectations. Such researchers also sometimes find themselves outside the community of educational researchers.

Despite these threats, and perhaps because of them, a strong community of health professionals do persevere in their work to have an effect on the education of future health professionals by supporting, developing and always engaging the teachers of those professionals.

REFERENCES

Amin, Z., Hoon Eng, K., Gwee, M., & Chay Hoon, T. (2006). Addressing the needs and priorities of medical teachers through a collaborative intensive faculty development programme. *Medical Teacher, 28*(1), 85-88.

Barlett, P., & Rappaport, A. (2009). Long term impact of faculty development programs: The experience of Teli and Piedmont. *College Teaching, 57*(2), 73-82.

Bland, C. J. (1980). *Faculty development through workshops.* Springfield, IL: C. C. Thomas.

Boucher, B., Chyka, P., Fitzgerald, W., Hak, L., Miller, D., Parker, R., et al. (2006). A comprehensive approach to faculty development. *American Journal of Pharmaceutical Education, 70*(2), 1-6.

Clark, G., Blumhof, J., Gravestock, P., Healey, M., Jenkins, A., & Honeybone, A. (2002). Developing new lecturers: The case of a discipline-based workshop. *Active Learning in Higher Education, 3*(2), 128-144.

Dearn, J., Fraser, K., & Ryan, Y. (2002). *Investigation into the provision of professional development for university teaching in Australia: A discussion paper.* A DEST commissioned project funded through the HEIP program. Retrieved from http://www.dest.gov.au/NR/rdonlyres/D8BDFC55-1608-4845-B172-3C2B14E79435/935/uni_teaching.pdf

Fidler, D., Khakoo, R., & Miller, L. A. (2007). Teaching scholars programs: Faculty development for educators in the health professions. *Academic Psychiatry, 31*(6), 472-478.

Foley, R. P., & Smilansky, J. (1980). *Teaching techniques: A handbook for health professionals.* New York: McGraw-Hill.

Frohna, A., Hamstra, S., Mullan, P., & Gruppen, L. (2006). Teaching medical education principles and methods to faculty using an active learning approach: The University of Michigan medical education scholars program. *Academic Medicine, 81*(11), 975-978.

Gall, M. D., Weathersby, R., & Dunning, B. B. (1971). *Higher cognitive questioning: A program for training preservice and inservice teachers in skills of higher cognitive questioning.* Beverly Hills, CA: Macmillan Educational Services.

Gibbs, G., & Coffey, M. (2000). Training to teach in higher education: A research agenda. *Teacher Development, 4*(1), 31-44.

Goody, A. (2007). *Report on the survey of foundations of university teaching programs.* Unpublished manuscript. Preparing Academics to Teach in Higher Education (PATHE). A project funded by the Carrick Institute for Learning and Teaching in Higher Education.

Hewson, M. (2000). A theory based faculty development program for clinician-educators. *Academic Medicine, 75*(5), 498-501.

Lang, F., Everett, K., McGowen, R., & Bennard, B. (2000). Faculty development in communication skills instruction: Insights from a longitudinal program with real-time feedback. *Academic Medicine, 75*(12), 1222-1228.

Light, G., & Calkins, S. (2008). The experience of faculty development: Patterns of variation in conceptions of teaching. *International Journal for Academic Development, 13*(1), 27-40.

Mahler, S., & Benor, D. (1984). Short and long term effects of a teacher training workshop in medical school. *Higher Education, 13*, 265-273.

Mathias, H. (2005). Mentoring on a programme for new university teachers: A partnership in revitalizing and empowering collegiality. *International Journal for Academic Development, 10*(2), 95-106.

McLaughlin, S. (2005). Faculty development. *Academic Emergency Medicine, 12*(4), 302.e1–302.e5.

McLean M., Cilliers F., & Van Wyk J. M. (2008). Faculty development: Yesterday, today and tomorrow. *Medical Teacher, 30*(6), 555-584. doi:10.1080/01421590802109834

Newland, M., Newland, J., Steele, D., Lough, D., & McCurdy, F. (2003). Experience with a program of faculty development. *Medical Teacher, 25*(2), 207-209.

Pawson, R., & Tilley, N. (1997). *Realistic evaluation.* London: Sage.

Pratt, D. D. (1992). Conceptions of teaching. *Adult Education Quarterly, 42*(4), 203-220.

Saroyan, A., & Frenay, M. (Eds.). (2010). *Building teaching capacities in higher education: A comprehensive international model.* Sterling, VA: Stylus.

Sheets, K. J., & Schwenk, T. L. (1990). Faculty development for family medicine educators: An agenda for future activities. *Teaching and Learning Medicine, 2*, 141-148.

Steinert, Y., Macdonald, M. E., Boillat, M., Elizov, M., Meterissian, S., Razack, S., et al. (2010). Faculty development: If you build it, they will come. *Medical Education, 44*(9), 900-907.

Steinert, Y., Mann, K., Centeno, A., Dolmans, D., Spencer, J., Gelula, M., et al. (2006). A systematic review of faculty development initiatives designed to improve teaching effectiveness in medical education: BEME Guide No. 8. *Medical Teacher, 28*(6), 497-526.

Steinert, Y., & McLeod, P. (2006). From novice to informed educator: The teaching scholars program for educators in the health sciences. *Academic Medicine, 81*(11), 969-974.

Steinert, Y., Nasmith, L., McLeod, P., & Conochie, L. (2003). A teaching scholars program to develop leaders in medical education. *Academic Medicine, 78*(2), 142-149.

Wenger, E. (1998). *Communities of practice: Learning, meaning and identity.* Cambridge, MA: Cambridge University Press.

Wilkerson, L., & Irby, D. (1998). Strategies for improving teaching practices: A comprehensive approach to faculty development. *Academic Medicine, 73*(4), 387-396.

World Federation Medical Education. (2000). WFME Task force on defining international standards in basic medical education. Report of the working party. *Medical Education, 34*, 665-675.

Olanrewaju Sorinola PhD Candidate
Faculty of Medicine
University of Warwick, UK

Tania Gerzina PhD
Faculty of Dentistry
The University of Sydney, Australia

Jill Thistlethwaite PhD
School of Medicine
University of Queensland, Australia

EDWINA ADAMS, PATRICIA LOGAN, DOREEN RORRISON
AND GRAHAM MUNRO

6. LOOKING AFTER YOURSELF

Lessons to Be Learned on Entering Academia

The development of a career as an academic can be a very rewarding experience, but many entering this career are unprepared for what the role actually entails. This lack of preparedness can bring unnecessary stress to new academics, delaying their achievement of career goals. In this chapter we aim to help reduce this unpreparedness by highlighting some common difficulties experienced by new academics. We provide context for the competing demands and outline key lessons to be learned from the experiences of those who have journeyed before you. The content of this chapter is derived primarily from the experiences of the authors (three of whom are from health professions) and supported by stories collected as part of their recent research project investigating the complexities of the development of an academic identity, "Transitions from practice to academia: How do those entering the academy from professional practice develop their identity as an academic?" (unpublished). The participants in the transition project were 12 Australian academics from two metropolitan and two rural universities.

Typically, the role of the academic requires participation in three areas – research, teaching, and another area sometimes called service or administration. These three areas compete for the individual's time and must be juggled to meet the job requirements. The challenge lies in knowing how much time and effort to put into each aspect of the role. For many, there is a risk that teaching will become all-consuming at the expense of the other areas, thereby compromising the career aspirations of the new academic and possibly raising work stress levels.

The Job Demands-Resources model of work stress and engagement highlights that all occupations have their job demands and resources (Bakker & Demerouti, 2007). Job resources, such as co-worker support, are the aspects of the job that help to achieve work goals and buffer demands. Job demands, such as work overload, are the physical or psychological costs to the worker. Excessive job demands can lead to poor health, exhaustion and withdrawal from the job (Bakker, Demerouti, & Schaufeli, 2003). Clearly, the balance of job demands and job resources will determine the level of stress that new academics encounter in their transition to academia, and will possibly determine their likelihood of staying. Here we address some key areas for consideration so that an understanding of what is required for a successful transition is attained. The concept of job demands and job resources is highlighted throughout the chapter.

S. Loftus et al. (Eds.), Educating Health Professionals:
Becoming a University Teacher, 61–70.

THE INFLUENCE OF UNIVERSITY FUNDING ARRANGEMENTS

The means by which a university is funded and attains its competitive standing has a direct impact on the work of an academic. Universities play two primary roles in a country's economic and social progress. One is to be a key part of national research and innovation, and the other is to provide quality degree-level qualifications (Department of Education and Employment Workplace Relations [DEEWR] Review of Australian Higher Education, 2008, p. xi). In an academic role one is expected to contribute to both these aspects of the university.

Across the Western world university funding is variable, but generally funding is derived from government sources, student fees and research income. Government funding is often linked to some form of policy and/or performance rating to determine the level of funding. These policies and performance indicators influence the mission and objectives of universities and therefore the work environment for academics.

As an example, Australian universities are funded primarily by government funds and student contribution fees. Since the 1980s the level of government funding has decreased substantially (Marginson, 2001). At the same time, there has been an increase in student numbers and a corresponding increase in student-to-staff ratios (King, 2001; Marginson, 2001; Winefield, Boyd, Saebel, & Pignata, 2008). In the 2008 Review of Australian Higher Education report (DEEWR, p. vii), student-to-staff ratios were described as "unacceptably high", but meanwhile there is a push to increase the proportion of the population obtaining a higher education qualification (p. viii). To offset the declining income of Australian universities, a rise in postgraduate fee-paying courses and in the number of international students has occurred because of the more favourable student fee structure (King, 2001; Williams, 2010). Shell (2010) reported the Organisation for Economic Co-operation and Development average for international student enrolments in tertiary education as 7.3%, but the average university in Australia derives 15% of its income from international student fees. University funding in Australia has directly influenced the number and type of students entering university and the workload for academics. The Australian situation is not unique, with reports of universities in most developed countries experiencing major reductions in government funding, leading to increased stress and work pressure on academics over the past two decades (Kinman & Jones, 2008; Winefield et al., 2008).

Research funds are another means for universities to acquire income, and as a consequence, academics employed in research universities are required to meet specific individual research output targets annually. Success in obtaining research grants is an indicator of research performance for the university and is linked to a university's credibility. A university's international and national ranking can influence its market share of student enrolments. Research output of the institution is measured primarily through the total grant acquisition as well as the number and quality of publications.

Journal quality can be measured in a number of ways. For example, journal impact factors are based on how often articles are referenced in other works. In the

United Kingdom, the Research Assessment Exercise (2008, http://www.rae.ac.uk/) determined a research quality level profile for each higher education institution, so that funding bodies could determine their level of research funding. In Australia, the Australian Research Council controls a similar tool, the Excellence in Research for Australia (http://www.arc.gov.au/era/). This initiative uses peer-reviewed publications as an indicator by assessing the proportion of the publication's content relating to a specific field of research and the impact of the journal on influencing research in the specific area (http://www.arc.gov.au/era/faq.htm).

KEY ISSUES AND LESSONS FOR THE NEW ACADEMIC

Having discussed the general context in which academic practice lies, we now move into specific areas that are important to understand when you enter academia.

Your Entry Point into Academia

There are two primary pathways to enter an academic position. The traditional entry point is to have completed an undergraduate degree with first class honours, followed by a PhD and then postdoctoral research experience. The other is to have an undergraduate degree, commonly a Master's degree, and extensive occupation-specific experience.

In the authors' unpublished research, *Transitions from Practice to Academia*, an analysis of stories of academics from both pathways found three common strong themes: teaching, research and time. The key difference, when considering the groups individually, was the ranking of these themes and therefore the priorities and/or stressors in the participants' work life. As a new academic it is important to be aware of these demands, the influence of your entry point on your career progress, and how to prioritise your work appropriately.

An outstanding difference between the two pathways and one that affects the new academic's identity and academic standing is whether he or she has a doctoral qualification. None of the authors of this chapter had a doctoral qualification at their entry point to academia, and we found that gaining this qualification was crucial to our career progression. The respondents in our study who entered from a health field reported similarly, with some indicating that they did not feel they were an academic until they had attained a doctoral qualification. The challenge lies in completing a degree that typically takes 3–3.5 years full-time or 6–7 years part-time while working in a position that carries a series of new and demanding responsibilities. We strongly recommend that if you enter academia without a doctoral qualification this achievement must become a top priority.

Lesson 1 – completing a doctoral degree should be a key priority if you don't already have one

For new academics without a doctoral qualification there are several factors that make it a primary focus. The doctoral qualification is the entry qualification as an independent researcher and is therefore necessary if you work in a university with research performance requirements. The skills, knowledge and understandings gained from a doctoral qualification help to develop the ability to critique and to independently gain knowledge in new areas. Achievement of these capabilities helps in your role as a teacher. Good teachers can take a critical and reflective stance in their work and have a sound, current and constructive understanding of the area in which they are teaching. A doctorate also allows the supervision of higher degree research students, an activity that contributes to your potential for promotion within the university.

Teaching

Quality teaching is a core aspect of academic work that all new academic staff members need to address. Workers entering the academy from health-related fields often have some teaching experience through educating new staff or being responsible for student work placements. Academics from a research background frequently work as tutors during their postgraduate studies. Yet regardless of background, except for those with a formal teaching qualification and experience, teaching at university was identified in our research as a major challenge.

One of the key challenges identified by participants was being "thrown in at the deep end". Participants reported being required to prepare their program in a very short space of time and with little support. Many found that they were unprepared to teach: they didn't know what made a good teacher or a good learning environment. The following vignettes highlight the "sink or swim" concept that many new academics experienced.

I quickly identified that I was struggling with the teaching aspect. (Cath)

They gave me 3 weeks preparation time which still didn't prepare me as I didn't really know what I was doing ... I had no previous teaching experience and there were no existing materials ... you know, things like designing assessments, trying to get things like that right, I didn't really know what I was doing. (Ruth)

I had 3 weeks to write all the lectures ... it was overwhelming – I was just terrified that I would never get it done. (Wendy)

That first year when you come in is the hardest, when you are teaching subjects for the first time ... I felt like in a way I was left to fend for myself a lot of the time. (Carly)

Although the first year is difficult, substantial improvement is usually made by the second year through commitment, seeking advice, and reflection. The following exemplifies the development and improvement made by one research participant. A number of difficulties were encountered in the first year of teaching, so this participant undertook a course of study in higher education and sought feedback from more experienced teachers. The participant recounted that a student who had experienced both the first and second year of teaching said, "You're so much better than you were last year", which was encouraging for the new academic.

Another key challenge is that of being misinformed about the time it takes to prepare for teaching. Actual teaching in the classroom might occupy only 10–12 hours of your week, but for every hour face-to-face, 3–4 hours of development time are required. It takes time to prepare an engaging lecture, a meaningful practical, or an appropriately challenging tutorial. Furthermore, you need time for detailed subject outline development and assessment design. Subject outlines usually have set formats to meet quality assurance guidelines, and strict publication deadlines. Assessments need to be carefully planned so that students invest in deep learning processes, while also minimising the risk for plagiarism. As well, there is student consultation time (face-to-face or more commonly via email), marking, result recording, teaching team meetings and assessment committee preparation and attendance. What appears to be only two days of your working week can rapidly occupy four days, even when classes are not in session, particularly if you are responsible for developing new resources.

Lesson 2 – don't underestimate the time it takes for the role of teaching

Time is also an issue when first learning the technologies associated with higher education. The use of distance education has become a focus of many institutions over the past decade (King, 2001; Ewell, 2010), bringing additional challenges to academics. Mastering technology for off-campus teaching and learning can add to the work demands. Delivery of the subject using tools such as chat rooms, forums or electronic responses to students can be more time-consuming than teaching in the classroom. More frequently these same tools are used in on-campus delivery and therefore need to be learned regardless of the mode of delivery. Well used, technology can facilitate more inclusive participation of students and can create some efficiency for the teacher when mastered.

Lesson 3 – embrace the technological skills required for teaching

The completion of a tertiary teaching course to better prepare academics is mandatory in most Australian universities, although our respondents differed greatly in their opinion of the value of such courses. Commonly, completion is required within the first year, during which time the new academic has already commenced developing teaching materials, writing assessment tasks and performing the teaching. In other words, new academics are well on their way performing teaching duties before they receive any guidance. Working in this manner means that new academics need to work it out themselves, which is often far more time-consuming and can be fraught with mistakes.

A good mentor early in your career can be a means to improve your teaching and overcome the possible shortcomings of teaching preparation. One of the most commonly reported problems in our study was that new academics had limited or no support for their teaching. Participants reported a hesitancy to ask for assistance for fear of being thought incapable of doing their job, or because other academics appeared too busy to ask them for help. These quotes highlight this issue:

A little bit of mentoring would be nice. (Carly)

I could have asked around but there's always that tendency to not do that because you don't want to look silly. (Cath)

Although finding a mentor or seeking advice from those more experienced may not be easy, it is an effective way to save you from falling into common pitfalls such as cramming too much content into a single class. One participant recollected having made the content far more detailed and complex than necessary in the first subject taught. In the Job Demands-Resources model (Bakker & Demerouti, 2007) described in the introduction to this chapter, co-worker support is a resource that helps to buffer job demands and therefore helps individuals to achieve work goals more effectively.

The art of teaching was found to be a challenge by many of the participants. Again, in this situation a mentor or someone with more experience can be of assistance, especially if that person can give the time to come into the classroom and provide constructive feedback on your teaching. One participant reported having a mentor come to peer-review her teaching of a class that she described as "particularly bad", with students who were difficult to handle, but the tips and hints provided by the mentor were very helpful. As academics who have had to learn the hard way, we would encourage all new academics to find someone they respect and ask them to give a little of their time. It can make a substantial difference to have some help in the early stages of teaching at university.

Lesson 4 – find a trustworthy teaching mentor early in your career

Another means to improve your teaching quality would be to complete a postgraduate degree in higher education – but we would caution you before taking that path. Although education that supports the quality of teaching and learning is an advantage, it takes time away from your other academic duties. A major consideration is whether the completion of such a course is viable given your multiple work demands. For instance, if part of the higher degree requires a research project on an aspect of your teaching that leads to a peer-reviewed publication, improves teaching and learning quality, and raises your understanding in an area of teaching, it is a worthwhile option. Several needs have been met – improvement of teaching quality, demonstration of scholarship, and research output.

We are not saying that teaching quality should be ignored, as teaching is core business for all universities. But we encourage you to consider the balance of what you do. A quote from one research participant clearly shows the dedication to quality in teaching and the informed decision-making prior to undertaking the additional study:

I realised when I did my education degree it was for myself; it was not for anybody else. I thought if I was teaching, I really needed to know what I was doing – basically, rather than going in and using my own views of teaching that were really a product of my own experience as a student. So I really needed to do that education degree and I feel a lot better equipped to do my job having done that. (Yolanda)

Remember, students are entitled to a quality education and you have a professional duty to provide this. Governments worldwide also consider quality teaching and learning to be priorities of universities, and over the last several decades have increasingly imposed quality assurance audits on universities (Breakwell & Tytherliegh, 2010; Ewell, 2010). A later chapter in this book addresses standards in health professional education.

Below is a list of teaching lessons learned by research participants, which provide helpful insights for new academics:

Lesson 5 – as a teacher you need to be in situational control and not let the students control you

Lesson 6 – prepare students for your expectations (matched to their level of study) and they will rise to the challenge

Lesson 7 – provide context/relevance to your lessons

Lesson 8 – don't cram too much content; work with principles/concepts so that students can apply them

Lesson 9 – the more that students interact with lesson material, the more they will remember

Research

Our purpose in this section is to raise two salient points based on our own reflections and those of the research participants in the context of workload balance. As already discussed, research is a major component of the research university and therefore is an important aspect of the academic role. Further discussion of this important topic is presented elsewhere in this book.

Our first point is to raise awareness that research and research output make a substantial demand in an academic role. More often than not, research competes with teaching, and finding a balance is necessary. It is important to be aware of this from the earliest stage of your career, to reduce any unpreparedness or misconceptions of the demands of the role. Being aware of the importance of research is one thing, but the most important message here is to find and sustain a balance among the competing demands of an academic role.

Lesson 10 – teaching and research activity can compete, but keep them balanced

Our second point is that research will affect your career path. If research is a crucial part of your university's promotion system, there is no point in trying to gain a promotion without having produced the output required. Cretchley (2009) conducted a study of science and engineering academics in Australia to compare the priorities and behaviours between research and learning and teaching. The results overwhelmingly indicated far greater professional rewards for research activity than for learning and teaching. Goldsworthy (2008) found these sentiments echoed by academics in law, reporting that enormous weight was given to research performance for appointments and promotion. Researchers in the United Kingdom found similar priorities, with 90% of respondents reporting a significant increase in the pressure to publish over the preceding few years (Kinman & Jones, 2008). Most workplaces hold annual performance reviews, and it makes the experience much less stressful if you know you have met the requirements for your review. Annual reviews can also influence your ability to apply for promotion.

Our advice is that early in your career you find and join an established research team with interests similar to yours. Actively participate in the team so that you can be a co-author of publications and grants. Teamwork is important because it helps to make the workload manageable and you learn valuable lessons from your peers. The support you gain from a team is a job resource that helps to buffer the job demands. Such teams are increasingly supported by the academy and are encouraged to attract and mentor early career researchers.

Lesson 11 – join a research group to initiate or broaden your research skills

A few key quotes from our research participants emphasise the importance of this part of the academic role:

> I think you can be an excellent teacher but you are not going to get anywhere in academia unless you publish. (Dexter)

> There are the external forces there about the relationship between research output and funding and ranking of journals and all that definitely influences what happens. (Yolanda)

> I am going into my third year now and I still haven't established my proper research and I'm struggling with that. (Ruth)

Time

Time in general (not just with teaching), and being time-poor, constitute a major theme that emerged from our research, and one that is identified in other research. One of the participants in our research study thought she would be able to "come in, blissfully teach and be able to talk theories and that kind of thing, and then have lots of time to collect data and research and write up papers" (Mary). Unfortunately that was not the case for the participant, nor is it for academics in general.

Kinman and Jones (2008) reported that occupational stress among academics has increased worldwide, with heavy workloads, time pressure and resource constraints being the primary stressors. The authors evaluated the level of wellbeing of United Kingdom academics and found that 66% of respondents worked more than 45 hours per week, with 68% reporting they did not have sufficient time to prepare for classes. These academics often worked evenings and weekends to manage their workload.

In a recent longitudinal study of Australian academics from 12 universities using the Job Demands-Resources model, Boyd et al. (2011) identified the most influential factors on occupational stress and wellbeing from a series of focus groups. The job demands were work pressure (or time pressure) and academic workload, whereas resources were job autonomy and procedural fairness. The authors noted that at the time of their study government funding and baseline levels of research funding were reduced, while student-to-staff ratios were increased. These factors had most likely increased job demands and influenced their results.

Participants in our research concurred with findings from the literature.

I am working until 10 o'clock at night trying to get these lectures together and in a big panic and never having anything properly prepared. (Ruth)

The issue is really what is going to be achieved … it is never going to be achieved in the hours we have, not 37 hours, not even if we were paid 70 hours per week. (Mary)

Another factor drawing on your time is the third aspect of the academic's role, often referred to as service. This can take many forms and is often last on the list of priorities. There is a broad interpretation of what constitutes this third dimension. It might be participation in university committee work such as learning and teaching, ethics or research committees. It could also be outside the university, such as on professional accreditation bodies or district committees. These broader activities are viewed as either contributing to the university as a whole or raising the university profile while you engage in outside professional activities. Our advice is that until you are comfortable with the teaching and research roles, participate only to the level of involvement that you can manage easily.

The matter of reconciling the time constraints of academia is not easy to resolve. Our counsel is to find efficiencies in the way you work, find support in as many areas as you can and be thoughtful about the priorities you allocate. There will be competing demands for your time, but for a successful career path you as an individual must be strategic in the way you work. It is also important to have a healthy work–life balance.

Lesson 12 – plan and prioritise your workload, keep a work–life balance

A CAREER IN ACADEMIA

Although there are increased demands on academics, there are still some important satisfying features that help to buffer the demands. A high degree of job autonomy,

69

intellectual stimuli, opportunities to use initiative, teaching and supervision all bring job satisfaction (Boyd et al., 2011; Kinman & Jones, 2008). These factors reflect why the authors of this chapter have enjoyed their academic careers and hope that the lessons presented in this chapter help you in your transition to academia.

REFERENCES

Bakker, A. B., & Demerouti, E. (2007). The job demands-resources model: State of the art. *Journal of Managerial Psychology, 22*(3), 309-328.

Bakker, A. B., Demerouti, E., & Schaufeli, W. B. (2003). Dual processes at work in a call centre: An application of the job demands-resources model. *European Journal of Work and Organisational Psychology, 12*(4), 393-417.

Boyd, C. M., Bakker, A. B., Pignata, S., Winefield, A. H., Gillespie, N., & Stough, C. (2011). A longitudinal test of the job demands-resources model among Australian university academics. *Applied Psychology, 60*(1), 112-140.

Breakwell, G. M., & Tytherleigh, M. Y. (2010). University leaders and university performance in the United Kingdom: Is it 'who' leads, or 'where' they lead that matters most? *Higher Education, 60*(5), 491-506.

Cretchley, P. (2009). Are Australian universities promoting learning and teaching activity effectively? An assessment of the effects on science and engineering academics. *International Journal of Mathematical Education in Science and Technology, 40*(7), 865-875.

Department of Education and Employment Workplace Relations. (2008). *Review of Australian Higher Education* [Online]. Retrieved from
http://www.deewr.gov.au/highereducation/review/pages/reviewofaustralianhighereducationreport.aspx

Ewell, P. (2010). Twenty years of quality assurance in higher education: What's happened and what's different? *Quality in Higher Education, 16*(2), 173-175.

Goldsworthy, J. (2008). Research grant mania. *Australian Universities Review, 50*(2), 17-24.

King, S. P. (2001). The funding of higher education in Australia: Overview and alternatives. *The Australian Economic Review, 34*(2), 190-194.

Kinman, G., & Jones, F. (2008). A life beyond work? Job demands, work-life balance, and wellbeing in UK academics. *Journal of Behaviour in the Social Environment, 17*(1/2), 41-60.

Marginson, S. (2001). Trends in funding Australian higher education. *The Australian Economic Review, 34*(2), 205-215.

Shell, T. (2010). Moving beyond university rankings: Developing a world class university system in Australia. *Australian Universities Review, 52*(1), 69-76.

Williams, R. (2010). Research output of Australian universities: Are the newer institutions catching up? *Australian Universities Review, 52*(1), 32-36.

Winefield, T., Boyd, C., Saebel, J., & Pignata, S. (2008). Update on national university stress study. *Australia Universities Review, 50*(1), 20-29.

Edwina Adams BAppSc, MAppSc, PhD
The Education For Practice Institute, Charles Sturt University, Australia

Patricia Logan PhD
The School of Biomedical Sciences, Charles Sturt University, Australia

Doreen Rorrison PhD
Adjunct Lecturer, School of Teacher Education, Charles Sturt University, Australia

Graham Munro MHSM, BHSc, CCP
The School of Biomedical Sciences, Charles Sturt University, Australia

DAVID PRIDEAUX, IRIS LINDEMANN AND ANAISE COTTRELL

7. COMMUNITY AND WORKPLACE EXPECTATIONS OF GRADUATES IN THE HEALTH PROFESSIONS

There is no doubt of the need for a well-educated health professional workforce in the increasingly interdependent global world of the twenty-first century. In economically developed nations, aging populations and increase of chronic and so-called lifestyle diseases associated with poor diet and inactivity have resulted in demands for more and differently educated health professionals. Economically developing countries face issues of workforce shortages, underserved populations and inequity of access to healthcare. This is exacerbated by the global mobility of health professionals. Almost everywhere the rapid technological advances in healthcare are moving at rates which are not consistent with growth of resources to fund them.

Starfield (2007) has commented that the predominance of chronic and lifestyle illnesses in the twenty-first century has meant that healthcare delivery has had to shift from the specific disease orientation of the twentieth century teaching hospital to the multi-morbidity, person-focused, co-ordinated, community-based care of the twenty-first century. This causes major tensions in allocation of scarce resources in health systems. It also causes tensions where health professionals receive most of their clinical education in large teaching hospitals. Health professionals in the twenty-first century require new competencies that will prepare them for effective practice in the new care settings.

NEW CAPABILITIES EXPECTED

The changing health system has created strong drivers for reform in educational institutions offering health professional education. As a consequence, education has undergone significant transformation. Industrial and politically motivated forces, such as the need for a competitive workforce internationally and the need for employees to be flexible to meet rapidly changing work environments, have had a strong influence. Educational institutions, including universities, have become increasingly responsive to workplace and community needs in the effort to ensure that graduates are employable and can contribute to society both personally and professionally.

Of note has been the recent drive worldwide towards defining and embedding "generic skills" or capabilities into educational programs. Although often called generic skills, a better descriptor is generic attributes, qualities or capabilities, as these terms embrace not only skills but also abilities and personal attributes. Catalogues of generic capabilities have been developed to be applied to almost all

S. Loftus et al. (Eds.), Educating Health Professionals:
Becoming a University Teacher, 71–82.

professions and workplaces. These capabilities are defined as those attributes that allow graduates to participate fully in applying their knowledge and skills in changing work environments. The definition of generic capabilities has been especially important to health professional education, as it has initiated stronger recognition of the skills in communication, problem-solving and teamwork that have always taken second place to the professional and content-focused skills (Australian National Training Authority, 2003). These capabilities are now integrated into curricula across a wide range of programs and the intention is for them to be firmly embedded as key aspects of training for future healthcare professionals.

What makes a work-ready graduate? Hager, Holland, and Beckett (2002) have defined eight key competencies applicable to a wide range of work settings. These are communication, teamwork, problem-solving, initiative and enterprise, planning and organising, self-management, learning, and technology skills. A range of personal attributes have also been identified as keys to employability, including loyalty, commitment, honesty and integrity, reliability, personal presentation, common sense, positive self-esteem, sense of humour, balanced attitude to work and home life, ability to deal with pressure, motivation and adaptability (Business Council of Australia, & Australian Chamber of Commerce and Industry, 2002). The Australian National Training Authority (2003) has expanded generic skills to include basic skills in literacy and numeracy, as well as people-related skills such as communication and teamwork, conceptual/thinking skills such as problem-solving and organisational skills, personal skills and attributes such as innovation and enterprise, and community-related skills such as citizenship skills. Hager et al. (2002) further to identify personal value attributes such as ethical practice, persistence, integrity and tolerance. It is clear that employers are seeking both interactive and personal attributes from graduates. In considering the future needs of the health workforce, the World Health Organization (WHO) has identified broader capabilities including a commitment to patient-centred care, partnering and quality improvement, skills in information and communication technology, and the ability to incorporate a public health perspective into work (WHO, 2005).

Although the identification and explicit inclusion of key graduate capabilities in programs is a positive step towards ensuring that graduates have optimal opportunities to contribute within their professional spheres, this alone will not provide the education required to develop future health graduates. Hager et al. (2002) have warned of the danger of treating generic capabilities as single entities. In the real work setting, capabilities are rarely used alone and are usually utilised in an integrated and applied manner to perform work tasks within a specific context. The integrated use of generic capabilities is highly relevant to work life and to specific work settings, and needs to be explicitly included in educational programs.

A recent critique of the more narrow competency-based approaches to health professional education has focused on tacit knowledge (Australian Medical Council, 2010). Tacit knowledge can be subconscious and is gained through experience and interaction with other health professionals in clinical settings. Tacit knowledge may well be the source of the commitment, judgement and responsiveness especially relevant to health professionals.

Within health systems, the arena of interprofessional education provides a clear example to illustrate the above. The skills and attributes that promote interprofessional collaboration have been identified as critical for the delivery of safe, high-quality patient-centred care. Despite an apparent match between the interprofessional workforce skills desired by the health system and the graduate attributes promoted by higher education, health professional education is failing to provide effective training in collaborative practices. Educational practices that encourage students explicitly to develop communication and teamwork skills within interprofessional contexts are needed to build the foundation for a workforce which is capable of working interprofessionally. Matthews et al. (2011) have indicated that embedding interprofessional education as a core component of all health professional curricula and practice standards is a requirement for enabling graduates to be key interprofessional team players. Thus Hager et al. (2002) were correct in arguing that just teaching generic skills or narrow competencies is not enough.

Harvey (2000) argued that it is critical for higher education to embrace a responsive approach and to emphasise employability as an outcome of producing lifelong learners. However, this may currently be occurring at a cost. Other capabilities that are essential to this discourse must not be ignored. Concerns have been raised that the focus on work-ready skills has diverted attention from research-based skills such as lifelong learning, curiosity, dealing with uncertainty, and an inquiry-based approach to problems. This is seen by some as a risk to academic quality and freedom. The reduced focus on research skills and attributes also defies a growing need for health professionals to be "information literate", capable of providing services within evidence-based and best-practice parameters. This continues to be a cause of tension, especially within higher education institutions as health professional programs grapple with the increasing demands placed on their curricula.

Academic institutions are increasingly required to provide evidence of outcomes to justify their directives and funding. One key emerging area for health professional training lies within an institution's mission to be responsive to its communities and for graduates to emerge from training with a sense of social responsibility (Biggs & Wells, 2011; THEnet, 2011). A great deal of work has already been done to identify what graduates who are equipped to become agents of change in their communities would look like. Within health professional programs, graduates not only need to be competent in knowledge encompassing broad definitions of health, but also need a commitment to high-quality and equitable healthcare. Values underpinning this work include equity, quality, relevance, efficiency and partnerships, with graduates not only providing quality healthcare in areas of high health need but also becoming advocates for change within the health system to achieve greater equity of access to healthcare (THEnet, 2011).

So where does this leave our communities? The education systems and service provision industries have played a key role in directing health professional programs through regular investigations into expectations of graduates. Industry bodies have a strong voice in government and educational institutions are responsive to the funding initiatives that result from new government policy. The consumer is often forgotten in the planning of education and services (Newman, 2009) and there are no standardised tools for measuring consumer satisfaction with the health system or outcomes achieved (Duckett, 2008). There is some evidence, however, that provides clues to consumer expectations of graduates. Benson, Quince, Hibble, Fanshawe, and Emery (2005) and Sivamalai (2008) provide examples of research which demonstrate that patients expect more than practitioners who knows their profession. Consumers expect practitioners to be competent in interpersonal communication and professional skills and to work respectfully. Most health consumer complaints relate to clinical practice, communication problems, interpersonal skills and ethical issues (Newby & McBride, 2004; Duckett, 2008). Consumers expect informed practitioners who communicate well, offer a holistic view of health, collaborate with other professionals for the wellbeing of the end users, and who offer time for promoting good health and education (Yura-Petro & Scanelli, 1992; Oermann & Templin, 2000).

Wiseman (2005) has provided evidence that consumer and health professional expectations of graduates are similar, thus giving confidence that industry views may represent community views. This finding should not, however, become an excuse for ignoring the voices of consumers, as it cannot be taken for granted that health professionals are detecting consumers' needs accurately. Authentic consultation is important for legitimising policy decisions. Internationally, there are powerful examples of how working with communities to address priority health needs can meet demand and improve health outcomes. For example a rural medical school in the Philippines has developed processes to select students preferentially from local populations and has based its curriculum on the community's expressed priority health needs. The health outcomes have been dramatic, including plummeting infant mortality rates (Cristobal & Worley, 2011). Similarly, in South Africa, the *UNITRA Community Health Partnership Project* has brought together the university, the health service and the community as foundation partners in the development of curriculum and education for local medical graduates. There are benefits for the local community in that students contribute through service learning and remain within the local area as practitioners to continue to serve (Westburg, 2007). There may be lessons here for more developed nations to be more inclusive of consumer needs in order to make a difference to health outcomes.

INTERDEPENDENCE AND SYMBIOSIS

The central tenet of the education of health professionals for a new century is the interdependence of health professional providers and health systems. This was certainly a strong feature of the first period in the evolution of health professional education defined by Frenk et al. (2010) as lasting from the beginning of the twentieth century until the 1960s. Student doctors and student nurses in particular provided a basic workforce in the large teaching hospitals. Students were expected to learn and supply essential services at the same time.

The interdependence started to break down in the second period of health professional education, from the 1960s onwards, at the precise time that the education of many health professionals was being taken out of teaching hospitals and located in universities. Despite the strengthening of formal associations between universities and teaching hospitals, the interests of health systems and university-based health professional education providers began to diverge. Service and efficiency became the priorities of health systems as they moved to fill the gaps provided by their former student workforces and as they responded to government concerns for meeting increasing demand. Reducing hospital waiting lists and emergency service waiting times became predominant issues. On the other hand, the priorities of universities were teaching and research. New pedagogies such as problem-based learning required increased time commitment from health professional education staff, as did the establishment of research projects and careers. Health professional educators themselves no longer provided services in clinical contexts. In nursing, for example, clinical educators employed by universities accompanied or visited students in clinical settings, with no clear role in patient care in those settings.

The re-establishment of the interdependence of health professional education and health systems, albeit in a different form, is the key to the third period of health professional education, from the turn of the century onwards. Cowen et al. (2008) described an ideal health system as having an organisational chart with patients and their caregivers at the top, and health organised through patient-centred, collaborative multidisciplinary teams providing a sound focus for both health service and education aims.

Such interdependence is illustrated by the concept of symbiosis which has emerged from community-based approaches to health professional education (Prideaux, Worley, & Bligh, 2007). Symbiosis is defined by a "win-win" relationship between health professional education providers and health services. Students receive enriched clinical experiences and excellent clinical teaching and learning opportunities from health services in return for a contribution to those services by students, graduates, and the university's presence in the system.

Evidence for the success of symbiotic clinical education has come through the Parallel Rural Community Curriculum (PRCC) in rural South Australia. Medical students from Flinders University are placed in comprehensive rural general practices and small rural hospitals for an entire year of core clinical education and are expected to cover the same academic and clinical content as their peers based in urban teaching hospitals. They relocate and live in small rural communities. More recently, the approach has been extended to other Australian and international medical schools in Australia and to other health professions such as nursing and paramedics.

Research findings have indicated superior clinical and written examination performance from students in the PRCC, and demonstrated that they can cover the same specialist content as students in city hospital-based contexts (Worley, Esterman, & Prideaux, 2004; Worley, Strasser, & Prideaux, 2004). Thus students in the PRCC receive good clinical teaching and learning opportunities. Furthermore, they make a significant and valued contribution to the general practices and the hospitals in which they are located, especially after the first three months of placement (Worley & Kitto, 2001). This has been achieved though taking meaningful roles in the healthcare team, developing longer-term professional relationships with patients and practice staff, undertaking patient-based care with decreasing levels of supervision, participating in after-hours and on-call service, and being involved in health and community programs. Students have addressed community concerns about the lack of health workforce capacity by demonstrating a commitment to undertake rural practice on graduation and have been part of a whole-university approach to improving the delivery of healthcare in the towns and regions in which they are placed (Worley, Prideaux, Strasser, Magery, & March, 2006; Roberts et al., 2012).

ACHIEVING SYMBIOSIS OR INTERDEPENDENCE

Research indicates that the key to achieving the concept of symbiotic education lies in relationships that provide the context and complexity for learning. Four relationships have been defined in the PRCC in South Australia (Worley, 2002):

- A personal–professional relationship
- A health professional–patient/client relationship
- A university–health service relationship
- A government–community relationship.

The Personal–Professional Relationship

One of the most important learning experiences for health professional students in meeting community and workplace expectations is reconciling their personal principles with the professional expectations of a health professional in a work environment. Moving from a university environment, where students are largely responsible for their own performance, to a work environment that depends on complex team relations with other staff, professional and ethical relations with patients and clients, and community expectations about the conduct of health professionals requires some adjustment. The key to achieving that adjustment is long placements. These provide greater opportunities for health professional students to get to know their clinical educators in work environments and, importantly, to observe how their supervisors deal with the difficult processes of reconciling their own interests with their professional and community expectations.

Research has highlighted the importance of the time factor. Tolhurst, Adams, andStewart (2006) demonstrated the importance of providing time for students to develop good social relationships in rural health settings. Oswald, Alderson, and Jones (2001) illustrated that time is important in the development of good relations with patients and clients in community-based settings, and Worley and Kitto (2001) demonstrated the importance of time in developing relationships within the working environments of health services.

The Health Professional–Patient/Client Relationship

Hoffman and Donaldson (2004) introduced the concept of 360° learning. With patients or clients at the centre of learning, students have access to all of the health professionals involved in patient care. Thus they have potential mentors and learning facilitators all around them. Nevertheless, the service demands for patient care in contemporary health systems are heavy, and facilitation of student learning must become an integral part of care, not an addition to it. Bleakley and Bligh (2008) argued in the medical education context that clinical learning should move from the "primacy" of the doctor-student relationship to the patient-student relationship. The patient becomes the primary educator of the student, with the doctor or health professional as the facilitator of learning.

Walters and her colleagues have demonstrated how this can be achieved for medical students in general practice by adopting "parallel consulting". Students see patients in parallel with general practitioners in separate rooms. The initial consultation is with the patient alone while the general practitioner consults with another patient. Patient, student and general practitioner then come together for a joint consultation. There is evidence to show that the general practitioners focus more on learning about history-taking and contextual factors in the joint sessions as these enrich the learning experiences that the students gain from the patients (Walters, Prideaux, Worley, Greenhill, & Rolfe, 2009). Importantly, parallel consulting enables the general practitioners to see the same number of patients in a consulting session as they would in the absence of students (Walters, Worley, Prideaux, & Lange, 2008). Walters, Prideaux, Worley, and Greenhill (2011) were also able to demonstrate that in the year-long PRCC program the general practitioners were able to move their facilitation of student learning from the student-as-observer role, through approaches in which the general practitioners took responsibility for both the patient consultation and the facilitation of student learning, and ultimately to a model akin to the patient-centred approach of Bleakley and Bligh (2008). The concept of parallel consulting or parallel patient and client care should be applied across the education of all health professionals.

The University–Health Service Relationship

Future health professionals require clinical learning that is authentic and supported. Authentic learning has been defined as learning that is constructivist, inquiry-based and of "real work value" (Newmann, Marks, & Gamorgan, 1996).

It is the role of the health service in the university-health service relationship to provide this.

Health professional students should be enabled to make an effective work contribution as members of healthcare teams. They need to engage in and add value to real work activities. They should do this at the same time as constructing their own learning under the facilitation, guidance and mentorship of the experienced health professionals in the team. Health services and health workplaces provide needed opportunities for what Hoffman and Donaldson (2004) have described as "hot" and "cold" action. Hot action represents the opportunities for learning while actively participating as a member of a healthcare team. Cold action represents opportunities to step out of direct action, for reflection and review of learning goals under experienced guidance and supervision.

The role of the university or health professional education provider is to deliver support for authentic learning. Health professional students require organisational, affective and teaching support (Dornan, Hadfield, Brown, Boshuizen, & Scherpbier, 2005). Information communication technology has facilitated the access of students to resources, study guides and supplementary materials even when they are located in diverse healthcare environments away from their universities. The universities also have an obligation in supporting the staff of the health service, both in their development as health professionals and in their roles as teachers and learning facilitators.

The Government–Community Relationship

This chapter began with reference to the constrained nature of contemporary health services as they are required to deal with increasing chronic care burdens, aging populations, staffing shortages and underserved populations. Hence the relationship between governments and health services, the imperatives to meet health priority needs, and the expectations of communities for well-educated and effective health professionals are significant. Health professional education, and in particular, curriculum content, needs to be oriented to priority health outcomes. This will equip health professional students to make a contribution to these outcomes and to respond to community expectations as members and learners in healthcare teams.

An example of this has been the Australian Government's investment in Rural Clinical Schools and University Departments of Rural Health. This has enabled health professional students to gain substantial clinical experience and learning in regional, rural and remote Australia where there are significant and ongoing workforce shortages and an increasing incidence of health problems. Students have been able to contribute in these locations by participating in real work situations as members of healthcare teams while learning and gaining the essential workforce and community capabilities outlined here. Furthermore, there is evidence from the Rural Clinical Schools of both intention and actual return of students to rural practice after graduation (Veitch, Underhill, & Hays, 2006; Worley et al., 2008; Stagg, Greenhill, & Worley, 2009; Roberts et al., 2012).

Priority health problems need to become the very substance of health professional education so that universities, providers and their health professional students can make a contribution to their alleviation. This is an essential part of meeting the community and workplace expectations for health graduates.

CONCLUSION

Communities and workplaces will expect more of health professional graduates in the healthcare systems of the twenty-first century. The increasing burden of disease associated with aging populations and lifestyle factors will demand it. Universities and other providers will need to deliver a new generation of work-ready graduates who are patient- or client-centred safe practitioners, who can continue to learn in the workplace and who can thrive in team-based and interprofessional environments. These graduates will need a commitment to ethical practice which they can maintain throughout their careers.

Sustained, relevant and supported clinical experience is the key to meeting the expectations. This will need to be underpinned by greater interdependence and symbiosis between health systems and education providers. Health professional students require opportunities to contribute to the work of healthcare teams while learning the essential capabilities for practice. Furthermore, the curriculum of health professional education needs to be transformed. It must address the priority health concerns of health services and enable health professional students to contribute to their alleviation. Health professional students and graduates must be part of the solution, not part of the problem.

REFERENCES

Australian Medical Council. (2010). *Competence-based medical education: AMC consultation paper.* Canberra: Australian Medical Council. Retrieved from http://www.amc.org.au/images/publications/CBEWG_20110822.pdf

Australian National Training Authority. (2003). *Defining generic skills report.* Adelaide, National Centre for Vocational Education Research Ltd. Retrieved from http://www.ncver.edu.au/publications/1361.html

Benson, J., Quince, T., Hibble, A., Fanshawe, T., & Emery, J. (2005). Impact on patients of expanded, general practice based, student teaching: Observational and qualitative study. *British Medical Journal, 331*(7508), 89. doi:10.1136/bmj.38492.599606.8F

Biggs, J. S. G., & Wells, R. W. (2011). The social mission of Australian medical schools in a time of expansion. *Australian Health Review, 35*(4), 424-429. doi:10.1071/AH10970

Bleakley, A., & Bligh, J. (2008). Students learning from patients: Let's get real in medical education. *Advances in Health Sciences Education, 13*(1), 89-107. doi:10,1007/s10459-006-9028-0

Business Council of Australia, & Australian Chamber of Commerce and Industry. (2002). *Employability skills for the future.* Report for Department of Education Science and Training & Commonwealth of Australia. Retrieved from http://www.dest.gov.au/sectors/training_skills/publications_resources/other_publications/

Cowen, M. E., Lakshmi, K., Halasyamani, D. M., Hoffman, D., Polley, T., & Alexander, J. A. (2008). Organisational structure for addressing the attributes of the ideal healthcare delivery system. *Journal of Healthcare Management, 53*(6), 407-419.

Cristobal, F., & Worley. P. (2011). Transforming health professionals' education. *The Lancet (Correspondence), 377*(9773), 1235-1236. doi:10.1016/S0140-6736(11)60494-7

Dornan, T., Hadfield, J., Brown, M., Boshuizen, H., & Scherpbier, A. (2005). How can medical students learn in a self-directed way in the clinical environment? Design-based research. *Medical Education, 39*(4), 356-364. doi:10.1111/j.1365-2929.2005.02112.x

Duckett, S. (2008). The Australian health care system: Reform, repair or replace? *Australian Health Review, 32*(2), 322-32. doi:10.1071/AH080322

Frenk, J., Chen, L., Bhutta, Z. A., Cohen, J., Crisp, N., Evans, T., et al. (2010). Health professionals for a new century: Transforming education to strengthen health systems in an interdependent world. A Global Independent Commission. *The Lancet, 376*(9756), 1923–1958. doi:10.1016/50140-6736(10)61854-5

Hager, P., Holland, S., & Beckett, D. (2002). *Enhancing the learning and employability of graduates: The role of generic skills.* B-Hert Position Paper no. 9. Melbourne: Business/Higher Education Round Table. Retrieved from http://www.bhert.com/publications/position-papers/B-HERTPositionPaper09.pdf

Harvey, L. (2000). New realities: The relationship between higher education and employment. *Tertiary Education and Management, 6*(1), 3–17. doi:10.1080/13583883.2000.9967007

Hoffman, K. G., & Donaldson, J. F. (2004) Contextual tensions of the clinical environment and their influence on teaching and learning. *Medical Education, 38*(4), 448-454. doi:10.1046/j.1365-2923.2004.01799.x

Matthews, L. R., Pockett, R. B., Nisbet, G., Thistlethwaite, J. E., Dunston, R., Lee, A., et al. (2011). Building capacity in Australian interprofessional health education: Perspectives from key health and higher education stakeholders. *Australian Health Review, 35*(2), 136-140. doi:10.1071/AH10886 0156-5788/11/020

Newby, L., & McBride, T. (2004). *Bringing in the consumer perspective: A final report.* Melbourne: Health Issues Centre Inc. and Resolution Resource Network. Retrieved from http://health.vic.gov.au/__data/assets/pdf_file/0009/319635/finalrpt_consumer_perspective.pdf

Newman, L. A. (2009). The health care system as a social determinant of health: Qualitative insights from South Australian maternity consumers. *Australian Health Review, 33*(1), 62-71.

Newmann, F. M., Marks, H. M., & Gamorgan, A. (1996). Authentic pedagogy and student performance. *American Journal of Education, 104*(4), 280-312. Retrieved from http://www.jstor.org/stable/1085433

Oermann, M., & Templin, T. (2000). Important attributes of quality health care: Consumer perspectives. *Journal of Nursing Scholarship, 32*(2), 167-172. doi:10.1111/j.1547-5069.2000.00167.x

Oswald, N., Alderson, T., & Jones, S. (2001). Evaluating primary care as a base for medical education: The report of the Cambridge Community-based Clinical Course. *Medical Education, 35*(8), 782-788. doi:10.1046/j.1365-2923.2001.x

Prideaux, D., Worley, P., & Bligh, J. (2007). Symbiosis: A new model for clinical education. *The Clinical Teacher, 4*(4), 209-212. doi:10.1111/j.1743-498X.2007.00188.x

Roberts, C., Daly, M., Kumar, K., Perkins, D., Richards, D., & Game, D. (2012). A longitudinal placement and medical students' intentions to practise rurally. *Medical Education, 46*(2), 179-191. doi:10.1111/j.1365-2923.2011.04102.x

Sivamalai, S. (2008). Desired attributes of new graduate nurses as identified by the rural community. *Rural and Remote Health, 8,* 938. Retrieved from http://www.rrh.org.au/articles/showarticlenew.asp?ArticleID=938

Stagg, P., Greenhill, J., & Worley, P. S. (2009). A new model to understand the career choice and practice location decisions of medical graduates. *Rural and Remote Health, 9,* 1245. Retrieved from http://www.rrh.org.au/articles/showarticlenew.asp?ArticleID=1245

Starfield, B. (2007). Global health, equity and primary care (Commentary). *Journal of the American Board of Family Medicine, 20*, 511-513. doi:10.3122/jabfm.2007.070176

THEnet (Training for Health Equity Network). (2011). *THEnet's social accountability framework Version 1*. Monograph 1 (1 ed.). Brussels: The Training for Health Equity Network. Retrieved from http://www.thenetcommunity.org/files/articles/Monograph%20print%20quality%20feb%201.pdf

Tolhurst, H. M., Adams, J., & Stewart, S. M. (2006). An exploration of when urban background medical students become interested in rural practice. *Rural and Remote Health, 6*, 452. Retrieved from http://www.rrh.org.au/articles/showarticlenew.asp?ArticleID=452

Veitch, C., Underhill, A., Hays, R. B. (2006). The career aspirations and intentions of James Cook University's first cohort of medical students: A longitudinal study at course entry and graduation. *Rural and Remote Health, 6*, 537. Retrieved from http://www.rrh.org.au/articles/showarticlenew.asp?ArticleID=537

Walters, L., Prideaux, D., Worley, P., & Greenhill, J. (2011). Demonstrating the value of longitudinal integrated placements to general practice preceptors. *Medical Education, 45*(5), 455-463. doi:10.1111/j1365-2923.2010.03901.x

Walters, L., Prideaux, D., Worley, P., Greenhill, J., & Rolfe, H. (2009). What do general practitioners do differently when consulting with a medical student? *Medical Education, 43*(3), 268-273. doi:10.1111/j.1365-2923.2008.03276.x

Walters, L., Worley, P., Prideaux, D., & Lange, K. (2008). Do consultations in general practice take more time when practitioners are precepting medical students? *Medical Education, 42*(1), 69-73. doi:10.1111/j.1365-2923.2007.02949.x

Westburg, J. (2007). Making a difference: An interview with Khaya Mfenyana. *Education for Health, 20*(1), 1-8. Retrieved from http://www.educationforhealth.net/publishedarticles/article_print_22.pdf

Wiseman, V. (2005). Comparing the preferences of health professionals and members of the public for setting health care priorities. *Applied Health Economics and Health Policy, 4*(2), 129-137.

World Health Organization (WHO). (2005). *Preparing a workforce for the 21st century: The challenge of chronic conditions*. Geneva: World Health Organization. Retrieved from http://www.who.int/chp/knowledge/publications/workforce_report/en/

Worley, P. (2002). Relationships: A new way to analyse community-based medical education? (Part 1). *Education for Health, 15*(2), 117-128.

Worley, P., Esterman, A., & Prideaux, D. (2004). Cohort study of examination performance of undergraduate medical students learning in community settings. *British Medical Journal, 328*, 207. doi:10.1136/bmj.328.7433.207

Worley, P., Martin, A., Prideaux, D., Woodman, R., Worley, E., & Lowe, M. (2008). Vocational career paths of graduate entry medical students at Flinders University: A comparison of rural, remote and tertiary tracks. *Medical Journal of Australia, 188*(3), 177-178.

Worley, P., Prideaux, D., Strasser, R., Magery, A., & March, R. (2006). Empirical evidence for symbiotic medical education: A comparative analysis of community and tertiary-based programmes. *Medical Education, 40*(2), 109-116. doi:10.1111/j.1365-2929.2005.02366.x

Worley, P., Strasser, R., & Prideaux, D. (2004). Can medical students learn specialist disciplines based in rural practice? Lessons from students' self reported experience and competence. *Rural and Remote Health, 4*, 338. Retrieved from http://www.rrh.org.au/articles/showarticlenew.asp?ArticleID=338

Worley, P. S., & Kitto. P. (2001). Hypothetical model of the financial impact of student attachments on rural general practices. *Rural and Remote Health, 1*, 83. Retrieved from http://www.rrh.org.au/articles/showarticlenew.asp?ArticleID=83

Yura-Petro, H., & Scanelli, B. R. (1992). The education of health care professionals in the year 2000 and beyond : Part 1: The consumers view. *The Health Care Supervisor*, March, 1-11.

David Prideaux Dip T (Prim), BA (Hons), MEd, PhD
School of Medicine
Flinders University, Australia

Iris Lindemann BSc, BNutDiet, MEd, APD
School of Medicine
Flinders University, Australia

Anaise Cottrell BIntStud, LLB(Hons), GDLP
School of Medicine
Flinders University, Australia

JOY HIGGS

8. PROFESSIONAL SOCIALISATION

This chapter deals with what it means to become a member of a profession and how this process or journey occurs. There are four key issues that will be addressed in this chapter to explore the topic of professional socialisation:

What is a profession?
What are the goals of professional socialisation?
How can professional socialisation be interpreted?
How can professional socialisation be pursued and facilitated?

Before we can talk about how a person becomes a member of a profession we need to understand what is meant by four key terms: professional, professionalism, profession and professional practice (see Figure 8.1). These comprise the goals and expected outcomes of the socialisation process. At its most positive and widely beneficial, the goal of professional socialisation is to develop and shape capable and accountable members (of professions) who contribute constructively to the services provided to society by these professions and who contribute to the foundations, growth, critique and health of the professions (as in healthy learning organisations). To achieve these outcomes a key issue is understanding what constitutes a profession, remembering that both the construct and the reality of a profession are socially and historically constructed phenomena influenced by multiple interests and forces including self-regulation by professional bodies and external monitoring through higher education influences, government policies and regulations and market forces.

A *profession* is a self-regulated occupational group having a body of knowledge, an inherent culture and a recognised role in serving society. Professions operate under continual scrutiny and development, and are … accountable and guided by a code of ethical conduct in practice decisions and actions. Membership of a profession requires completion of an appropriate (commonly degree-based) intensive educational program (Higgs, McAllister, & Whiteford, 2009, p. 102).

A *professional* or *professional practitioner* is a member of a profession who practises in that profession and provides services to individuals and communities.

Professional is a multi-meaning term. As well as a noun (as above) it can be used adjectivally to refer to a mode of behaviour and standard of conduct, in

S. Loftus et al. (Eds.), Educating Health Professionals:
Becoming a University Teacher, 83–92.

which case it can be and often is used formally to reflect the expected behaviour of professionals. The term is often used more informally in common language to refer to something like respectful and sound conduct by any worker (e.g. "a very professional plumber") and sometimes a notion of status or payment category (e.g. a professional athlete).

Being (a) *professional* and demonstrating *professionalism* (or professional behaviour) means acting in ways that demonstrate the standard of conduct required of members of a profession (in general) such as ethical and humanistic behaviour and the duty of care to clients expected by society and by professional associations. And, it means being competent and acting professionally in the enactment of the roles and responsibilities of a member of the specific profession.

We expect professionals to be knowledgeable, competent, safe, critical and preferably, able to engage with their clients in a people-centred manner. They need to be up-to-date, profession-specific, quality service providers. In serving the needs of individuals, groups and society (consider for instance the nursing of a patient, teaching a class of school children, building a bridge across a river), professionals need to work for both the individual and common good as well as for "their pay packets". At the very least we expect of them technical and discipline-specific competence, at best we want them to have a social conscience and to contribute to the good of society.

Professional practitioners need to be sound, responsible and capable decision makers, advisors and information managers, critically appraising information, knowledge and strategies used in practice, not simply adopting the latest research findings uncritically. Clients expect them to critique alternative options to best address the client's situation and needs. Professionals are expected to use their professional judgement and decision-making abilities against an up-to-date knowledge base in this critical-practice approach, similar to the notion of the reflective practitioner developed by Schön (1987). Importantly, such critique should not just be about the work of others but also about the work, the knowledge, the preparation, the motivations and the effects of one's own practice. Further, being critical means adopting a critical perspective to the status quo. This means that working with status quo knowledge and practices in an unquestioning manner is not appropriate or professional. Such non-critical behaviour fails to address issues of contextualisation, alternatives to hegemonic practices, preferences of practitioners and clients for non-dominant practices, problematics associated with protocols and standardised practices, and the value of forms of evidence beyond propositional, scientific and research knowledge. Being critical requires professionals to challenge the assumptions, motivations, values and interests that underlie professional practice as well as workplace practices and cultures. And, it requires them to contribute to the practice discourse about the need for change and new directions in practice to enhance practice and the service the profession provides to society and their clients.

Being constructive change agents and demonstrating duty of care in relation to the services provided to clients is part of the expectation that professionals demonstrate social responsibility. During professional socialisation novices encounter dialogues and experiences which challenge, extend or affirm their entry values and interests or motivations. Topics such as social responsibility, professional ethics and codes of professional conduct typically form part of professional education curricula and are faced personally during workplace learning experiences.

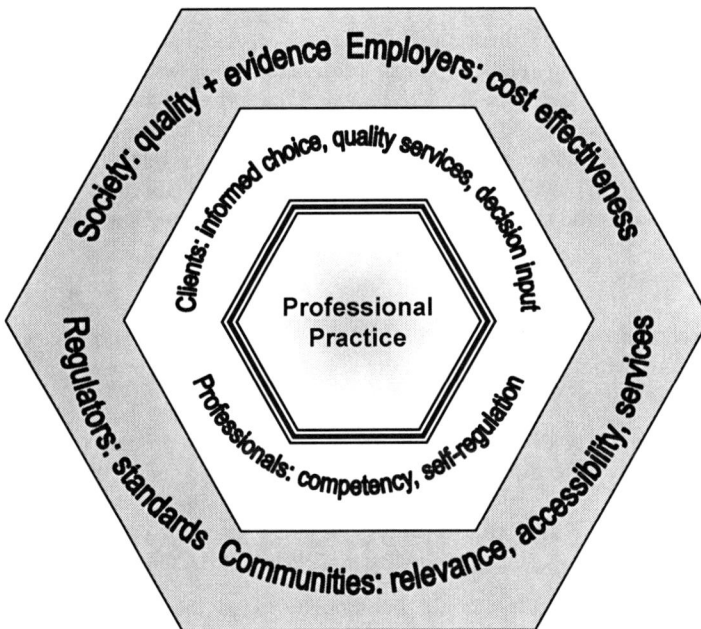

Figure 8.1. Stakeholders expectations of professions and professional practitioners

(Outer ring: external stakeholders, Inner ring: internal stakeholders)

Professional practice refers both to the general notion of practice that is professional, as well as the particular form of social practice – its scope, culture, norms, knowledge base, code of conduct and set of practices – of a given profession. *Practice models* come in many shapes and forms: technical-rational, empirico-analytical, evidence-based, interpretive, and critical emancipatory models, for example (Higgs, 2011).

85

Professional practice is arguably one of the key contextualised social practices operating in society today and so it is desirable that an important part of current literature framing our understanding of professions is social theory. Through social theory we can understand professions as bounded sets of social practices. Schatzki (2010) defines professions as social phenomena that are composed of organised activities of doings and sayings in time and space conducted by many people. Practices are timespace events that emerge, persist then dissolve through activities and are inseparably linked to material arrangements such as workloads, contracts, budgets and professional gadgets. Past practices influence current and in turn, future practices.

Bourdieu's (1986) theoretical framework provides an interpretation of the sociology of human relations where professions exist within fields of practices. These fields are spaces for social interaction that provide conflictual spaces where practices occur and people act in relation to particular rules. The notions of field, interest and habitus are related: interests influence the products of real life games (Bourdieu, 1984) while habitus is the product of socialisation and predisposes people to value and seek out some things more than others (Bourdieu, 2000).

PROFESSIONAL SOCIALISATION

The section above places the culture of professions and professionalism at the core of this discussion. Acculturation is the primary purpose and process of professional socialisation, thus:

> *professional socialisation* refers to the acculturation process (through entry education, reflection, professional development and engagement in professional work interactions) by which individuals develop both the expected capabilities of the profession and a sense of professional identity and responsibility. (Higgs, McAllister, & Whiteford, 2009, p. 102)

Professional socialisation could be thought of as the individual's journey in becoming a member of a particular profession, a unique social group, and learning to be part of the culture of that group with all its privileges, requirements and responsibilities. In addition, professional socialisation could be taken to mean the way in which a profession, through its educators, practitioners and leaders socialises or inducts new members.

Becoming a professional requires "mastery of a complex body of skills and knowledge" (Cruess, Johnston, & Cruess, 2004, p. 74). We can see this as a process of helping newcomers to the profession learning to "walk the walk" and "talk the talk", and I would add "think the think" – or learn how to reason – as expected (by the profession, society and clients) of those who are accorded the status, privileges, recognition and custom of professionals. Yet there are two provisos we need to make in this context and process.

First, it is individual professional practitioners who are responsible for their own actions. Part of this responsibility is the development of their unique professional identity (i.e. their individual beliefs, values, style and sense of professional self) and practice model that is informed by stakeholder expectations, and professional codes of conduct. This identity is also informed by the personal ethics, worldview, career and life journeys of the individual practitioners.

Second, it behoves those guiding and shaping the acculturation of novices to do this well, in the wider interests of society and of the particular interests of the emerging practitioners. Professional socialisation is not a place for brainwashing, powerplays and restrictive practices; it needs to embody the best spirit of professionalism. The (potentially) mixed positive and negative purposes and outcomes of professional socialisation are reflected in the following viewpoint:

> Professions are like social movements. They recruit only certain types of persons, they develop highly elaborate ideologies and supra-individual values, they have their own mechanisms of socialization and they often attempt to proselytize and bring new persons into the fold. (Denzin, 1968, p. 376)

A key dimension of professions and professionalism is the matter of control of, and standards for, practice. This is reflected in the role of professions (particularly professional associations) in self-regulation, the external regulation of the conduct of members of professions through government acts and regulatory authorities, various levels of practice accreditation (of individuals, practices/companies and institutions) plus self-accreditation and external accreditation (by professional associations, councils and governments) of professional education courses.

The role of regulatory authorities is a typical (if not universal) distinguishing feature of professions. This is supported by Bourdieu (1979) who expands upon the idea to include National Standards, Registration and National Educational Standards. Increasingly higher education is being regulated at professional, national and international levels. This regulation is linked to the global demands for accountability, marketability and cross boundary enrolment transference alongside market-driven educational strategies, technology-enabled educational products and opportunities plus national and international market alliances. The impact of all of these initiatives is to place a very high emphasis and workload on regulation of higher education and also, in many instances, of the workplace and practice arenas. In combination, since professional socialisation occurs through and for both education and work/practice arenas, the increasing level of regulation can result in professional socialisation emphasising conformity, risk management, narrow bands of evidence and regulated services, rather than professional identity, professional judgement and tailored services for individual clients.

Any program that seeks to facilitate the journey of others, typically novices or newcomers, to achieve readiness for membership of a profession, needs to be built on a rich understanding of the nature, practice, identity and roles in society of the given profession. Such programs need to go far beyond the simple teaching of knowledge, skills and attitudes of that profession; these are atomistic and disassociated bits of what makes up that profession and of what the novice needs to learn.

Instead, a whole culture of learning is required comprising a curriculum frame of reference, a learning environment that is informed by the professional practice culture, and learning opportunities to engage in the profession's practice world. These are core ingredients of a rich socialisation process. And educational goals must include the development of capabilities required for an unknowable future such as practice epistemology (an understanding of the practice's knowledge and the capacity to generate such knowledge) and professional identity building skills, self-critique and reflexivity. These dimensions of learning programs built around professional socialisation clearly identify that the responsibility for learning is shared between learners and teachers (including academics, practice role models, workplace learning educators and peers).

PROFESSIONAL SOCIALISATION AS PROCESS

Professional socialisation as an acculturation process occurs through entry education, reflection, professional development and engagement in professional work interactions. Through these processes and experiences novices learn what it means: to be a member of their professional community, to understand the way their professional culture operates, to develop the expected capabilities of the profession and to generate a sense of professional identity and responsibility that will enable them to be recognised and capable members of that community.

During immersion in the culture of their profession and workplaces, and through this acculturation novices develop an understanding of:

- professional codes of conduct and boundaries delineating acceptable from professionally inappropriate or taboo behaviours
- professional, legal and ethical sanctions associated with professional conduct transgressions
- the roles and responsibilities of members of the profession
- the role relationships between members of the same and related professions, the public and other people encountered during their work
- the professional work context, including the goals, roles and procedures of that system. (Cant & Higgs, 1999)

Professional socialisation does not occur in any one specific context (Cant and Higgs, 1999). Instead it is both a formal and informal part of an ongoing journey for individuals and their evolving community engagement with multiple individuals. For individuals there is a period of anticipatory socialisation resulting from multiple life and learning experiences prior to commencing tertiary education and prior to entering the workforce. During this time, expectations about future roles and work are created and the emerging practitioner's identity and capabilities start to evolve.

Professional education can take multiple paths including transitions from vocational education training (e.g. associate degrees in TAFE colleges in Australia) to university degrees, undergraduate tertiary education courses, graduate entry programs at masters and doctoral level building on first degrees through colleges (such as in USA) or universities. This path diversity produces a range of graduates and graduate backgrounds which can provide individuals and professions with rich preparation for practice futures. Across these paths novices' professional development is influenced by many people including teachers, curriculum developers, workplace educators, professional role models, clients and peers.

In both the academic and workplace settings learners become immersed in their communities of practice and their learning is grounded in the way these communities operate. In essence, each practice community and practice preparation community (including the professional entry curriculum environment) shapes students' learning, their sense of what is expected of a member of their particular profession and what is expected of them in their workplaces and work roles. Students graduating from these programs should have acquired a professional identity, the expected practice competencies as determined by their professional bodies, the capacity to critique and develop themselves as practitioners and professionals, and relevant graduate learning outcomes. These outcomes include the ability to apply theoretical knowledge in practice situations, provide rationales for clinical decisions, communicate effectively with clients and staff and have a lifelong learning approach to their careers (Adamson, Harris, Heard, & Hunt, 1996). Importantly, graduate learning outcomes need to be embedded in disciplinary teaching and not be seen as added-in learning goals; the achievement of these outcomes requires student engagement in learning (Murdoch-Eaton & Whittle, 2012). Similarly, Crebert et al. (2004) reported that workplace learning (particularly, collaboration and team work) is important in promoting the development of generic skills.

Learning in the workplace as well as the grounding of learners' whole education in preparation for practice, are key foundations of successful professional education. Workplace learning is particularly powerful since it directly situates learners' learning in the physical, cultural, social and personal setting of the workplace and the profession, as well as the interprofessional and institutional settings that comprise the workplace. And, it places learners (even while under supervision of a workplace learning educator or experienced practitioner) in a position where their decisions, actions and professional relationships have real life-influencing consequences. They assess and treat clients, and although their supervisor typically retains the legal responsibility for overall client care and observes client outcomes, what the learners do really matters (Roe-Shaw, 2004). This heightens the reality of their learning and deepens and broadens their experience and understanding of what their practice involves, what professional identity they are building, what practice model choices they are facing and how what they say, think and do impacts on the wellbeing of their clients.

Students often encounter gaps between the expectations of the university and the realities of the workplace. Similarly, as students their level of responsibility and range of work is often more restricted than the expectations they face after graduation. To some extent these gaps are unavoidable. For instance, the consequences of actions in classroom simulations with fellow students are not as great as with ill or disabled clients in clinical settings (Roe-Shaw, 2004).

The educational preparation of new graduates is influential in shaping their experiences of their early employment. Hummell (2007) studied allied health graduates' first year of employment. Her participants highly valued their clinical placements and their university subjects with direct clinical application because these subjects assisted successful integration into the workplace.

Educational programs need to consider what goals and outcomes to target and how extensively to prepare the expected 'work-ready' graduates. How can this be done and how is this responsibility shared across the educational institution, the profession, the workplace (employers and practitioners), workplace educators, and, of course, the students? At times inadequacies in professional preparation are linked to educational deficiencies, such as isolation of academics from the real world, lack of clinical or teaching expertise of clinical educators, inadequate resourcing or patient access in clinical settings, and clinical systems that are unprepared for or unsupportive of student education (Roe-Shaw, 2004). Educators and workplaces need to address such barriers to quality clinical education in sharing the task of producing competent future healthcare employees. Similarly, students should be active agents in their education and take an important role in ensuring the quality of their clinical education experience and outcomes.

Reality shock for new graduates is commonly linked to educational preparation limitations since curricula cannot hope to cover all relevant graduate knowledge, capabilities and situations (including clinical conditions, workplace regulations, and team or leadership approaches). Workplace educators are highly influential in shaping the quality of student learning on placements. They organise placement programs and access to patients, facilitate students' learning and supervise their practice, provide constructive feedback and assess students' performance.

Roe-Shaw's (2004) New Zealand study of professional socialisation of physiotherapists found the greatest level of reality shock was reported by graduates who had not experienced increasing workload levels and complexity during student placements. They entered the workforce expecting high levels of support from experienced physiotherapists, light caseloads and a limited level of responsibility. They were shocked to discover that workplace reality involved high direct client caseloads with limited supervision or mentoring, and complex non-client work tasks such as meetings, ward rounds, patient note writing, team meetings and family meetings.

Hummell (2007) found that clinical placements which incorporated a graded increase in client workloads, responsibility and accountability and a graded decrease in direct supervision in combination with effective support contributed to graduates' smooth transition into the workplace and a reduced level of reality shock. Participants in Hummell's research reported that particularly in the final year of the course, university subjects which addressed the realities of initial employment, including the complexity of work roles, managing work stressors and seeking supervision/mentoring, reduced their reality shock and facilitated their initial workplace transition.

A key aspect of professional socialisation is the way that students develop working relationships with other practitioners and team members from a range of professions. Professional socialisation involves learning to work in practice communities. The term communities of practice was developed by Lave and Wenger

(1991) to describe a theory of social learning, that places learning "in the context of our lived experience of participation in the world" (Wenger, 1998, p. 3). Communities of practice are dynamic and flexible as people arrive and leave, and as they become more or less central to the practice of the group. Some communities of practice are formally established and managed, others are more organic and evolve, developing shared purposes based on interests or passions.

Underpinning this theory are four premises: (i) that people are social beings, (ii) that knowledge occurs in relation to valued enterprises, (iii) that knowing results from participating and pursuing ability in these enterprises, and (iv) that learning produces meaningful knowledge. Although these premises have been critiqued and extended they do connect social practice and learning by framing learning as social and relational participation (Hughes, Jewson, & Unwin, 2007). Two key concepts related to communities of practice (Lave & Wenger, 1991) are:

- *situated learning,* which views learning as part of an activity in the world, in that agent, activity, and the world mutually constitute each other
- *legitimate peripheral participation* which relates to the contention that for newcomers to a practice community, learning through activity happens legitimately from the periphery towards the core of the community of practice as they become full practitioners integral to the maturing of the field of practice.

Professional socialisation involves both learning through practice communities and learning to be part of communities of practice. In her research on collaboration in healthcare Croker (2011) found that most health professionals engage with multiple practice communities in their work (for example, their discipline team, their local work area group such as in a ward, their broader professional association). Newcomers need to learn how to relate across each of these groups and communities.

CONCLUSION

In a book on the education of health professions the notion and practice of professional socialisation holds a central place. Students can learn about their profession, they can learn the skills and knowledge of their profession and they can graduate and gain the status of their profession. But, without experience of their profession and an induction into the culture of the profession and without gaining a professional identity they have not really become members of the profession; they have not been socialised into it. Online learning about the profession is insufficient for professional socialisation and preparation for practice.

For both educators and students or novices, understanding of professional socialisation and the capacity and willingness to engage in this process is a necessary part of preparing for and supporting professional entry and for gaining professional membership. This chapter has examined what needs to be learned to pursue, support and enhance the process of professional socialisation for the benefit of individual professionals, the profession and the society that professionals serve. In the context of the health professions the socialisation process is particularly pertinent since fostering the wellbeing of patients and the betterment of communities is the key goal of healthcare and the ultimate goal of health professional education.

REFERENCES

Adamson, B., Harris, L., Heard, R., & Hunt, A. (1996). *University education and workplace requirements: Evaluating the skills and attributes of health science graduates*. Sydney: The University of Sydney Printing Service.

Bourdieu, P. (1979). *La distinction: Critique sociale du jugement*. Paris: Les Editions de Minuit.

Bourdieu, P. (1984). *Questions de sociologie*. Paris: Les Editions de Minuit.

Bourdieu, P. (1986). The forms of capital (R. Nice, Trans.). In J. G. Richardson (Ed.), *Handbook for theory and research for the sociology of education* (pp. 241-258). New York: Greenwood Press.

Bourdieu, P. (2000). *Esquisse d'une théorie de la pratique*. Paris: Editions du Seuil.

Cant, R., & Higgs, J. (1999). Professional socialisation. In J. Higgs & H. Edwards (Eds.), *Educating beginning practitioners: Challenges for health professional education* (pp. 46-51). Oxford: Butterworth-Heinemann.

Crebert, G., Bates, M., Bell, B., & Patrick, C.-J. (2004). Developing generic skills at university, during work placement and in employment: Graduates' perceptions. *Higher Education Research & Development 23*(2), 147-165.

Croker, A. (2011). *Collaboration in rehabilitation teams*. Unpublished PhD thesis, Charles Sturt University.

Cruess, S. R., Johnston, S., & Cruess, R. L. (2004). "Profession": A working definition for medical educators. *Teaching and Learning in Medicine, 16*(1), 74-76.

Denzin, N. (1968). Pharmacy - Incomplete professionalization. *Social Forces, 46*(3), 370-384.

Higgs, J. (2011). *Practice-based education: Enhancing practice and pedagogy*. Final report for ALTC teaching fellowship, Australian Learning and Teaching Council, Australia.

Higgs, J., McAllister, L., & Whiteford, G. (2009). The practice and praxis of professional decision making. In B. Green (Ed.), *Understanding and researching professional practice* (pp. 101-120). Rotterdam, The Netherlands: Sense.

Hughes, J., Jewson, N., & Unwin, L. (Eds.). (2007). *Communities of practice: Critical perspectives*. London: Routledge.

Hummell, J. (2007). *Allied health graduates' first year of employment*. Unpublished PhD thesis, The University of Sydney, Australia.

Lave, J., & Wenger, E. (1991). *Situated learning: Legitimate peripheral participation*. Cambridge: Cambridge University Press.

Murdoch-Eaton, D., & Whittle, S. (2012). Generic skills in medical education: Developing the tools for successful lifelong learning. *Medical Education, 46*(1), 120-128.

Roe-Shaw, M. (2004). *Workplace realities and professional socialisation of recently graduated physiotherapists in New Zealand*. Unpublished PhD thesis, University of Otago, New Zealand.

Schatzki, T. (2010). *The timespace of human activity*. New York: Rowman & Littlefield.

Schön, D. A. (1987). *Educating the reflective practitioner: Toward a new design for teaching and learning in the professions*. San Francisco, CA: Jossey-Bass.

Wenger, E. (1998). *Communities of practice: Learning, meaning, and identity*. Cambridge, MA: Cambridge University Press.

Joy Higgs AM PhD
The Education For Practice Institute
Charles Sturt University, Australia

PETER O'MEARA AND SUSAN FURNESS

9. EDUCATION IN THE EMERGING PROFESSIONS

Universities are huge multidisciplinary enterprises of learning and scholarship that have evolved from the traditional biblical Tower of Babel (Kaghan & Phillips, 1998). The reality is very different, with both students and academics facing the challenges of how to both create new knowledge and impart it to a new generation of students and future professionals.

Beyond the traditional disciplines of science, the humanities, law and theology, and arguably medicine, universities now provide education and training to a large range of professions that are relatively new to the university sector. These new disciplines reside throughout the university, in Faculties of Business, Health, Education, and in other pockets of universities. Some of these new disciplines have thrived, while others are in fragile states of development. For instance, those in the paramedicine discipline sometimes continue to experience a challenge being recognised within ambulance services and other workplaces as university-educated health professionals. One manifestation of this is the continuing difficulty of promoting an academic career as a strong option for practising paramedics.

Part of the explanation for this is the relatively high remuneration of paramedics in industry compared to university salaries, but another factor is that the discipline is still undertaking the journey from vocational training to higher education (Joyce, Wainer, Piterman, Wyatt, & Archer, 2009). Furthermore, there remains a strong drive from within government and the community to solve long-term workforce challenges with short-term "solutions" that may involve a return to apprentice-style training programs.

Despite the wide dispersion of the new disciplines throughout the university, individuals within them can still feel isolated, neglected and in some ways misunderstood. Each wave of emerging professionals face challenges as they seek to educate entrants for their respective professions and form productive relationships with industry and their own profession; sometimes these challenges are similar across disciplines, while at other times particular disciplines face unique challenges. A consistent phenomenon is that they can all feel like the "new kids on the block", who need to earn the respect and recognition of their predecessors, while maintaining credibility within their field of practice.

In this chapter we identify and discuss the major issues that confront students in the emerging professions as they enter the hallowed halls of the university. Although much of the literature relied upon here emanates from the nursing and

S. Loftus et al. (Eds.), Educating Health Professionals:
Becoming a University Teacher, 93–102.

allied health professions, the chapter explores issues through the perspective of paramedicine, one of the most recent entrants to the higher education sector. That profession has emerged quickly since the first university conversion programs in the mid-1990s, to the point where half of Australia's universities offer entry-level paramedicine programs in every State and Territory. The most common structure of these programs is the traditional three-year bachelor's degree, but there are a smaller number of popular double degrees with nursing, a handful of shorter postgraduate conversion degrees and one combined master's degree with a Bachelor of Health Science.

The chapter is divided into four sections:

1. Key issues for emerging professions
2. Industry and professional expectations
3. Theory and practice tensions
4. Future challenges and actions.

KEY ISSUES FOR THE EMERGING PROFESSIONS

Having established some of the general context in which academic practice lies, we now move into more specific areas that are important to understand when practitioners of an emerging discipline enter academia.

One of the major challenges that the emerging professional programs initially face is the recruitment and retention of academic staff from disciplines that often have a limited pool of suitably qualified people. Although most professions can draw from established trainers who have the qualifications and experience to teach basic vocational skills, many battle to recruit those who have the necessary qualifications and track records to meet the standard qualification frameworks for appointment at university level. For example, a lecturer in a university is expected to undertake teaching and research without the need for close supervision.

In contrast to industry-based training programs, which can be limited to teaching a limited range of occupational competencies that are stable and unchallenged, university education requires academics to develop curricula from research evidence and to participate in the scholarship of their discipline. They are expected to contribute to a successful research program, publish findings, and obtain competitive funding. There is also a requirement to supervise research students. These expectations are largely premised on the academic model of the established disciplines, even though many of the emerging disciplines do not fit this set of assumptions (Crane, O'Hern, & Lawler, 2009). In the paramedicine discipline, as in many professions in previous years, academic staff members generally enter academia without a doctoral qualification or an established scholarly track record. This has a major impact on those individuals, who can struggle to meet these new expectations, while the profession and industry may lack an adequate appreciation of the challenges confronting transitioning clinicians.

Even at a junior level, academics are generally expected to meet stringent qualification and skills requirements. In the case of appointment of a lecturer in an established field, it is not at all unusual to expect applicants to meet the following requirements:

- Hold a PhD degree in the discipline
- Demonstrate experience in teaching at a tertiary level
- Have experience in the co-ordination of a tertiary level subject
- Show evidence of a record of research within an area compatible with the interests of the discipline
- Have experience in the supervision of honours and postgraduate students
- Demonstrate well-developed oral and written communications skills
- Have evidence of the ability to work as a member of a team.

Senior lecturers are typically expected to make a significant contribution to the discipline at the national level, including original contributions that expand knowledge or practice in their discipline. Crucially, senior lecturers should be able to demonstrate they are established and productive researchers with a significant track record of publications and competitive research income in their research field. These requirements can be frustrating, both for the universities attempting to establish a teaching program in the emerging disciplines and for those professionals who have a desire to enter academia. Of course, the challenges for academics from the emerging disciplines hoping to progress to the professoriate are even greater.

The reality is that there is only limited recognition of vocational or industry qualifications and experience within universities. Appointment to junior academic positions is relatively easy for industry-trained professionals with some tertiary qualifications, provided they are prepared to accept a decrease in remuneration and understand that they are at the bottom of the career ladder as novice academics (Beres, 2006). This is not always an easy reality for aspiring academics or the profession to understand and accept. In some cases, universities recognise this tension and offer clinical loadings to help bridge the gap between junior academic remuneration and higher salaries in industry.

Closely linked to this issue is the requirement that in addition to teaching, academics are expected to undertake and publish research. This is a major departure for teachers from industry and the vocational sector; consequently, few potential entrants into academia have the necessary skills to attract research funding, undertake research and publish the results without major support from universities and their more established peers. In response to these types of requirements, course accreditation for occupational therapy programs in the United States have required all full-time faculty to have a master's degree since 2008 and a doctoral qualification from 2012 (Fain, 2011). Many other disciplines are following similar paths as they seek to establish themselves as legitimate professions.

This is a far cry from the situation in newly emerging disciplines such as paramedicine, where "academics" have until recently been recruited with "front-line" experience, limited teaching experience and no research training at all. Universities, industry and the profession have a responsibility to support those individuals in making their transition into the academy. This support can take the form of mentoring, continuing professional practice opportunities, and support for emerging researchers. Something as simple as access to some data for research can make an immense difference to a novice academic striving to complete a research degree or get a scholarly paper accepted for publication.

In at least some cases, emerging disciplines have expected that the transfer of education from industry to the universities would be little more than a transfer of existing programs from industry-based training schools to a university campus (O'Meara, Tourle, Madigan, & Lighton, 2011). Little regard was given to the curriculum or to the pedagogical changes necessary to satisfy university requirements, or to how these would ultimately change the professions. As a result of this naivety in industry and the emerging professions, new academics often share elements of this culture shock when they are faced with university expectations that their curriculum should be based on an established body of evidence. When they arrive in the universities they can also be shocked by the degree of internal and external change taking place, the workload implications of developing new teaching materials, and the relentless demands of administration and committee work. On top of these day-to-day challenges, new academics must come to terms with a workplace that both allows high levels of autonomy and demands accountability.

In the case of paramedicine at least, no great account was taken of the changing characteristics and expectations of students (Boyle, Williams, Cooper, Adams, & Alford, 2008). While university students tend to be younger than those in many vocational education programs, their demographic profiles vary enormously, with a wide mix of gender, age, and ethnicity. Universities and individual academics are required to cope with a wide range of student needs and expectations. Likewise, the emerging professions and industry are faced with the challenge of adapting to changes in the educational and career expectations of students and graduates. One Australian study of paramedic and nursing/paramedic students (O'Meara et al., 2011) aimed to determine the initial career intentions of full-time paramedic students and to identify the key factors that influenced their career choices. The authors found that these students were more likely to seek employment with organisations when their personal and professional needs were met through positive recognition of graduate attributes, provision of attractive working conditions, opportunities for further education, recognition of personal needs, and the projection of the paramedic as a health professional.

INDUSTRY AND PROFESSIONAL EXPECTATIONS

Because of their different perspectives, the expectations of industry and the emerging professions can differ from those of academic staff and universities. One result is that there may be lingering tensions about course content and the standards of new graduates entering the workforce. Are they "work-ready"? Accreditation processes can potentially become battlegrounds for different perspectives on what is expected of university programs and the staff involved in teaching and research. With most of the newer professions having emerged from the vocational education training sector, it is very easy for there to be a continuing emphasis on occupational competencies. This emphasis can occur apart from the development of a broader professional framework that locates educational programs within a broader philosophical context that values scholarship and the generation of knowledge and independent thought (O'Meara, 2011a).

Associated with the difficult challenge of breaking away from a vocational mind-set, and sometimes the lack of respect for "education" in the workplace, are the challenges that individuals face when making the transition to academia. In the emerging professions, the drive for a continuing "hands-on" role is strong. Although there are good reasons why continuing professional practice is desirable, the strong views associated with the concept may be result of the ingrained "guild" or apprentice-based history of specific occupations. There is arguably a lingering suspicion about the values embodied in higher education and a perverse desire to see retention of the legitimacy of the former route to practice. This is particularly evident in some of the dialogue around the transfer of nursing to universities over the last 20 to 30 years. As recently as 2007, the then Commonwealth Minister of Health, Tony Abbott, seriously advocated for the return of nursing education to hospitals (O'Keefe & Armitage, 2007). Although this call for a return to "traditional" nursing education may have been driven by financial concerns related to the escalating cost of clinical education, the nursing profession strenuously opposed a return to a hospital-based education that no longer reflects the reality of where many nurses now practise.

One vexed question concerns the extent to which professionals should maintain their "currency" in their discipline through continuing practice and continuing education activities. From the outside, the answer may be obvious, along with the conviction that such continuing practice should be easily achieved. However, the day-to-day pressures of academic life and the need to develop a research track record to ensure a productive career path make this problematic for many emerging academics (Pickering, 2006). Others will experience problems gaining access to continuing practice opportunities because of rigid organisational and industrial boundaries. In one novel case, an Australian paramedic academic resorted to veterinary nursing practice to maintain clinical skills (Madigan & Smith, 2010).

A lack of awareness and support from both industry and universities exacerbates the daunting challenges that academics from the emerging professions face when making their transitions to academia. A cynical view of universities suggests that they are more interested in the income from popular undergraduate courses than in good staff development or recognition of professional status (Kenny, 2008). Nor does industry necessarily have any particular interest in supporting or recognising those who have moved into academia. A good example of this is the difficulty academics can face as "outsiders" when they seek to undertake field research in their own industry. Nursing academics from higher education institutions are forced to negotiate competing external agendas when they undertake research, despite the pivotal role that nursing academics play in the development of nursing research (Segrott, McIvor, & Green, 2006). There is little doubt that academics in the emerging disciplines are left with a feeling of fighting a losing battle on two fronts in these circumstances.

THEORY AND PRACTICE TENSIONS

With the transfer of education to the university, emerging professional programs face the challenge of determining how to integrate a set of existing occupational competencies with the educational requirements of the university system. Teaching practical skills without reference to theory and the evidence base is no longer acceptable. Almost all professional programs undertaken in universities draw on a mixture of supporting sciences and discipline-specific knowledge and skills. One of the challenges for the emerging professions is that students, and in some cases established practitioners, call into question these foundational knowledge domains. Despite existing evidence in the literature (Nettleton, Litchfield, & Taylor, 2008), there appears some degree of confusion or lack of clarity about how these educational elements contribute to the graduation of "work-ready" professionals.

The accreditation of paramedic programs in Australia and New Zealand is currently administered by the Australasian Council of Ambulance Authorities with some input from Paramedics Australasia (Council of Ambulance Authorities, 2010). However, there remains some continuing tension between supporters of the former in-house training programs, with their strong emphasis on specific occupational competencies, and university programs that require a broader range of graduate attributes that have some commonality with the other health professions (Council of Ambulance Authorities, n.d.).

A counter-argument to this position can be advanced, based on Benner's pedagogical theories that universities can only produce novices, and that a more overt integration between occupational competencies, clinical evidence and the supporting sciences would be more likely to facilitate the transition from novice to beginning practitioner (Willis, Williams, Brightwell, O'Meara, & Pointon, 2010).

One of the substantive criticisms of at least some emerging professions is that they lack distinctive signature pedagogies, such as those that are well established in the long-standing professions, to define what counts as knowledge (Shulman,

2005). It can be hard for new professions to articulate all of their nuances to "outsiders" who see only the surface layers and therefore miss those deeper layers such as professional dispositions (Willis, Pointon, & O'Meara, 2008; Willis et al., 2010). In the case of the paramedic profession, it has been argued that there is a lack of a "*sustained and cohesive discourse*" on significant aspects of paramedic education for practice (Willis et al., 2010). In common with other recently emerging disciplines before them, this has resulted in the adaptation of research evidence from near disciplines such as nursing and medicine to inform teaching (Lazarsfeld-Jensen, 2011). Nursing has grappled with these challenges in its transition from hospital-based training to colleges of advanced education to university education, the turbulence of a generational change in their scope of practice, and a simultaneous shift in culture and power relationships (Boychuk Duchscher, 2001; Boychuk Duchscher & Cowin, 2004).

Perhaps one of the biggest challenges for emerging professions relates to their capacity to shape a professional identity that moves beyond traditional images of sub-professional occupations reliant on others for leadership and legitimacy. This is a particular challenge for paramedics in the United States, where paramedics work under the medical licence of physicians and there are few university-level programs available (National Highway Traffic Safety Administrator, 1996; Sayre, White, Brown, & McHenry, 2002). In contrast, recent decades have witnessed the emergence of the allied health professions that have succeeded in establishing their own place within the educational and professional landscape.

This continuing challenge is particularly acute for the emerging professions that are yet to demonstrate a history of independent scholarship. Paramedicine is again a good example of a profession that remains in the early stages of academic and professional development. As a profession, it is yet to build and disseminate a body of knowledge that is based on robust evidence combined with informed debate and discussion (Tippett, Clark, Woods, & Fitzgerald, 2003; Snooks et al., 2008). One observation of ambulance services and paramedicine is that there is a tendency to ignore or dismiss other options that do not fit with established patterns of practice, such as the evidence that endotracheal intubation might not always be the best option for managing airways (Deakin et al., 2008). Encouraging more research within the profession and evidence-based decision making is a challenge that is shared across all the emerging professions. If the questions are not asked, researched, and published, potential improvements and resolutions of these situations will never see the light of day (O'Meara, 2011b).

FUTURE CHALLENGES AND ACTIONS

Even when emerging professions have made their first successful step into the university sector, their challenges are far from over. Efforts to sustain the transition of individuals and professions are ongoing. This is amply demonstrated in the case of nursing, with some sections of the community and the political elite continuing to question whether the profession belongs in the university or would be better located in the vocational education sector (O'Keefe & Armitage,

2007). To counter these arguments that some professions should step back in time it is incumbent on the professions themselves, industry groups and universities to ensure ongoing success through support for the emerging professions. Because of some historical and cultural barriers it can sometimes be difficult for emerging professions to strongly support their scholarly members. Despite these barriers, they can be supportive through the provision of opportunities for academics to continue to practise professionally, the establishment or expansion of professional registration arrangements that recognise the non-clinical roles of academics in the professions, and the participation of members in research activities.

Industry also has a responsibility, to say nothing of self-interest, to support the emergence and future vitality of the new health professions and their graduates. This can be facilitated through the provision of high-quality professional placements and through making staff available for practical and specialist lectures to students. Industry also has an obligation to support current and future academics through the provision of research opportunities to the institutions and departments that are teaching their future employees.

The literature strongly supports the notion that universities have a responsibility to play their role in this enterprise through strong support mechanisms, communication of clear expectations and the mentoring of new academics as they make their personal transition to academia (Siler & Kleiner, 2001).

In the longer term, each new discipline will be judged against its own objectives and how members take their place in the academy alongside the established professions. Some professions will be happy to work with others as "adjunct professionals", whereas others will aspire to greater professional autonomy. In some ways, success will be symbolised when members of the emerging professions fill senior positions within universities and influence policy within their own spheres and more widely in related domains of public policy.

REFERENCES

Beres, J. (2006). Staff development to university faculty: Reflections of a nurse educator. *Nursing Forum, 41*(3), 141-145.

Boychuk Duchscher, J. (2001). Out in the real world: Newly graduated nurses in acute-care speak out. *Journal of Nursing Administration, 31*(9), 426.

Boychuk Duchscher, J., & Cowin, L. (2004). The experience of marginalization in new nursing graduates. *Nursing Outlook, 52*(6), 289-296.

Boyle, M., Williams, B., Cooper, J., Adams, B., & Alford, K. (2008). Ambulance clinical placements – A pilot study of students' experience. *BMC Medical Education, 8*(19). doi:10.1186/1472-6920-8-19

Council of Ambulance Authorities. (2010). *Guidelines for the assessment and accreditation of entry-level paramedic education programs.* Adelaide: Council of Ambulance Authorities Inc.

Council of Ambulance Authorities. (n.d.). *Paramedic professional competency standards.* Adelaide: Council of Ambulance Authorities Inc.

Crane, B., O'Hern, B., & Lawler, P. (2009). Second career professionals: Transitioning to the faculty role. *Journal of Faculty Development, 23*(1), 24-29.

Deakin, D., Clarke, T., Nolan, J., Zideman, A., Gwinnut, C., Moore, F., et al. (2008). A critical reassessment of ambulance service airway management in prehospital care: Joint Royal Colleges Ambulance Liaison Committee Airway Working Group. *Emergency Medicine Journal, 27,* 226-233.

Fain, E. A. (2011). Bridging the gap: Helping more practitioners become academics. *American Occupational Therapy Association, 16*(3), 9-12.

Joyce, C. M., Wainer, J., Piterman, L., Wyatt, A., & Archer, F. (2009). Trends in the paramedic workforce: A profession in transition. [Letter to the Editor]. *Australian Health Review, 33*(4), 533-540.

Kaghan, W., & Phillips, N. (1998). Building the tower of Babel: Communities of practice and paradigmatic pluralism in organizational studies. *Organization, 5*(2), 191-215.

Kenny, J. (2008). Efficiency and effectiveness in higher education: Who is accountable for what? *Australian Universities Review, 50*(1), 11-19.

Lazarsfeld-Jensen, A. (2011). *Fast track: Evidence-based strategies for optimising short-term paramedic internships.* Bathurst: Charles Sturt University.

Madigan, V., & Smith, B. (2010). How vets can assist paramedics in improving patient care – A humorous but thoughtful tale of nightshift. *Response, 37*(1), 21-23.

National Highway Traffic Safety Administrator. (1996). *Emergency medical services agenda for the future.* National Highway Traffic Safety Administrator.

Nettleton, S., Litchfield, A., & Taylor, T. (2008). *Engaging professional societies in developing work-ready graduates.* Paper presented at the 31st HERDSA Annual Conference, Rotorua.

O'Keefe, B., & Armitage, C. (2007, 19 September). Hospital nurse training "a waste". *The Australian.* Retrieved from http://www.theaustralian.com.au/higher-education-old/business-education/hospital-nurse-training-a-waste/story-e6frgcp6-1111114448959

O'Meara, P. (2011a). So how can we frame our identity? *Journal of Paramedic Practice, 3*(2), 5.

O'Meara, P. (2011b). The maturation of the paramedic profession through international scholarship. *International Journal of Paramedic Practice, 1*(2), 2-3.

O'Meara, P., Tourle, V., Madigan, V., & Lighton, D. (2011). Getting in touch with paramedic student career intentions. *Health Education Journal.* doi:10.1177/0017896911406962

Pickering, A. M. (2006). Learning about university teaching: Reflections on a research study investigating influences for change. *Teaching in Higher Education, 11*(3), 319-335.

Sayre, M. R., White, L. J., Brown, L. H., & McHenry, S. D. (2002). The national EMS research agenda executive summary. *Annals of Emergency Medicine, 40*(6), 636-643.

Segrott, J., McIvor, M., & Green, B. (2006). Challenges and strategies in developing nursing research capacity: A review of the literature. *International Journal of Nursing Studies, 43*(5), 637-651.

Shulman, L. (2005). Pedagogies of uncertainty. *Liberal Education, 91*(Summer), 18-25.

Siler, B. B., & Kleiner, C. (2001). Novice faculty: Encountering expectations in academia. *Journal of Nursing Education, 40*(9), 397-403.

Snooks, H., Archer, F., Clarke, T., Dale, J., Hartley-Sharpe, C., Janes, D., et al. (2008). What are the highest priorities for research in pre-hospital care? Results of a review and Dephi consultation exercise. [Special report]. *Journal of Primary Health Care, 6*(4), Article No. 990320.

Tippett, V., Clark, M., Woods, S., & Fitzgerald, G. (2003). Towards a national research agenda for the ambulance and pre-hospital sector in Australia. *Journal of Emergency Primary Health Care, 1*(1-2), Article No. 990007.

Willis, E., Pointon, T., & O'Meara, P. (2008). *Paramedic education: Developing depth through networks and evidence-based research:* Australian Learning & Teaching Council Discipline-Based Development Initiatives. ISBN 978-0-7258-1132-7.

Willis, E., Williams, B., Brightwell, R., O'Meara, P., & Pointon, T. (2010). Road-ready paramedics and the supporting sciences curriculum. *Focus on Health Professional Education, 11*(2), 1-13.

Peter O'Meara BHA, MPP, PhD
La Trobe Rural Health School
La Trobe University, Australia

Susan Furness Dip Hlth Sc Nursing, Dip Amb Para, Grad Dip Emerg Health, MHSc
La Trobe Rural Health School
La Trobe University, Australia

MEGAN SMITH AND TRACY LEVETT-JONES

10. PROVIDING CLINICAL EDUCATION

Working across Sectors

In this chapter we provide a background on the topic of clinical education for teachers who are new to health professional education. A unique facet of clinical education is that the learning experiences for students occur in both academic settings and the workplace. The connections and boundaries between these two settings of education fundamentally shape the practice of clinical education. The language of clinical education is often couched around the notions of relationships and partnerships, reflecting the dependence on participation in the education of future health professionals shared by teachers located in both academic and clinical environments. Few would contest the importance of building, negotiating and sustaining relationships as fundamental concerns for all involved in providing clinical education. However, the partnerships that span these two sectors and the experiences of negotiating these partnerships are complex and dynamic.

This chapter sets the scene for those working across educational and health service sectors by providing a broad understanding of the issues in clinical education, considering each sector and specifically looking at the intersections where the practices of the sectors meet. We bring together the many threads of discussion prevalent in the consideration of clinical education today. Rather than providing a how-to guide for the organisation and conduct of clinical education we instead explore some of the factors that shape and determine how clinical education is conducted and how the wider context of clinical education influences the nature of education that is undertaken. We use the lenses of stakeholders such as educators, students and managers involved in clinical education and explore their experiences of working across sectors and the issues that arise as a result. We then reflect upon how these issues are being addressed and how they will influence the ongoing provision and conduct of clinical education.

CLINICAL EDUCATION AND ITS ROLE IN EDUCATING HEALTH PROFESSIONALS

Clinical education is largely accepted as integral to the education of beginning health professionals. Although many issues related to the conduct of clinical education are debated, the tradition of students needing to gain practical experience with real clients as an element of their "education" is rarely contested. Clinical education provides students with the opportunity to develop the ability to cope with the complexities of real-world practice (Higgs, 1992; Cooper, Orell, & Bowden,

S. Loftus et al. (Eds.), Educating Health Professionals:
Becoming a University Teacher, 103–112.
© 2013 Sense Publishers. All rights reserved.

2010). It is accepted that beginning practitioners are not capable of providing safe and effective levels of healthcare without some exposure to actual practice. The value placed on clinical education is reflected in the amount of time that students spend undertaking clinical education as a component of their courses. For example, across the range of health professions, students completing 3 and 4 year degrees typically undertake 800-1000 hours of clinical education, depending on the discipline accreditation requirements. This corresponds to approximately 23-25 weeks of placement. It is difficult to generate estimates of the proportion of time devoted to clinical education, as clinical education is increasingly spread throughout the year and is undertaken during both term and break time. It would be reasonable to conclude, however, that there is a ratio of 1:3 clinical to academic teaching.

The role of clinical education can be seen as providing students with the opportunity to apply the theory gained in academic settings to the clinical environment, allowing students to develop the skills and knowledge necessary for professional practice. A deepening theoretical and research-based understanding of learning through experience reveals that clinical education is not just the application of theory to practice but a more complex process of learning about practice through and from contextual experiences (Billett, 2004; Eraut, 2004; Newton, Billett, Jolly, & Ockerby, 2009; Grealish & Smale, 2011).

The emphasis in clinical education has always been on the acquisition of discipline-specific skills and knowledge and achieving professional competence, and it has been increasingly acknowledged that students are socialised into a profession through work experiences (Ajjawi, Loftus, Schmidt, & Mamede, 2009), with students being exposed to existing workplace cultures. Recently, attention has also been paid to the contribution of workplace-based experiences to the development of generic capabilities for work that prepare students to function in real-world contexts (Cooper et al., 2010).

Clinical education has a clear purpose for students in preparing for their future work practice. There is value vested in clinical education for other stakeholders, however, as well as for students and their learning. For example, managers of health services interested in ensuring future workforce needs have a vested interest in promoting clinical education in their facility, with a view to ensuring an ongoing supply of staff to achieve health service objectives. Although it might not be immediately obvious to clients, they also have a vested interest in the quality of healthcare that results from the quality of student learning and practice during clinical education experiences (Prideaux et al., 2000).

RELATIONSHIP BETWEEN THE EDUCATION AND HEALTH SERVICE SECTORS

In the introduction we positioned our discussion of clinical education from the perspective of the sectors involved. In health professional education these sectors are broadly (a) the health service sector, providing healthcare to clients, and (b) the education sector, responsible for the education of professionals capable of providing health services. The two sectors are often implicitly assumed to be synonymous with the public hospital system and universities, but changes to both health service and education sectors have seen a broadening of the scope of clinical education to include, in the case of health services, greater emphasis on primary and Aboriginal healthcare settings, rural and remote locations, non-government organisations and community-based placements. In the case of education, preparation of health professionals is undertaken in vocational training institutes as well as universities. For example, in Australia, education of enrolled nurses and allied health assistants is undertaken in the Technical and Further Education (TAFE) sector.

The sectors currently involved in clinical education also need to be acknowledged as broader than local relationships. Contemporary clinical education involves students undertaking placements in international as well as local settings, and clinical education might therefore be more appropriately regarded as a global enterprise (Kinsella, Bossers, & Ferreira, 2008). Clinical education is further complicated by the engagement of education providers in the provision of healthcare in university-operated clinics established for the purpose of providing a location for clinical placements while concurrently providing health services. The engagement of universities in health service provision has a number of benefits, including the supply of placements for students as well as the opportunity for universities to positively engage with their local communities. Such engagement can include opportunities to undertake clinical research that is relevant and valuable for local communities. There are also a number of inherent challenges in these arrangements, such as the university being able to ensure the continuity and quality of health service provision (Higgs, Pope, Kent, O'Meara, & Allan, 2010).

The provision of clinical education requires the sectors involved to work collaboratively; the relationship between the education provider and the health service providing placements for students is integral to the success of the education process. Although there are examples where individual universities form exclusive relationships with individual health service providers for the provision of placements, in the contemporary context of clinical education it is more common to see complex webs of relationships between several education providers and health services. Grealish and Smale (2011) observed that nursing "clinicians today are confronted by students from different tertiary providers, with different curricula, and different levels of preparation" (p. 52), which can introduce tensions for the health service provider in being able to schedule and manage clinical placements. Likewise, education providers are managing a number of diverse relationships in ensuring access of their students to clinical placements. A key factor that has been driving this complex clinical placement environment, both in Australia and globally, has been the rapid expansion in the number of education providers in the field of health professional education and the consequent increase in the number of students, both being driven by the predicted shortfall in the future health workforce (World Health Organization, 2006; National Health Workforce Taskforce, 2008).

There are fundamental differences between the education and health service sectors that shape but also create barriers for optimal clinical education practice. For example, Newton et al. (2009) have drawn attention to the two sectors as separate and divided communities with different philosophies, cultures and purposes. These authors argue that the education and health service sectors might be considered as "parallel universes" (after Melia, 1984), with the important distinction between them being that education serves to develop practice through academic rigour and underpinned by sound theoretical practice, whereas the health service sector is focused on the unwell and "getting the work done" (Newton et al., 2009, p. 317). Hodkinson (2005) acknowledged the differences between the sectors but argued that the distinctions have been exaggerated and that there are important similarities across the sectors. For example, both sectors are committed to health provision, and students are learning for the same purpose regardless of the sector. The reality, however, is that although clinical education of significant concern to education providers, the education of students is peripheral to the everyday work of the health service.

The notion of communities of practice (Wenger, 2000) may be applied to help develop an understanding of the nature of clinical education and the sectors involved. Lave and Wenger (1991) introduced the concept of communities of practice to refer to "groups of people who share a concern or a passion for something they do and learn how to do it better as they interact regularly" (Wenger, 2006). In the context of clinical education, the shared concern of the education and health service sectors is developing a workforce that is safe and competent for practice. Wenger (2000) proposed that boundaries exist between communities of practice, which "arise from different enterprises; different ways of engaging with one another; different histories, repertoires, ways of communicating, and capabilities" (p. 232), and that these boundaries can create difficulties and opportunities for those trying to work at the boundaries or those who cross them. Rather than portraying the education and health service sectors as separate universes, these ideas raised by Wenger suggest that we should look to the boundaries as opportunities for the sectors to work together more productively. However, there are distinctive differences between the day-to-day functions and nature of the two sectors that need to be unpacked and acknowledged to facilitate the conduct of clinical education, as we describe in subsequent sections.

WORKING ACROSS SECTORS: BROKERING RELATIONSHIPS AND NEGOTIATING PARTNERSHIPS

A number of key stakeholders work across the sectors in the conduct of clinical education. Wenger (2000) used the term "brokers" to apply to those who work across the boundaries that exist between communities of practice and we have drawn upon this notion in our discussion in the previous section. In clinical education the stakeholders, and therefore brokers, are students, teachers, practitioners, professional bodies, and managers of the organisations involved. These stakeholders must engage with their own as well as the other sector or, in the case of students, need to function and perform in both sectors. In the next section we explore the experiences of these stakeholders as brokers and identify the key issues that might be addressed in developing clinical education partnerships.

Students as Brokers

A critical group that must work across sectors is the student group. Students need to contend with the difference between the sectors as they move from learning in the academy to learning in practice environments. It is well documented that students confront differences between what they have been taught in education settings and what they see enacted in the workplace (Newton et al., 2009). Melia (1984) identified that students responded to the paradox they observed in workplaces by "fitting in" and developing ways of practising that met the expectations of the two sectors, raising important questions about how students would reconcile potentially conflicting practices in their future work. Levett-Jones and Lathlean (2009) also noted that students were unwilling to question poor practices and often conformed to dominant work practices as strategies to enhance their sense of belonging and their acceptance by the clinical team. They further suggested that the interpersonal relationships forged between students and the educators with whom they worked on a regular basis exerted a significant influence on students' sense of belonging, their learning and their willingness to confirm or question practice.

In the two sectors, students are faced with differences in the methods by which they are taught and how they learn. Grealish and Smale (2011) observed that students' experiences of teaching and learning in educational institutions tended to be structured, concrete and, at times, relatively passive. In contrast, learning in the workplace requires students to learn through doing, to be more active and opportunistic, using episodes that are not always planned in an environment that does not exist primarily for the purpose of their learning (Hodkinson, 2005; Cooper et al., 2010). Students are required to transfer the knowledge acquired in one setting to the other and to adapt to this new type of learning, often in a very short period of time.

Students also experience a contrast in the way assessment occurs between the two sectors. In education settings, assessment methods are usually single tasks that retrospectively assess knowledge or material learned over an extended period of time. In contrast, clinical assessment in the workplace is usually a process of ongoing evaluation, repeated over a number of learning and assessment cycles (Smith, 2010). Students are exposed to complex discourses of assessment in clinical settings used by members of the profession who believe that they hold a gate-keeping responsibility for their profession and that the onus is to ensure students are suitable for their chosen career (Harman & McDowell, 2011).

Cooper and associates (2010) have argued that it is essential for education providers to prepare students for their clinical education experience in relation to the learning context and to help them develop the skills required in the workplace, such as workplace literacy, motivation, learning to work with others, observing and reflecting upon the work practices of others, and self-awareness, if they are to successfully negotiate both sectors. We would add that the responsibility for student preparation for clinical experiences should involve both sectors working collaboratively to ensure that students transition smoothly into the clinical environment and are able to learn effectively.

Clinical Educators as Brokers

Clinical educators, like students, function at the critical point where the two sectors meet. Many roles of clinical educators have been identified beyond just teaching. They include managing placements, counselling students and assessing students' achievement of competency; educators must juggle these roles in the context of their everyday work as practitioners (McAllister, Higgs, & Smith, 2008). Clinical educators are foremost clinicians, and although education providers undertake activities to prepare educators for their clinical education role, educators consistently report that they feel under-prepared and lacking in confidence, especially as assessors and when working with students who are experiencing difficulties (McAllister, Bithell, & Higgs, 2010). Educators supervising students from different universities need to contend with differing expectations which add to the complexity of being prepared to provide clinical education (Grealish & Smale, 2011). The full explanation for why clinical educators feel under-prepared for their role is likely to be multi-factorial, and indeed it has been observed that there is a lack of understanding about what educators need and want (Health Workforce Australia, 2010).

Working at the intersection between sectors, however, clinical educators can take action to improve the situation for all the stakeholders. Suggested approaches that have emerged from collaboration include common discipline assessment forms, co-ordinated calendars, proposals for the development of core competencies, co-ordinated educator training programs and, most importantly, dialogue about the needs of educators and working towards a shared understanding to optimise the strategies educators are using. Collaboration in the form of conjoint positions, in which staff are employed across both sectors, is another positive contemporary approach. A further development through collaboration can be the shared engagement in research to identify and develop a pedagogy for education in clinical settings. A number of studies have been undertaken to identify the characteristics of effective clinical teaching, with several studies particularly highlighting the importance of the supervisory relationship (Irby, 1994; Kilminster & Jolly, 2000; Yeates, Stewart, & Roger Barton, 2008). There is scope to develop this research further, as clinical education is clearly recognised as needing particular educational approaches.

Managers as Brokers

The final group of stakeholders who work across sectors are those involved in the management of clinical education. In this group we include those responsible for clinical education at an organisation wide-level. Cooper and associates (2010) referred to work-integrated learning (of which clinical education is one form) as the new higher education enterprise; we would add that it is also the new health service enterprise. A key consequence of the growth in demand for clinical placements in the health sector has been the development of interest in clinical education as an education and health service leadership and management concern. Both sectors have responded positively, and clinical education is increasingly viewed as more than just the task of placing students in a clinical setting. The system-wide impact of clinical education is becoming recognised, with initiatives being implemented to address challenges to the sustainable supply of clinical placements.

In Australia this has been revealed in the politicisation of clinical education. In 2008 the Council of Australian Governments (COAG) established Health Workforce Australia (HWA) to address the challenges of providing a skilled, flexible and innovative health workforce to meet the future needs of the Australian Community (HWA, 2010). A key element of this initiative was funding investment in building the capacity for clinical training in the health professions. Among the series of measures employed, there have been initiatives requiring the health service and education sectors to work collaboratively in developing the capacity for clinical training (for example, Clinical Placement Networks established in Victoria). The Australian initiative reflects similar situations internationally, where there are formal connections between health and education in building the health workforce, such as in the United Kingdom (Bithell, Bowles, & Christensen, 2010) and the British Columbia Academic Health Council in Canada, (http://www.bcahc.ca/).

Although the HWA initiative addresses some of the key concerns raised previously in regard to clinical education, such as the provision of funding (McAllister, 2005), related changes to the clinical education context in Australia are influencing the landscape for those involved. The demand for and access to funding for clinical education has commodified clinical education to some extent. An agenda regarding the costs versus benefits of clinical education has always been present, but the current climate has opened a dialogue about the need for payments to pass from universities to health service providers for clinical placements. Although there is evidence that students can contribute positively to service provision and do not always lead to costs for the hosting organisation (Rodger, Stephens, Clark, Ash, & Graves, 2011), the issue of the costs of clinical education remains prevalent and unresolved. The expectation for payments for placements is not solely a response to HWA but also reflects the increased demand and the response by some universities to gain access to placements through monetary guarantees to health services. The effect of this marketing of clinical education is unclear at this stage, but questions need to be asked regarding equity of access to placement experiences for all students who are being educated to join the health workforce, the relationship of payments to quality, and the impact of payments on the traditional relationships and shared responsibility for clinical education. One of the factors that will be debated in the future political agenda of clinical education is the time required in clinical education. As Cross (2011) noted, "the accreditation of health professional curricula must take into account the nexus between competence and time (hours) spent in clinical because funding for clinical placements based on hours will continue to shrink" (p. 57).

A parallel factor impacting on those working across sectors at the enterprise level is a changing view of education: the movement from a view of providing students with a broad education in a profession to a view dominated by reference to vocation and an increasing emphasis on education to meet workforce needs. The positive impact of this development on clinical education is that it fosters positive connections between education providers and health services as the workforce and its preparation becomes a common interest leading to shared dialogue. This is particularly beneficial when both sectors agree on the importance of clinical education leading to the education of students becoming part of the core business of health services. However, it also has the effect of encouraging workplaces to raise expectations of new graduates entering the workforce. This in itself can be positive, particularly with regard to the identification of, and agreement on, shared practice standards. Professional bodies and academics argue that it is also important that research and theoretical considerations are significant in leading future workforce practices, and that education providers have an important voice in establishing what can reasonably be achieved in the preparation of new graduates, rather than merely being responsive to workplace expectations.

CONCLUSION

We have reviewed some of the key issues in clinical education that are revealed by looking at the intersection between the two sectors involved, educational institutions and health services. We have identified that the key stakeholders involved in clinical education, students, educators and managers, need to broker the differences between the sectors in order to successfully achieve effective clinical education. For those working across the sectors these distinct differences between the contexts, mostly related to purpose, give rise to particular challenges for students, educators and staff managing clinical placements. However, as Wenger (2000) has noted, working between sectors also offers great opportunities. Clinical education has always relied on relationships between universities and clinical settings and this will remain unchanged. Future strong collaborations between stakeholders will be needed in the provision of clinical education informed by shared understanding and dialogue.

REFERENCES

Ajjawi, R. L., Loftus, S., Schmidt, H. G., & Mamede, S. (2009). Clinical reasoning: The nuts and bolts of clinical education. In C. Delany & E. Molloy (Eds.), *Clinical education in the health professions* (pp. 107-129). Sydney: Churchill Livingstone Elsevier.

Billett, S. (2004). Workplace participatory practices: Conceptualising workplaces as learning environments. *The Journal of Workplace Learning 16*(6), 312-324.

Bithell, C., Bowles, W., & Christensen, N. (2010). Issues in design and management of fieldwork education. In L. McAllister, M. Paterson, J. Higgs, & C. Bithell (Eds.), *Innovations in allied health fieldwork education* (pp. 61-73). Rotterdam: Sense.

Cooper, L., Orell, J., & Bowden, M. (2010). *Work integrated learning: A guide to effective practice.* London: Routledge.

Cross, W. (2011). Developing the health workforce: What constitutes clinical education? *Contemporary nurse: A journal for the Australian nursing profession,* 56-58. Retrieved from http://ezproxy.csu.edu.au/login?url=http://search.ebscohost.com/login.aspx?direct=true&db=a9h&AN=66 646260&site=ehost-live

Eraut, M. (2004). Informal learning in the workplace. *Studies in Continuing Education, 26*(2), 247-273.

Grealish, L., & Smale, L. A. (2011). Theory before practice: Implicit assumptions about clinical nursing education in Australia as revealed through a shared critical reflection. *Contemporary Nurse: A Journal for the Australian Nursing Profession, 39*(1), 51-64.

Harman, K., & McDowell, L. (2011). Assessment talk in design: The multiple purposes of assessment in HE. *Teaching in Higher Education, 16*(1), 41-52. doi:10.1080/13562517.2010.507309

Health Workforce Australia. (2010). *Clinical supervisor support program – Discussion paper.* Retrieved from http://www.hwa.gov.au/publications/discussion-papers

Higgs, J. (1992). Managing clinical education: The educator-manager and the self-directed learner. *Physiotherapy, 78*(11), 822-828.

Higgs, J., Pope, R., Kent, J., O'Meara, P., & Allan, J. (2010). University clinics. In L. McAllister, M. Paterson, J. Higgs, & C. Bithell (Eds.), *Innovations in allied health fieldwork education: A critical appraisal* (pp. 85-93). Rotterdam: Sense.

Hodkinson, P. (2005). Reconceptualising the relations between college-based and workplace learning. *Journal of Workplace Learning, 17*(8), 521-532.

Irby, D. M. (1994). What clinical teachers in medicine need to know. *Academic Medicine, 69*(5), 333-342.

Kilminster, S., & Jolly, B. C. (2000). Effective supervision in clinical practice settings: A literature review. *Medical Education, 34,* 827-840.

Kinsella, E. A., Bossers, A., & Ferreira, D. (2008). Enablers and challenges to international practice education: A case study. *Learning in Health and Social Care, 7*(2), 79-92.

Lave, J., & Wenger, E. (1991). *Situated learning: Legitimate peripheral participation.* Cambridge: Cambridge University Press.

Levett-Jones, T., & Lathlean, J. (2009). 'Don't rock the boat': Nursing students' experiences of conformity and compliance. *Nurse Education Today, 29*(3), 342-349.

McAllister, L. (2005). Issues and innovations in clinical education. *International Journal of Speech-Language Pathology, 7*(3), 138-148.

McAllister, L., Bithell, C., & Higgs, J. (2010). Innovations in fieldwork education. In L. McAllister, M. Paterson, J. Higgs, & C. Bithell (Eds.), *Innovations in allied health fieldwork education* (pp. 1-13). Rotterdam: Sense.

McAllister, L., Higgs, J., & Smith, D. (2008). Facing and managing dilemmas as a clinical educator. *Higher Education Research & Development, 27*(1), 1-13.

Melia, K. M. (1984). Student nurses' construction of occupational socialisation. *Sociology of Health & Illness, 6*(2), 132-151. doi:10.1111/1467-9566.ep10778231

National Health Workforce Taskforce. (2008). *Health education and training. Clinical placements across Australia: Capturing data and understanding demand and capacity.* Retrieved from http://www.ahwo.gov.au/documents/Education%20and%20Training/Clinical%20placements%20across %20Australia%20-%20Capturing%20data%20and%20understanding%20demand%20and %20capacity.pdf

Newton, J. M., Billett, S., Jolly, B., & Ockerby, C. M. (2009). Lost in translation: Barriers to learning in health professional clinical education. *Learning in Health & Social Care, 8*(4), 315-327. doi:10.1111/j.1473-6861.2009.00229.x

Prideaux, D., Alexander, H., Bower, A., Dacre, J., Haist, S., Jolly, B., et al. (2000). Clinical teaching: Maintaining an educational role for doctors in the new health care environment. *Medical Education, 34*(10), 820-826.

Rodger, S., Stephens, E., Clark, M., Ash, S., & Graves, N. (2011). Occupational therapy students' contribution to occasions of service during practice placements in health settings. *Australian Occupational Therapy Journal, 58*(6), 412-418. doi:10.1111/j.1440-1630.2011.00971.x

Smith, M. (2010). Assessment of clinical learning. In K. Stagnitti, A. Schoo & D. Welch (Eds.), *Clinical and fieldwork placements in the health professions* (pp. 171-185). South Melbourne: Oxford University Press.

Wenger, E. (2000). Communities of practice and social learning systems. *Organization, 7*(2), 225-246.

Wenger, E. (2006). *Communities of practice: A brief introduction.* Retrieved from
http://www.ewenger.com/theory/

World Health Organization. (2006). *The world health report 2006: Working together for health.*

Yeates, P. J. A., Stewart, J., & Roger Barton, J. (2008). What can we expect of clinical teachers? Establishing consensus on applicable skills, attitudes and practices. *Medical Education, 42*(2), 134-142.

Megan Smith PhD
School of Community Health
Charles Sturt University, Australia

Tracy Levett-Jones RN PhD
The School of Nursing and Midwifery
The University of Newcastle, Australia

SECTION 3: TEACHING AND RESEARCH

STEPHEN LOFTUS AND ANTHONY MCKENZIE

11. THINKING ABOUT CURRICULUM

Curriculum has been attracting a lot of attention in recent years. Not too long ago there were complaints that the idea of curriculum was neglected in higher education (e.g. Barnett & Coate, 2005) with more attention being paid to pedagogy and to the activities that foster teaching and learning. This has changed. There is now a substantial and growing literature on various aspects of curriculum. In this chapter we focus on some of the key aspects of curriculum that we believe are important for a new academic teacher, without attempting to be exhaustive. An overarching theme is integration, meaning that an integrated approach is needed to meet the many different demands placed on a curriculum.

A common misconception is to confuse curriculum with syllabus. Syllabus is merely the content of the course whereas curriculum can be defined as the whole educational experience. Curriculum thus includes the syllabus but goes much further. Barnett and Coate (2005) discussed curriculum along three axes: knowing, doing and being. The students who graduate from our courses must know a body of knowledge, although it might be more accurate to say that they must know several bodies of knowledge and, even more importantly, know how these bodies of knowledge are related to each other. Our students must be able to do particular tasks. For example, in most health professions, students must become capable of assessing patients (sometimes called clients) in the way expected of their profession. An occupational therapist's assessment of a disabled person living in her own home will be quite different from the assessment performed by a paramedic of a victim of a car crash on the roadside, although there will be some similarities. In some professions, such as dentistry, a great deal of the curriculum must be devoted to the investment of time and effort required to provide students with the opportunity to master many complex practical tasks to a high degree of technical proficiency, a learning process that needs to mesh with development in other areas of the curriculum. As well, our students need to become and be different people. They must be professional, be ethical, be critical, be reflective, and also be lifelong learners. The curriculum must enable and encourage all this to happen and in a manner that co-ordinates these axes so that the curriculum forms a whole. As mentioned above, a theme that can be seen to run through much of the current interest in curriculum is integration.

One form of integration that is now widely accepted is constructive alignment (Biggs & Tang, 2011). This means that the various parts of the curriculum must support each other in a coherent and cohesive manner. The simplest version of constructive alignment divides the curriculum into three parts, the learning objectives, the learning and teaching activities that fulfil those objectives, and the assessments that allow us to know if the objectives have been fulfilled. A common

S. Loftus et al. (Eds.), Educating Health Professionals:
Becoming a University Teacher, 115–128.

error is to design an assessment that tests only recall of factual knowledge whereas the curriculum might claim to develop critical thinking in students. This is probably because it is relatively easy to design and mark assessments that measure factual recall. Designing and marking assessments that judge critical thinking is much harder; but if this is what we want students to do then this is what needs to be assessed. It is now well known that assessment drives student learning and that many students adopt a very strategic approach to a course. This means that they will concentrate on learning only whatever is needed to pass the assessments. If the assessments require only factual recall then this is what many students will engage in, despite efforts to encourage them to do anything else, such as becoming critical thinkers. It is important, therefore, when designing or reviewing a curriculum, to ensure that the parts of the curriculum are aligned and integrated and do reinforce each other.

Another aspect of integration is the values that underpin a curriculum. Fish and Coles (2005) explained that when designing or reviewing a curriculum it is important to avoid the temptation to rush into analysing the content knowledge. Rather, one should begin with articulating the professional values on which the curriculum is based. The argument is that the curriculum must allow these values to be clearly conveyed to students, with the intention that they will embrace those values in their own professional practice. The values relate to the becoming and being aspect of our students. We want our graduates to embody the values of our profession. If the values we subscribe to include empathy and ethicality then our graduates will need to be empathic and ethical, and must allow these values to underpin and drive their own professional behaviour. Simply knowing that these are the values of the profession is not enough. The curriculum thus needs to include many opportunities for students to see professional role models behaving in an empathic and ethical manner towards patients. Those role models are frequently the academic teachers of the course. It is important, therefore, for academic teachers to have the chance to articulate their own professional values so that these values can explicitly and implicitly inform the curriculum. Such values can then become part of the espoused or formal curriculum, not merely be implied as part of a hidden curriculum.

Much has been written in recent years about the so-called hidden curriculum (e.g. Hafferty & Castellani, 2009). The hidden curriculum includes those aspects of a course that are not explicit but implicit. These aspects can include the behaviour of professional role models and the attitudes they display towards patients. If a professional role model clearly shows antipathy towards patients, there is a chance that these attitudes can be picked up by students, who are often at an impressionable age and striving to form a professional identity of their own. Snyder (1971) claimed that student success was determined, in large part, by the ability of students to "position" themselves between the expectations of the formal curriculum and what was happening in the hidden curriculum. Snyder further suggested that some students, due to ethnicity or sociocultural background, may be ill-equipped to deal with the subtle differences between these different forms of curriculum and may struggle to position themselves appropriately. Even when students can position themselves they may be prone to cynicism because they are forced to live in a space where there are contradictions between the two curricula. For example, students are likely to become cynical if the formal curriculum emphasises the primacy of patient care but the hidden curriculum clearly privileges research activity above all else. It has been claimed, however, that dividing the curriculum in this way between the explicit and the hidden is an oversimplification and that there are other complex issues to be considered (Hafferty & Castellani, 2009).

Recognition of a hidden curriculum seemed to become important in medical education in the last decade of the twentieth century. That, according to Hafferty and Castellani (2009), was due to an emerging crisis of professionalism in which the medical profession, in particular, seemed to be losing its prestige and social status. The hidden curriculum was blamed for this crisis and the concept became a means of focusing attention on the issue. It was sometimes thought that by making the informal curriculum part of the formal curriculum the difficulties could be overcome. What was forgotten was that "there is always a latent to every manifest, an informal to every formal, and/or a backstage to every front stage" (p. 33). In other words, there will always be a hidden curriculum of some sort. Other variations on the theme of hidden curriculum include overt, societal, null, phantom, concomitant, and rhetorical curricula (Wilson & Wilson, 2007). The null curriculum, for example, focuses on what is not taught. If a formal curriculum espouses interprofessional care and education in its learning objectives but these appear nowhere else in the course, this is an example of a null curriculum. Hafferty and Castellani claimed that the traditional approach to curriculum development, which is to develop, deliver, assess and remediate, is too simplistic as it presumes that higher education is nothing more than a product to be delivered. They argued that education needs to be seen as a complex system which is emergent and self-organising, and that the various forms of curriculum mentioned above should be seen as intersecting social practices. Another perspective on this is that the various aspects of a curriculum are dialogical.

In a dialogical view it is accepted that entities interpenetrate each other in complex ways that defy simplistic cause–effect thinking. For example, the teaching of clinical reasoning has traditionally been restricted to highly procedural cause–effect thinking. There is a growing realisation that in a complex activity such as clinical reasoning, we need to explore different ways of knowing and different ways of thinking through problems. The cause–effect thinking of the scientific method can be combined with narrative thinking and narrative knowing from the humanities (Loftus, 2012). Hafferty and Castellani (2009) concluded that to better understand the hidden curriculum there needs to be more focus on institutional issues. These issues include the allocation of resources (what is allocated to research as opposed to teaching, for example), the selection of subjects that are compulsory for study and those that are optional, and how staff are rewarded and promoted (again often for research as opposed to teaching). Such inquiry can reveal the true values that underpin an institution. It is these values, in turn, that shape how a curriculum is designed.

A number of theoretical backgrounds have been advocated as useful lenses to provide a basis for an inquiry into curriculum. Atkinson and Delamont (2009) advocated using Bernstein's (2000) sociology of the curriculum. Bernstein often focused attention on boundaries, beginning with principles of selection and combination. He was concerned with questions such as: how are contents of knowledge identified as such, and how are they related to each other? For example, Bernstein identified the collection type curriculum, which can be contrasted with the integrated curriculum. Traditional medical schools have a curriculum that is characterised by the collection model. There is a collection of distinctive subjects with strong boundaries around them, with an emphasis on the separation between subjects. The preclinical subjects, as a group, are also sharply demarcated from the clinical subjects. Within each group the subjects are sharply demarcated from each other. Anatomy is distinct from physiology which is distinct from biochemistry. These preclinical subjects must also precede the clinical subjects. Atkinson and Delamont pointed out that the structure of a curriculum can impose a particular epistemological world view. The way knowledge is organised in a curriculum implies that this is the way the world itself is organised and that, therefore, knowledge of the world should be acquired in distinctive ways that match the structure of the curriculum. In this way, curriculum structure can "naturalise" particular ways of organising knowledge and professional practice so that they become normative. The traditional curriculum requires that the basic medical sciences must be mastered before a student can begin to see patients, and the implication is that this is the way things must be. With strong demarcation there is also strong framing. In Bernstein's terms, framing refers to the management of the pedagogical encounter, the order in which knowledge is presented and how it is presented. One outcome of this strong framing and a strongly demarcated curriculum is that the roles of teacher and student tend to become circumscribed and fixed within a clear and definite hierarchy. In contrast, the integrated model has more porous boundaries between subjects.

In an integrated model there is an underlying principle of synthesis. Instead of individual subjects dominating a curriculum there tend to be themes that draw on all subjects. The scientific method can be a theme used to organise the study of the cardiovascular system, for example. There will be input from all the basic medical sciences, as well as from clinicians and others such as ethicists. Problem-based learning is a well-known example of an integrated approach to curriculum. Students can be required to study a series of cases with a range of cardiovascular problems. The aim is to provide students with an overview of all relevant subjects that they can then apply to each case. In doing so, students are encouraged to see the links between different subjects and to understand how subject knowledge is applied to real-world cases. However, a word of warning is necessary. Sometimes the word "integrated" is used simply because it seems fashionable. We need to be careful that something described as integrated really is.

With the shift to more integrated curricula there are also other shifts. There is a move towards weak framing, with many ways of implementing pedagogy. Problem-based learning tutorials are dovetailed with traditional lectures and demonstrations. Students are encouraged to come together within informal learning groups, to support each other rather than compete as individuals in the traditional model. There are also changes in the expectations and roles of students and teachers. The old "expert–novice" relationship can give way to a more collegial joint pursuit of knowledge and capability. Ignorance is not necessarily seen as a reason for shame and humiliation but is understood as an opportunity to learn. One intention of the integrated approach is to bring about a shift towards more self-directed learning, so that students also become more critical consumers of knowledge and are willing and able to become lifelong learners. Atkinson and Delamont (2009) claimed that Bernstein's insights allow for specific predictions to be made. For example, in an integrated approach the identities and personal qualities of students become an explicit part of the educational project, whereas in a traditional collection curriculum these features are implied and presupposed and part of the hidden curriculum.

The work of other well-known scholars has also been used to shed light on the curriculum for health professionals. Brosnan (2009) argued that the work of Pierre Bourdieu (1988) can deepen our understanding of health professional education. Bourdieu explored the deep divisions that can exist between basic medical scientists, who are preoccupied with research in their fields, and clinicians who must balance research with patient care and teaching. Using these ideas, much of the curricular reform that has occurred in recent decades can be seen in a different light. Bloom (1988) claimed that there was often "reform without change" (p. 294), meaning that curriculum reform was being undertaken for a range of reasons that had little to do with improving education. Bloom claimed that the overwhelming focus on research activity prevented any meaningful curriculum reform. According to Vinten-Johansen and Riska (1991), the introduction of the social sciences into the curriculum in US medical schools was often a cosmetic exercise in response to threats of government intervention. Brosnan (2009) pointed out that in the UK, the newer medical schools have usually been the quickest to adopt a new and integrated curriculum and this may have been done as a means of symbolically differentiating themselves from the more established medical schools. Thus reform is undertaken for reasons organisational rather than educational. Brosnan also pointed out that curriculum reform is subverted when the underlying value system remains in place. One of the dominant values in Western medical schools has been and, in many cases, continues to be competent technical performance founded on a biomedical scientific basis. The less dominant value of providing care to human beings may be acknowledged but often plays a secondary role.

An attempt to bring about genuine curriculum reform that is currently exciting much interest is the application of threshold concepts. Threshold concepts are ideas that are held to be central to mastering a discipline (Cousin, 2006). There have been complaints for decades that the traditional collection curriculum, described above, is overstuffed with content. The newer integrated courses tend to have a core curriculum. Beyond learning this core, students are expected to direct their own learning. Threshold concepts are a means of conceptualising what must go into such a core. Proponents of the idea claim that threshold concepts have certain key features in common.

Threshold concepts are said to be transformative. Once grasped, they change people, and they change people forever. There is as much an ontological change as there is an epistemological change. For example, when learning to cope with complex, ill-structured conditions, such as chronic pain, it can come as a major revelation to some students to find that definitive cure is not always possible (Loftus, 2011). The simplistic cause–effect mechanistic thinking characteristic of many students when they begin turns out to be inadequate. They discover that managing rather than curing the complexity may be the only viable option. They may also come to appreciate that such complex management is often best done in a multidisciplinary partnership with other health professionals. Once this has been grasped, patients with complex, ill-structured problems are never seen simplistically again. This highlights another feature of threshold concepts: they are irreversible once learned. This can be a problem for teachers who can, in a sense, forget that they know such concepts. In such cases, the concept has become so embodied and so much a part of the experienced practitioner that there is little conscious awareness of it, even though it is used in practice every day. Such embodied and unconscious awareness is often referred to as intuition. Another characteristic of threshold concepts is said to be that they are integrative and expose relationships with other concepts that might not have been so obvious before. Related to this is another characteristic: threshold concepts are bounded, in that they are clearly demarcated. Cousin (2006) warned that some threshold concepts can be regarded as the exclusive property of a specific discipline, with the danger that they might be accepted uncritically. The implication is that curriculum design should always include the requirement for any concept to be questioned and challenged. Cousin advised that it is always best, therefore, to regard threshold concepts as provisional. Finally, threshold concepts tend to involve "troublesome knowledge". There may be a commonsense or procedural understanding of a concept that can interfere with the ability of students to grasp the concept in the deeper way that their teachers may expect. Many students may need to experience a liminal state before arriving at a fuller understanding of threshold concepts.

Meyer and Land (2005), the original proponents of threshold concepts, introduced the idea of liminal states. A liminal state is a transition phase in which students must spend time and effort grappling with their emerging understanding of a threshold concept. A liminal state can be an uncomfortable place to be and, rather than investing the time and effort to develop this understanding, there is a temptation for some students to substitute mimicry for mastery and only give the appearance of having mastered the concept. As Cousin (2006, p. 5) remarked, what can happen then is that "learning is the product of ritualised performances rather than integrated understandings". Threshold concepts have implications for curriculum design (Land, Cousin, Meyer, & Davies, 2005). These include the notion of "jewels in the curriculum" (p. 57). Threshold concepts often mark key transformative points in a curriculum; points at which students are more likely to struggle and teachers therefore need to pay more than usual attention to helping them achieve mastery. Another connected implication is "listening for understanding". Teachers must pay careful attention to students' misunderstandings and uncertainties and must be able to engage with students at the appropriate level. This can be difficult for teachers who may have difficulty remembering their own struggles to master threshold concepts and who may have had to deal with different misconceptions.

120

To this point we have surveyed some of the ideas and concerns to be found in the higher education literature relating to the teaching curriculum. We now widen our field of view to take account of our readers' experience of a university teaching role, whatever your particular institutional practices and underlying culture and practice philosophy (or pragmatic) might be. First, however, we clarify what we mean by these terms. Institutional practices are the things done to implement the teaching curriculum. Institutional culture here refers to the way these practices are more or less tacitly understood, valued and adopted by the staff community. Practice philosophy refers to the values, principles and theories underpinning curriculum practice. Practice pragmatic is a less complimentary term, referring to practices that have evolved in response to a need to just get things done, on time and on budget, rather than as an expression of a philosophy of practice. Practice philosophy and practice pragmatic can be thought of as two ends of a spectrum – what we would like to do at one end and what we have to do at the other, with many positions in between. In the health professions, common constraints on curriculum design are the requirements of accreditation bodies. One of our goals in this chapter is to encourage you to reflect on your curriculum and hopefully move your teaching practice toward the noble end of the spectrum.

CURRICULUM: AN IDEA FOR INTEGRATING TEACHING PRACTICE

As we have already seen, the term *curriculum* can conjure up a range of meanings for people. We now invite you to join us on a more self-reflective interrogation of the idea of curriculum. In the remainder of this chapter we consider these questions:

- How can I make use of the idea of curriculum in my approach to my teaching?
- Given the current state of affairs within the course I teach, is "curriculum" as an idea and a practice going to make me a better practitioner or enable me to contribute more to my course team?
- Will my students benefit?

In this section we draw on research being undertaken by the second author (AM). Education for the world of work is future-looking and goal-oriented, and this is expressed in different kinds of statements about what a course will deliver. We need to be alert to the differences and to use our words carefully. We need to distinguish between:

- The institutionally endorsed aspirational statements about curriculum in general
- The more specific formal objectives or learning outcome statements
- The actual capability of each graduating student.

An example of the first statement from an agricultural science course (but typical of many courses) is: "Provide industry-ready graduates possessing the confidence to thrive in professional practice" (CSU, 2010a, p. 5). An example of the second, from a course on midwifery, is: "To provide a supportive learning environment in which students can fully develop their potential to become midwives with a woman-centred focus; ... To utilise clinical opportunities that enhance the process of developing into practising midwives who have an empathic, holistic, and culturally sensitive approach to their work" (CSU, 2010b, p. 9). The most elusive kind of statement, however, is the final one, the actual capability/achievement of each graduating student, recognised in the award of a university degree. The difference is the space between intention and achievement.

Consider the award that will be granted to your students, if successful. If your course team was invited to describe how that award would be lived out in reality, demonstrated, validated by its recipients, what words would do? The language we use will reflect our practice philosophy, which will be informed more or less by our theory of curriculum. This is related to our underlying professional and personal values and how we integrate all these different levels of thinking about curriculum. In 1975, American educational theorist James B. Macdonald wrote on the nature and purpose of curriculum theorising. He closed his essay thus:

> It is a difficult task to formalize [the] diverse and wide ranging field [of curriculum theory]. Yet it is an exciting venture for persons whose dispositions lead them in this direction. There is an article of faith involved which is analogous to Dewey's comment that educational philosophy was the essence of all philosophy because it was "the study of how to have a world". Curriculum theory in this light might be said to be the essence of educational theory because it is the study of how to have a learning environment. (Macdonald, 1975, p. 12)

Macdonald here juxtaposed two ideas: *how to have a world* and *how to have a learning environment*. There is an underlying holism here that does not receive enough attention in studies of curriculum. If curriculum is a learning environment, it is the world or "space" in which educational transformations are enabled. Problem-based learning, referred to earlier, is just one such available model that can fill this space. This space is open for your course team to develop but it is constrained by the team's collective imagination and by the kinds of curriculum theory or models that they bring to bear on the curriculum design. Macdonald's concern about "how" to have a learning environment is potent because it asks that practitioners acknowledge the wider cultural, political, economic and administrative realities operating in a given situation – your institution, for example – and how they predispose the curriculum to take a particular form, the overall learning journey of students. There is still inadequate concern for the integrity and wholeness of this learning journey. A scan of contemporary literature on higher education reveals a notable emphasis on a still common modular approach – curriculum as building blocks, without glue, in a sense – and with little concern for the integrity and wholeness of the overall learning journey. The latter, holistic approach is what interests us here. This is reflected in the recent and growing interest in the way students experience their university studies within the larger, more holistic idea of "life at university" (see e.g. McInnis, James, Hartley, & University of Melbourne Centre for the Study of Higher Education, 2000; Pitkethly & Prosser, 2001). And yet a large question remains. What kind of theoretical perspective will be adequate to inform the design of an integrated, course-long, life-wide learning experience? The term "life-wide" is an attempt to draw attention to the importance of a holistic approach that embraces the whole person. Just how holistic and integrated do we want our students' experience to be?

The driving belief behind the second author's research project is that curriculum practice, the implementation of a learning environment design, will achieve more robust outcomes the more closely it mirrors or accommodates the way humans work, cognitively, socially, physically, emotionally, spiritually – "the big five". Let us spend a moment considering this idea. Its value, we believe, lies in its deliberate attempt to place concern for a holistic student learning outcome at the centre of the teacher's view of the curriculum challenge. This position has elegance and power as a design principle in a number of ways. First, in the context of education for the world of work, it seeks coherence between a *conception of curriculum* and a *conception of the goal of education for practice*.

Coherence is seen in a curriculum that aims to provide a holistic learning experience (spanning and integrating the big five) in order to graduate *novice rounded, grounded practitioners*. That is, the new graduates may still be novices in their professions but they are educationally well-rounded and yet firmly grounded in the real world of practice. In other words they have been educated holistically in order to practise holistically. Thanks to their professional formation (i.e. course) experience they are more likely to bring a holistic *thinking–doing–being habit* to their relations with their clients/patients. Another coherence is between a *conception of curriculum* and *the nature of human understanding*, which underpins all our knowing, doing, and being in the world. According to Bortoft (1996), scientific explanation is analytical, whereas understanding is holistic. Understanding is holistic because one understands as one grasps the interconnectedness, the relationships between phenomena and between ideas. The practice of a health profession in today's world needs such an ability in order to understand the complexities of the problems our patients bring to us, which can often defy simple scientific explanations.

Another sense of coherence in the curriculum is that teachers can explore the possibility of allowing their own experience of holistic meaning-making to guide their imagining of, and interventions in, their students' meaning-making as the students begin to grapple with complexity. As noted above, teachers may need considerable imagination to understand how students struggle with threshold concepts and how these students can become personally transformed by those same threshold concepts. We might think of curriculum, then, as one big *"what if?"* – as a talking point for the course team as it considers how to design an extended learning experience that brings the transformative potential of holistic meaning-making into one's way of living, as student, as person and as practitioner. If we want that kind of curriculum, how do we proceed? We will offer two responses. The first could be called a blueprint for transformative, collaborative curriculum practice which we call a curriculum of becoming. The second provides an important countervailing consideration.

The term *curriculum of becoming* was coined in the process of the second author's research into the question, how might Australian universities enact a "fit-for-greater-purpose" education? Greater purpose here picks up the points mentioned above concerning an education that is richer in a more complex, rounded, open-ended way than one designed to achieve simplistic, quantified, measurable outcomes. The *triple hologenesis model of curriculum renewal* (Figure 11.1) provides a concise bird's-eye view of this curriculum of becoming. The model emphasises three dimensions of higher education practice.

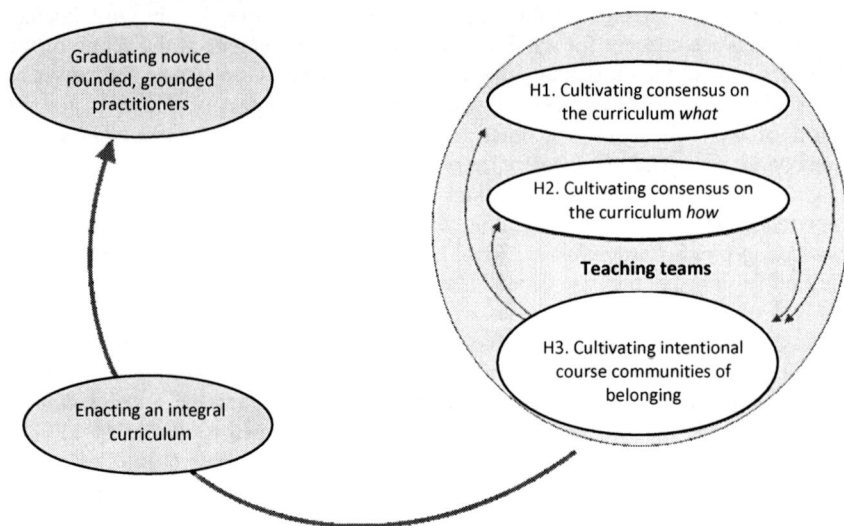

Figure 11.1. The triple hologenesis model of curriculum renewal
Source: McKenzie, Higgs, & Simpson (2012), p. 13 ©Common Ground Publishing.
Figure reproduced with the kind permission of Common Ground Publishing. Publisher permission required to re-publish; email support-roundup@commonground.com.au

According to the model, in a *curriculum of becoming*, curriculum transformation comprises three mutually dependent goals. Each goal can be seen as a "hologenesis"; that is, each goal has a particular emphasis but reflects the whole curriculum in its attempt to foster a rounded, grounded practitioner. First, going beyond what professional accrediting bodies might demand, the teaching team works to reach consensus on the curriculum *WHAT* (H1) – What constitutes a novice *rounded, grounded practitioner* for the target field of practice? One of the questions to be considered here concerns the values the course team wishes the students to accept as their own.

The second hologenesis concerns the course team's process of reaching consensus on the curriculum *HOW* (H2) – How to orchestrate the students' learning journeys to pursue their course-long metamorphosis into novice practitioners? One major problem confronting course teams today is the rapidly changing world of educational technology. This means that the pedagogy of the curriculum needs to be in a state of continuous improvement or else it becomes rapidly dated. As course teams continuously, and in good faith, problematise the curriculum *WHAT* and *HOW* together, they will take on the character of *a community of belonging* (H3) – the third hologenesis in the model – in which members need to bond as a community and develop a strong, shared commitment to the work as well as the welfare of the course team. In return, the course team has a strong commitment to each member and his or her capacity to contribute fully to its goals and activities. Course teams also can and perhaps should include students. Students too can be encouraged to start understanding and taking responsibility for the curriculum. It is out of this reciprocal relationship that the community can pursue its goals effectively, elegantly, responsibly.

Figure 11.1 invites us to see a course community, teachers and students together, continuously problematising the rounded, grounded practitioner ideal in the flux of practice within the profession concerned, against a fluid backdrop of 21st century complexity, whether it be economic, geo-political, ecological, cultural or existential/spiritual. "Enacting a university curriculum of becoming is a values-driven, hope-driven endeavour" (McKenzie, Higgs, & Simpson, 2012, p. 15). Underpinning all this are four critical dimensions of performance in any field of practice, which become essential dimensions of professional preparation. They are:

– *understanding and know-how*;
– *uncertainty dexterity* – the capacity to thrive in uncertainty;
– *social presence*;
– *sense of self* as the anchor for moral judgement and personal agency.

These dimensions need to be carefully interwoven throughout the course if students are going to graduate as novice, rounded, grounded practitioners.

This curriculum of becoming framework emphasises holistic learning experiences and outcomes. Concern for curriculum here implies concern for *the whole learning journey*, in the belief that the fragmented learning activities offered across a course are all elements of a larger "something", a learning experience that has some kind of emergent integrity, reaching towards the state of being whole. In this way of thinking the goal of the course team in designing and executing the curriculum is to provide a holistic learning experience in order to graduate students who are in the process of realising their potential, people working, to use Ron Barnett's phrase, "to become themselves in new ways" (2011, p. 14) – a holistic process/means to achieve a holistic outcome/end.

We hasten to add that the position we are developing here is not yet common practice, not yet even common theorising; but we see it as central to the teaching challenge. We now return to the elusive category we noted above: the *actual capability/ achievement of each graduating student, recognised in the award of a university degree*. Because we are arguing for a holistic conception of curriculum we need to consider more carefully *how* a curriculum might provide a holistic learning experience in order to graduate novice, rounded, grounded practitioners who are committed and able to *practise holistically* by bringing a holistic *thinking–doing– being habit* to their relations with their clients.

We invite you to imagine a graduate who has been working in her chosen field for some years. To make this exercise meaningful for you, it is the same field your own students will one day work in. Now, think of two dramatically different curricula purporting to prepare students for that field of practice. One of them follows the traditional modular approach – curriculum as building blocks without glue. The other endeavours to engage with the holistic conception of curriculum being presented here, which we call a "curriculum of becoming" framework because the term envelops the whole, emergent practitioner-person. Further let's suppose that your imaginary student would like to be just like the midwifery graduate mentioned earlier, who has "an empathic, holistic, and culturally sensitive approach to [her] work". In our view, a curriculum of becoming, which deliberately and carefully aims to cultivate novice rounded, grounded practitioners throughout the course learning journey, is far more likely to enable your imaginary practitioner to understand and realise her need for self-actualisation many years into her practice than a curriculum of building block construction would. This judgement has not been tested; indeed, the curriculum of becoming stands as an ideal to challenge us all to imagine new ways of teaching and learning. The point of this thought experiment is to raise awareness of the idea of a holistic practitioner and the idea that curriculum might have a role to play in nurturing such a quality of practice. We want to encourage new teachers in the health professions to seriously consider these ideas, as we believe they can deepen the conversation about curriculum.

The curriculum of becoming framework, as briefly introduced here, has potential to help course teams to reflect on their collective aspirations for their students and on their capacity to collaborate for their students' benefit. There is, however, a reservation we must declare (our countervailing consideration mentioned above). It arises from the nexus between a *conception of curriculum* and *the nature of human understanding*. The point is simply that, despite our best intentions, it is not possible to design every aspect of a curriculum and be confident that students will learn precisely what we want them to learn and in the way we want them to learn it. Education involves human transformation and this transformation is somewhat unpredictable because it requires students to interpret what we want them to learn.

The study of curriculum continues to develop. A number of disciplines can be used to inform such study and development. Barnett (personal communication), who has done much to reinvigorate the conversation about curriculum in recent years, states that he has drawn inspiration from the work of Martin Heidegger (1996). The authors of this chapter draw particular inspiration from work based on Heidegger's pupil and successor, Hans Georg Gadamer (1989). For example, Davey (2006) developed Gadamer's idea of *bildung* briefly defined as "cultural and educative formation" (p. 2). One of Davey's insights (p. 50) is that in education:

What is of importance is neither that which is transmitted per se nor that which is received but the transformative space which the processes of transmission and reception enable.

This is because we need to visualise the curriculum content "not as a body of set received works but as a cluster of issues, questions, and practices that over time have come to define a certain cultural practice" (p. 50).

A health profession is such a complex cultural practice. The education we provide needs to articulate and demonstrate how new practitioners are expected to engage with this practice so that they can continue it and, most importantly, develop it further. A carefully designed curriculum is central to providing the transformative spaces where this can occur.

CONCLUSION

In this chapter we have argued that curriculum is of central importance in the education of health professionals. It is a complex phenomenon, however, that can be studied and understood in a great variety of ways, some complementary and some opposed. We argue that a holistic and integrated approach to understanding curriculum is needed. The renewed interest in curriculum matters is encouraging, even though it can be daunting to new academics. Yet the field of curriculum has been exciting much scholarship and research in recent years and we encourage new academics to embrace the complexity and immerse themselves in the fascinations of curriculum.

REFERENCES

Atkinson, P., & Delamont, S. (2009). From classification to integration: Bernstein and the sociology of medical education. In C. Brosnan & B. S. Turner (Eds.), *Handbook of the sociology of medical education* (pp. 36-50). Abingdon: Routledge.

Barnett, R. (2011). *Being a university.* London: Routledge.

Barnett, R., & Coate, K. (2005). *Engaging the curriculum in higher education.* Maidenhead: Open University Press.

Bernstein, B. (2000). *Pedagogy, symbolic control and identity: Theory, research, critique.* London: Rowman and Littlefield.

Biggs, J., & Tang, C. (2011). *Teaching for quality learning at university: What the student does* (4th ed.). Maidenhead, UK: Open University Press.

Bloom, S. (1988). Structure and ideology in medical education: An analysis of resistance to change. *Journal of Health and Social Behavior, 29,* 294-306.

Bortoft, H. (1996). *The wholeness of nature: Goethe's way towards a science of conscious participation in nature.* Hudson, NY: Lindisfarne Press.

Bourdieu, P. (1988). *Homo academicus.* Cambridge: Polity Press.

Brosnan, C. (2009). Pierre Bourdieu and the theory of medical education: Thinking 'relationally' about medical students and medical curricula. In C. Brosnan & B. S. Turner (Eds.), *Handbook of the sociology of medical education* (pp. 52-68). Abingdon: Routledge.

Charles Sturt University. (2010a). *Bachelor of Agricultural Science: Course modification.* CSU Intranet.

Charles Sturt University. (2010b). *Postgraduate diploma in midwifery: Course review.* CSU Intranet.

Cousin, G. (2006). An introduction to threshold concepts. *Planet, 17,* 4-5.

Davey, N. (2006). *Unquiet understanding: Gadamer's philosophical hermeneutics.* Albany, NY: State University of New York Press.

Fish, D., & Coles, C. (2005). Medical education: Developing a curriculum for practice. Maidenhead: Open University Press.

Gadamer, H.-G. (1989). *Truth and method* (J. Weinsheimer & D. G. Marshall, Trans., 2nd revised ed.). New York: Continuum.

Hafferty, F. W., & Castellani, B. (2009). The hidden curriculum: A theory of medical education. In C. Brosnan & B. S. Turner (Eds.), *Handbook of the sociology of medical education* (pp. 15-35). Abingdon: Routledge.

Heidegger, M. (1996). *Being and time: A translation of Sein und Zeit* (J. Stambaugh, Trans.). Albany, NY: State University of New York Press. (Original work published in 1927).

Land, R., Cousin, G., Meyer, J. H. F., & Davies, P. (2005). Threshold concepts and troublesome knowledge (3): Implications for course design and evaluation. In C. Rust (Ed.), *Improving student learning – equality and diversity* (pp. 53-64). Oxford: OCSLD.

Loftus, S. (2011). Pain and its metaphors: A dialogical approach. *Journal of Medical Humanities, 32*(3), 213-230.

Loftus, S. (2012). Rethinking clinical reasoning: Time for a dialogical turn. *Medical Education 46*, 1174-1178.

Macdonald, J. B. (1975). Curriculum theory. In W. Pinar (Ed.), *Curriculum theorizing: The reconceptualists* (pp. 5-13). Berkeley, CA: McCutchan.

McInnis, C., James, R., Hartley, R., & University of Melbourne Centre for the Study of Higher Education. (2000). *Trends in the first year experience in Australian universities.* Canberra: Department of Education, Training and Youth Affairs.

McKenzie, A. D., Higgs, J., & Simpson, M. (2012). Being a university in the twenty-first century: Re-thinking curriculum. *Journal of the World Universities Forum, 4*(4), 1-18.

Meyer, J. H. F., & Land, R. (2005). Threshold concepts and troublesome knowledge (2): Epistemological considerations and a conceptual framework for teaching and learning. *Higher Education 49*, 373-388. doi:10.1007/s10734-004-6779-5

Pitkethly, A., & Prosser, M. (2001). The first year experience project: A model for university-wide change. *Higher Education Research & Development, 20*(2), 185-198. doi:10.1080/758483470

Snyder, B. R. (1971). *The hidden curriculum.* New York: Alfred A. Knopf.

Vinten-Johansen, P., & Riska, E. (1991). New Oslerians and real Flexnerians: The response to threatened professional autonomy. *International Journal of Health Services, 21*, 75-108.

Wilson, L., & Wilson, O. (2007). Leslie Owen Wilson's curriculum pages. Retrieved from http://www4.uwsp.edu/Education/lwilson/curric/curtyp.htm#covert0

Stephen Loftus PhD
The Education For Practice Institute
Charles Sturt University, Australia

Anthony McKenzie BA, DipEd, MSc(Hons)
The Education For Practice Institute
Charles Sturt University, Australia

JOY HIGGS AND EDWINA ADAMS

12. STANDARDS IN HEALTH PROFESSIONAL EDUCATION

Contextualising Standards Design and Implementation

Academic standards are not new to higher education. Universities seek to provide quality education. Today, we face increasing internal as well as external scrutiny in higher education, while at the same time the health sector, which is engaged in workplace learning aspects of health professional education, is also encountering ever-increasing demands for quality. This context provides the background for this exploration of standards in health professional education.

THE NATURE AND RATIONALE FOR ACADEMIC STANDARDS

Defining Academic Standards

Academic standards are expectations of levels of performance; they are benchmarks of quality and excellence in education. They imply that the means to achieve this performance will be in place, as well as the outcomes to be attained. Standards may relate to the performance of students and to the performance of educational institutions. For example, the UK Quality Assurance Agency for Higher Education provides the following definitions:

> Academic standards are "the standards set and maintained by institutions for their courses (programs and modules) and expected for their awards". (http://www.qaa.ac.uk/aboutus/glossary/pages/glossary-a.aspx#a3)

> "Threshold academic standards are the minimum acceptable level of achievement that a student has to demonstrate to be eligible for an academic award.[i] The Quality Code sets out expectations which higher education providers are required to meet to ensure that academic standards are set and maintained". (http://www.qaa.ac.uk/AssuringStandardsAndQuality/quality-code/ Pages/UK-Quality-Code-Part-A.aspx)

> A subject benchmark statement is a "published statement that sets out what knowledge, understanding, abilities and skills are expected of those graduating in each of the main subject areas (mostly applying to bachelor's degrees), and explains what gives that particular discipline its coherence and identity. The statements are consistent with the relevant generic qualification descriptors". (http://www.qaa.ac.uk/aboutus/glossary/pages/glossary-s.aspx #s7)

S. Loftus et al. (Eds.), Educating Health Professionals:
Becoming a University Teacher, 129–144.
© 2013 Sense Publishers. All rights reserved.

Quality Agendas and Standards

Standards occur as part of the quality imperative for higher education. It is a responsibility of universities to achieve high quality in the resourcing, provision and outcomes of higher education and to promote high-quality learning experiences for students. Other stakeholders, including university staff, employers, professional bodies and the community, also have a vested interest in high-quality experiences, engagement and outcomes of university education. Quality, then, refers to the attainment of *high quality*, meaning superiority with reference to the standards in the given field, as opposed to *the quality*, level or degree of excellence of something. Inherently, high quality contains dimensions of contextual relevance, fitness for purpose, and suitability. High-quality children's education would contain different parameters from those in university education, for instance. Quality is also referential and subjective, particularly when it relates to experience and perceptions. What may be perceived as high quality for one group or individual might not be so for others.

Quality is thus a response to influence and expectations. Evaluation of quality is therefore a complex and not easily evaluated endeavour. Quality cannot be assessed via a single dimension. From his extensive evaluation of quality assurance in Australia, Coates (2010) proposed a multi-dimensional framework as the most useful means for evaluating academic quality, because of the complexity of influences on the quality of learning. Factors such as student entry capabilities, teachers' experience and the institutional climate all impact on the quality of learning and teaching. Similarly, Ehlers (2009) identified a number of factors that influence interactions between teachers and learners, such as the skill of teachers, the abilities of students, the organisational context, values and structures.

The indicators of quality in a multi-dimensional framework must be valid, relevant to standards, non-trivial, assessable, and relevant to the university school/discipline, industry, professions and the broader community. In assessing attainments against the multiple indicators within such a framework, measures must be used that provide evidence of what is being achieved. The data provided as evidence should be based "on fact, on subjective feedback, or on objective assessment" (Coates, 2010, p. 8). A key factor in evaluating quality is recognising the importance of not just measuring outcomes, performance or infrastructure but also using such measures to enhance quality. Given the scope of the factors impacting on quality, a multi-dimensional approach is needed to effect positive change.

Within educational institutions the review and assurance of the quality of education is an ongoing endeavour, driven by internal accreditation processes, government-led quality review agendas, external accreditation requirements linked to professions, government targets and incentives. Consider, for example, the following statements by quality agencies in which they describe their agendas:

(The) Quality Assurance Agency for Higher Education: Our job is to uphold quality and standards in UK universities and colleges. We guide and check the quality of teaching, learning and assessment in UK higher education, because we want every student to have the best possible learning experience. (http://www.qaa.ac.uk/)

The Tertiary Education Quality and Standards Agency (TEQSA) is Australia's regulatory and quality agency for higher education. TEQSA's primary aim is to ensure that students receive a high-quality education at any Australian higher education provider.
(http://www.teqsa.gov.au/)

(In Australia) Mission-based Compacts are three-year agreements that show how each university's mission contributes to the Government's goals for higher education, and include details of major higher education and research funding and performance targets.
(http://www.deewr.gov.au/ HigherEducation/Policy/Pages/Compacts.aspx)

Academic Standards

Standards or expectations are framed by those who have an interest in higher education: students, families of students, educational institutions, professional bodies, regulatory authorities, quality assurance agencies, society and governments. All of these people and agencies have their unique perspectives on what interests should be served by higher education and what such education should realise. What value should be added through university education – to the individual student and to society? How should the student and society benefit from the costs (time, private moneys, public funds, resources and infrastructure) of higher education? In addressing these questions we see that standards are clearly a matter of accountability; they form part of the university's implicit and explicit contracts with stakeholders. When they articulate standards, universities are identifying what performance, resourcing and outcomes they are agreeing to provide.

Pursuing Quality Assurance and Standards

The time demands of external quality assurance and accreditation processes can be considerable and can compete with other university work requirements, especially if seen as simply an obligation. Quality assurance can be counterproductive if the processes are driven by checklists and targets that focus more on compliance than quality promotion and attainment. Staff involved in accreditation and quality assurance can become frustrated if different drivers/groups have competing targets, record-keeping demands and reporting strategies or forms. Moreover, there is the danger that standards (both minimal or "threshold" standards or aspirational "gold" standards) can be collapsed together and growth or improvement can be neglected in the problematic pursuit of standardisation or the achievement of (mere) "adequacy". There also needs to be room for viewing the pursuit of quality in the context of the stage of development, purpose and uniqueness of the course and institution in question.

Optimally, we argue, quality assurance should adopt the dual form and purpose of accountability and particularised development via enabling processes that foster curriculum frameworks for good education, risk management, benchmarking and continuous quality improvement. Standards can be pursued in quality–action cycles involving such phases as planning, implementing, reviewing and improving.

In health professional education, an important consideration is that academic standards cannot be limited to university-managed strategies. When we consider various approaches to professional education, including problem-based learning, practice-based education and work-integrated learning, each approach emphasises the key role of the world of practice and practitioners in the education of future health professionals. For this reason we need to consider the role of practitioners as role models of practice, and it is valuable to remember that academics are also seen as role models of professionalism and academic standards. The standards agenda needs to consider practice standards as well as educational standards, and practitioner educators need to be part of the pursuit of educational standards.

THE CONTEXT OF ACADEMIC STANDARDS

Standards in Higher Education – International Perspectives

Over the past two decades, increasing external quality assurance demands have been imposed on higher education worldwide (Westerheijden, Hulpiau, & Waeytens, 2007; Ewell, 2010). With external quality assurance, evaluation of the higher education institution's performance and outcomes is set and measured by an agency (e.g. a professional regulatory authority) outside the institution, whereas internal quality assurance processes are driven within the institution itself.

In general, the aims of quality assurance processes are to enhance learning (processes and outcomes) in higher education and to set benchmarks for the achievement of qualifications. For instance, recent trends in European higher education have been implemented to encourage the development of quality mechanisms and to promote quality cultures in European universities (Gvaramadze, 2008). In the U.S., Ewell (2010) has noted that the focus of quality assurance has changed from 20 years ago when it was largely on resources and process: now it requires institutions to provide evidence of learning outcomes and an examination of the levels of performance achieved by students.

External quality assurance processes are designed to stimulate change and bring improvement in courses, but there is a body of literature that questions the ability of the quality assurance process to achieve this aim. External monitoring has been identified as having less impact on quality than the internal self-evaluation process that takes place prior to the external audit (Berlin Communiqué, 2003; Stensaker, Langfeldt, Harvey, Huismann, & Westerheijden, 2010). The *Trends* series reports on the effectiveness and impact of the Bologna Process[ii] which has identified the need for a move away from "governmental actions" to that of internal quality assurance processes (Birtwistle, 2009, p. 58). The *Tuning Project*, developed in Europe in 2000 (http://www.unideusto.org/tuningeu/home.html), is an approach to evaluating and enhancing quality in European higher education, as well as providing guidance for design and implementation of curricula. Its members consider that the responsibility for quality lies within a university, and acknowledges that external agents can identify problems but are unable to create and implement quality within the institution.

The way quality assurance processes are designed is important for creating an environment where positive change to actual learning occurs. Huisman and Westerheijden (2010) questioned the ability of the 2005 European Standards and Guidelines to manage and enhance quality. The authors stated that the effect is only at the "meta-compliance level" and does not flow down to teachers and students. The need to comply with an extensive checklist stimulates a tick-box approach at the organisational level rather than promoting change in teaching and therefore outcomes in learning. Blackmur (2010) wrote that the guidelines for good practice in external quality assurance processes, created as part of a quality provision in cross-border education established by UNESCO in conjunction with the OECD and the International Network for Quality Assurance Agencies in Higher Education, are superficial and incomplete. Blackmur contested the assumption that a quality assurance process incorporating so-called best practice and peer audit will result in quality higher education outcomes, arguing that important aspects required for identifying higher education quality are absent in the current process.

Measures applied in quality assurance processes may fail to evaluate the effects of "quality" teaching and learning, such as whether students' attitudes change through their participation in a course. Higher education should promote citizenship, ethical and professional reasoning and behaviour. Birtwistle (2009) echoed this sentiment in his overview of the effect of the Bologna Process; he concluded that there is a fundamental need to judge the development and performance of students. Learning outcomes are proposed as a means for judgement of students' performance, but Birtwistle acknowledged that this strategy can only address to a degree this aspect of quality assurance.

The approach taken in quality assurance programs has a direct effect on the actual program outcome. Processes that employ a control (top-down) approach focused on bureaucratic documentation or atomisation of specific aspects of higher education fail to develop a quality culture within the institution. This approach reduces the potential to create positive change and improvement within the organisation (Ehlers, 2009; Stensaker et al., 2010).

Stensaker et al. (2010) reported that external quality assurance more often impacts on structural, organisational and managerial processes, while the desired improvement in teaching and learning is not realised. If, for instance, an external body sets minimum standards for the specific level of qualification and failure to achieve these requirements results in a loss of accreditation for the university, this process will not necessarily bring an improvement in teaching and learning. A combination of control (top-down) and enhancement (bottom-up) processes is required to result in a positive impact on teaching and learning (Ehlers, 2009; Stensaker et al., 2010).

Accountability for quality teaching and learning lies at a number of levels, for example, both at the teaching level and at management level in the provision of adequate resources. If positive outcomes to teaching and learning in higher education are to be achieved, a shared understanding of common goals and agreement to support them is required The development of a quality culture within the institution, where quality assurance principles are embraced by all those involved, has a greater positive impact than external scrutiny.

Australian Context for Standards in Higher Education

In 2008 the Australian Government commissioned an independent review of higher education in Australia with the aim to determine whether Australian higher education was "structured, organised and financed" to compete effectively in the global market (Department of Education and Employment Workplace Relations (DEEWR), 2008, p. xi). The final report noted dramatic changes to Australian higher education over the past 30 years and the need for further change to ensure a high-quality education system of world standing. Stronger accreditation and quality assurance processes, including a standards review, were recommended. The rationale for the standards review was that by "getting the standards right", the quality assurance process could better measure the effectiveness of higher education, thereby working towards enhancing quality.

Australian higher education has moved from a small number of publicly funded universities to a substantially greater number of providers (including private universities) that derive a large proportion of their income from sources other than government funding. The *2008 Higher Education Review* reported the proportion of Australia's 25–34 year olds with degree-level qualifications as 29%, which is less than the typical 50% goal set by other countries in the OECD. (p. xi). The review identified that changes to financing and regulation of higher education were required if Australia was to be an effective competitor in the global market.

Broadly, the Higher Education Review goals for reform in Australia by 2020 are to have a high-quality system with equitable entry, increased participation rates for 25–34 year olds, and adequate resourcing of higher education. To achieve this high-quality system, with increased participation rates from a greater diversity of student backgrounds (e.g. low socioeconomic, rural and remote) than previously accepted into universities, a more rigorous accreditation and quality assurance system with national benchmarking is required.

Currently, a proportion of Australian government university funding is determined by the institution's performance against agreed teaching and equity targets (http://www.deewr.gov.au/HigherEducation/Pages/IndicatorFramework. aspx). The quality of the student experience has a substantial impact on success rates, with a "stimulating and rewarding experience" being more likely to result in students completing their course of study and returning later in life for further education (DEEWR, 2008, p. 69). In line with this concept of quality education, the Review recommended that a set of comprehensive teaching and learning measures be developed to monitor the student experience (DEEWR, 2008).

Following the Higher Education Review, the Australian Qualifications Framework (AQF) Council undertook a review to strengthen qualification outcomes, improve pathways for students, enhance the recognition of Australian qualifications overseas and provide a mapping against international qualifications (AQF, 2009). In 2011 the national revised qualifications framework (AQF, 2011) was adopted for 14 qualification levels, providing reference points for accrediting Australian qualifications and for comparison against international qualifications.

The framework uses learning outcomes as the end point measure of the qualification, justifying the use of this measure to provide consistency and clarity for qualification levels. The qualification levels are described in a number of forms. *Level attributes* are key characteristics of a level, for example, duration. *Level criteria* are descriptors of context, for example, degree of complexity. Finally, there are three *learning outcome dimensions*: knowledge (what the graduate knows and understands), skills (what the graduate can do) and application of knowledge and skills (range of autonomy and complexity of what the graduate can apply).

As part of the reform to ensure quality teaching and learning in Australia's higher education sector, the Australian Universities Quality Agency and State accreditation bodies have been replaced by a national regulatory body. TEQSA was introduced in its quality assurance role in 2011 and took up its regulatory function in January 2012.[iii] TEQSA will register and evaluate higher education performance against the Higher Education Standards Framework (http://www.teqsa.gov.au/higher-education-standards-framework). This standards framework consists of:

– Provider Standards, comprising The Provider Registration Standards, The Provider Category Standards and The Provider Course Accreditation Standards
– Qualification Standards
– Teaching and Learning Standards
– Research Standards
– Information Standards.

As can be seen from this multi-dimensional framework, Australian higher education providers will be evaluated and monitored with considerable scrutiny.

AN EXEMPLAR: DEVELOPING PROFESSIONAL AND PRACTICE-BASED
EDUCATION STANDARDS AT CHARLES STURT UNIVERSITY (CSU)

The goals of CSU include enhancing the internal quality assurance process and strengthening preparation for external quality assurance (e.g. via TEQSA's Higher Education Framework). As part of this preparation, CSU's The Education For Practice Institute (EFPI) was asked to develop a set of educational standards for professional and practice-based education (P&PBE) (EFPI, 2011). The focus on professional practice-based education links with the University's mission to provide high-quality courses that have a professional basis.

A highly inclusive approach was taken in development of the standards. Initially, a literature review was conducted to determine the key aspects of the standards and rationale for the components. The first draft of the standards was produced from a working party established and led by EFPI. The working party included representatives from all faculties and the library. Two major iterations of the standards were later presented to the entire university for review and comment. Substantial feedback was obtained on both occasions. Thematic analysis of all comments was conducted and modifications to the standards were determined.

The CSU standards comprise a set of statements or criteria that identify characteristics of good P&PBE at the course level. The standards are holistic in approach and describe thresholds for course learning outcomes, teaching and learning activities, and infrastructure standards at course and university level. The aims of the standards are to:

– enhance the quality of education using a cycle (plan, implement, review and improve) of continuous quality improvement
– support course teams in curriculum development
– provide a common frame of reference across P&PBE undergraduate and graduate entry courses at CSU to help in course design, delivery and review
– describe the information required to be entered into course and subject profiles in the curriculum database
– provide a means for demonstrating accountability in the delivery of professional courses at CSU
– provide a means of reflection for course teams and individuals on their performance and contribution to the quality of CSU professional courses.

The P&PBE course standards encompass and identify good practices for P&PBE across the curriculum. Tables 12.1 (course goals), 12.2 (teaching and learning activities), and 12.3 (course infrastructure) are course-related. A fourth table, not included in this chapter, deals with the university-level infrastructure necessary for the P&PBE standards to be realised.

Table 12.1. Course goals and learning outcomes

Students will demonstrate by the completion of the course the following capabilities and attributes as expected of graduates entering their professional communities and workplaces

DIMENSIONS/MEANING	STANDARDS

PROFESSIONALISM AND CITIZENSHIP

Capabilities and attributes:
- Accountability, ethical conduct
- Trustworthiness, respect, dedication
- Commitment to professional values
- Lifelong learner
- Social inclusion, diversity acceptance
- Contribution to society's wellbeing
- Commitment to quality
- A global perspective of practice
- Understanding of financial, social and environmental sustainability
- Reflective practitioner

1. Demonstrate commitment, and an ability to undertake lifelong learning through reflection, self-evaluation and self-improvement.
2. Exhibit qualities and behaviours consistent with professional values informed by social justice, global citizenship, Indigenous and cultural competencies and inclusion principles.
3. Explain how practice is informed by knowledge of continuous quality improvement, sustainability and global trends in practice.

PROFESSIONAL JUDGEMENT

Capabilities and attributes:
- Critical reflection, analytical
- Constructive criticism of own practice
- Flexibility, ability to manage change
- Problem-solving capability
- Creativity
- Ethical decision making ability
- Practise according to the law

4. Demonstrate critical and creative decision making and problem solving that is context-relevant.
5. Make work-related decisions that are aligned with professional values, standards and ethics and address legal requirements.
6. Demonstrate accountability by being able to report and articulate the basis for professional decisions and actions.

COMMUNICATION AND INTERACTIONS

Capabilities and attributes:
- Communication according to professional values and boundaries
- Supportive communicator
- Cultural competence (particularly in relation to Indigenous and multicultural Australia)
- Confidentiality
- Team worker
- Collegiality and collaboration

7. Demonstrate ethical, respectful, supportive & culturally competent communication consistent with professional practice codes.
8. Demonstrate proficient and professional communication, through a variety of delivery media/modes to specialist and non-specialist audiences.
9. Demonstrate teamwork, leadership, collegiality, conflict management and professional conventions at the level of an emerging professional.

137

Table 12.1. (continued)

DIMENSIONS/MEANING	STANDARDS
INFORMATION LITERACY	
Capabilities and attributes:	10. Demonstrate an ability to critique new information and determine its relevance to a given situation.
– Ability to access new information	
– Ability to judge information applicability to a specific work setting	
– Synthesise information from multiple sources	11. Demonstrate efficacy in the use of information and communication technologies as part of:
– Produce reports and presentations utilising multiple forms of media	a) learning b) professional practice.
PROFESSION COMPETENCE AND WORK READINESS	
Capabilities and attributes:	12. Demonstrate the discipline-specific technical capabilities of a beginning practitioner or professional.
– Profession knowledge	
– Profession skills	
– Ability to integrate theory with practice	13. Integrate discipline, practical and social knowledge and skills in contemporary professional practice.
– Knowledge of and ability to work within relevant legislation	
– Competence in safe work practices and knowledge of relevant OH&S policies	14. Demonstrate an understanding of legal and ethical requirements and the boundaries in which to work.
– Competence in discipline/ profession knowledge and skills	15. Recognise and respond appropriately to unsafe practice.
– Initiative	16. Demonstrate an ability to plan and manage workloads.
– Ability for independent work	

Table 12.2. Learning and teaching activities and processes

The focus of these learning and teaching strategies are on professional socialisation and learning to learn and perform in communities of practice.

DIMENSIONS	STANDARDS
CURRICULUM DESIGN (planned content, learning activities and assessment)	17. The formal curriculum reflects PBE goals (dimensions making up Table 12.1) and good practice. 18. Curriculum mapping is in place with: a) constructive alignment of P&PBE goals, learning activities and assessment b) a range of learning opportunities relevant to preparation for practice c) relevant sequencing of learning activities and content (particularly theory and practice). 19. Relevant stakeholders such as students, industry partners and community partners are involved in curriculum design.

Table 12.2 (continued)

DIMENSIONS	STANDARDS
CURRICULUM REVIEW (continuous quality improvement)	20. The curriculum is regularly reviewed internally to ensure the PBE standards are addressed. 21. The curriculum is subject to external scrutiny to ensure that external expectations of professional education are addressed. 22. Relevant stakeholders including students, industry partners and community partners are involved in curriculum review.
RISK MANAGEMENT OF THE CURRICULUM	23. Staff in WPL placements ensure a relevant balance between student learning and client services priorities and appropriate levels of student supervision. 24. Relevant processes are in place to manage risks (legal, health, safety, environment, values, ethics, reputation) for students, site, university. 25. Recognise and address the risks inherent in any mal-alignment between the hidden and planned curricula.
(ACTUAL) PBE TEACHING AND LEARNING ACTIVITIES	26. Teaching methods activities (lectures, learning materials etc.) explicitly demonstrate relevance of content to practice (i.e. the practice of the students' future profession/occupation or a broad work arena e.g. business). 27. Strategies other than teacher–led learning and assessment activities (e.g. self-directed and peer learning/ assessment). 28. Learning activities include considerations of and/or opportunities to engage with relevant stakeholders and CSU's communities (rural and regional Australia; Indigenous Australians; professions, industries and students; national and international institutions, scholars and researchers) through responsiveness, partnerships, ethical reciprocity and inclusiveness in relation to these communities. 29. Distance students have learning activities to develop practice skills, cultural capabilities, interactive skills, professional identity etc. 30. Assessment activities that accurately evaluate and promote learning related to the goals in Table 12.1 and identify the need to take action (e.g. with failing students).
INCLUSION OF WIL/WPL ACTIVITIES	31. Provide WPL activities to gain real-world and/or simulated experiences to develop sound decision making in practice. 32. Provide WIL strategies (e.g. simulations, e-learning, visits by industry partners and clients) to bring the practice world into the classroom. (E-learning is of particular value to distance students.) 33. Assessment methods promote learning as well as evaluating students' practice ability.

Table 12.3. Learning and teaching infrastructure

DIMENSIONS	STANDARDS
STAFFING (numbers, expertise)	34. Skilled staff that can provide effective learning to a diverse range of students are available and in appropriate numbers. 35. Staff collectively have a range of expertise and experience including relevant theoretical and scholarly knowledge and relevant professional experience. A whole course approach is required to achieving and improving the standards.
STAFF SUPPORT AND DEVELOPMENT SYSTEMS	36. Staff have support for quality teaching e.g. workloads that provide adequate time for teaching, curriculum development and career advancement. 37. Staff development opportunities/systems are in place to enhance teaching.
STUDENT SUPPORT SYSTEMS	38. Learning support schemes are available to students to develop their learning skills, information literacy, etc. and to remediate learning difficulties. 39. Systems and schemes are in place to support students' and their participation in learning opportunities (e.g. WPL placements).
ON-CAMPUS WORKPLACE LEARNING ENVIRONMENTS	40. To enable students to gain relevant work experience either to complement real-world experience or where real-world workplace learning is not feasible, the school/faculty provides alternative learning opportunities e.g. via simulated learning and workplaces or university clinics/farms etc. These strategies provide for: - developing practice skills & knowledge of the occupation - developing professional identity - learning to work in practice communities - developing relevant interaction and social capabilities - developing professional decision making & self-appraisal. 41. Resources create an up-to-date practice-relevant setting that enables students to experience their practice world e.g. - real/simulated clients - practice workloads - real/simulated interactions with practice communities, clients and local communities. 42. Staff provide sound role models for the occupation/profession/discipline.
LEARNING RESOURCES	43. Resources available to staff and students to promote student practice-based learning are: - relevant to P&PBE goals/outcomes (See Table 12.1) - accessible and sufficient (in numbers) - current quality.

IMPLEMENTING THE CSU P&PBE STANDARDS IN CURRICULA

As discussed above, when working towards quality enhancement of teaching and learning, a greater effect can be achieved if the change comes from within the institution itself. External regulators can impose levels of achievement but these may not bring about the desired change to the quality of teaching and learning. The aim of the course-level P&PBE standards developed for CSU profession-specific courses is to provide a means for internal quality enhancement for a course.

Using the Standards to Review Curricula

Course reviews are a regular occurrence in universities, often attached to policy that mandates the frequency of these reviews. The method for undertaking the course review is not always clearly defined, and this is where a framework such as the CSU P&PBE course standards can be used as a quality enhancement agent. The design and proposed use of the CSU standards as a quality review cycle instrument evaluating performance from a multi-dimensional framework aligns with Coates' (2010) multi-dimensional framework for evaluating academic quality as described above.

The CSU P&PBE standards evaluate performance from multiple aspects and provide measurable standards that have been extensively reviewed by the CSU community in relation to applicability across the range of disciplines. The four tables comprising CSU's P&PBE standards can be used as a means by which course teams can evaluate and frame their curriculum. A series of questions based on these standards can be used as a simple but effective method to prompt course evaluation and review. This process aids in supporting a culture of quality enhancement because a grass-roots approach is taken. With this approach, those in the course team have ownership for what is to be changed and how to make the change. The types of questions and possible means for review are presented.

- Question one: *What is the course aiming to achieve?* This can be assessed by reviewing the dimensions of Table 12.1 and their related meanings. These are key components of professional practice and therefore should be the goals that a practice-based course aims to develop in their learners. Are these goals present in curriculum statements and activities? Does assessment provide evidence of the achievement of the 16 learning outcomes (listed as standards in Table 12.1)? If all the goals (dimensions) are not part of the present course, this informs the course team as to where change to the curriculum may be required. Similarly, if the 16 learning outcomes are not well represented in a course, identification can provide the direction for future change.
- Question two: *How is the course addressing the desired learning goals?* A review of the course against the dimensions and standards in Table 12.2 will provide a framework for evaluating the teaching and learning activities and processes in the course. For example, investigating the types of teaching activity used in a subject or the risk management processes for the course

141

might indicate where any difficulties may lie. The standards described in Table 12.2 can provide a strategy to improve any identified issues.
- Question three: *How well is the course supported at course level to achieve the teaching and learning goals?* Table 12.3 of the standards defines standards for local infrastructure to support quality teaching and learning. An evaluation of the course context against these standards helps to determine whether there are issues adversely impacting on the course quality. For example, if a course has poor student employment rates post-graduation, review of the workplace learning environments and up-to-date resources may be part of the solution.

As indicated above, learning is influenced by a range of factors and therefore a multi-dimensional frame of reference is required to adequately evaluate quality. Finding where current course strengths exist or where deficiencies or missed opportunities in a course may lie is an important step, but equally important is the need to create a plan for prioritising and implementing changes. One method for such planning is to set targets based on the following factors: the relative importance of the deficiency/opportunity to the course, the level of urgency in addressing the identified risk, and the feasibility of addressing the risk. The severity of risks will influence the priority for support, correction or enhancement. In other words, a plan should be made to enhance quality over a cycle of time, depending upon the importance of the need for improvement.

Incorporating the Standards into Curricula

As an example of how the P&PBE standards have been used, in 2011, the four CSU Faculties and the EFPI jointly funded five teaching fellowships focused on enhancing teaching and learning by using the standards. The funds awarded to successful applicants provided staff with teaching relief to conduct their project. As well, a staff member from the EFPI mentored the successful teaching fellows for the year of their fellowship.

A brief description of the projects conducted by the 2011 fellows is provided to demonstrate the range of possibilities associated with employing the standards in curricula. Project 1 used the course goals (Table 12.1) and teaching activities (Table 12.2) as a framework for creating a new Masters professional entry coursework program. Project 2 developed three new workplace learning subjects for a course that previously was without such subjects. The rationale for including these subjects was to bring a greater depth of practice understanding and decision making into the course. The P&PBE standards were used as a framework to determine how the subjects would be structured and their overarching aims. Project 3 evaluated the degree of practice relevance of a masters coursework program by using the course goals (Table 12.1) and teaching activities (Table 12.2) as a framework for review. Project 4 was part of a larger program creating an online Faculty-based quality assurance instrument. The P&PBE standards were incorporated in this instrument. Project 5 developed a process for a course review that required evidence of attaining a specific set of professional accreditation standards. The course goals (Table 12.1) were used as the framework for mapping the professional accreditation standards in the course.

CLOSING STATEMENTS

In this chapter we have reflected upon academic standards and the quality agenda facing higher education. An example of P&PBE standards that are highly relevant to health professional education was provided to illustrate how standards can be used to enhance curricula and students' education.

NOTES

[i] Course expectations are spelt out in qualifications frameworks. In the UK this refers to the "formal structure identifying qualification levels in ascending order and stating the requirements for qualifications to be awarded at each one". (http://www.qaa.ac.uk/aboutus/glossary/pages/glossary-q.aspx#q3)

[ii] http://www.ond.vlaanderen.be/hogeronderwijs/bologna/

[iii] Under the *Tertiary Education Quality and Standards Agency Act 2011* (http://www.teqsa.gov.au/)

REFERENCES

Australian Qualifications Council. (2009). *Strengthening the AQF: An architecture for Australia's qualifications consultation paper.* [Online]. Retrieved from http://www.aqf.edu.au/

Australian Qualifications Council. (2011). *Australian qualifications framework* [Online]. Retrieved from http://www.aqf.edu.au/

Berlin Communiqué. (2003). [Online] Retrieved from http://www.bologna-bergen2005.no/Docs/00-Main_doc/030919Berlin_Communique.PDF

Blackmur, D. (2010). Does the emperor have the right (or any) clothes? The public regulation of higher education qualities over the last two decades. *Quality in Higher Education, 16*(1), 67-69.

Birtwistle, T. (2009). Towards 2010 (and then beyond) – the context of the Bologna Process. *Assessment in education: Principles, policy & practice, 16*(1), 55-63.

Coates, H. (2010). Defining and monitoring academic standards in Australian higher education. *Higher Education Management and Policy, 22*(1), 1-17.

Department of Education and Employment Workplace Relations. (2008). *Review of Australian Higher Education* [Online]. Retrieved from http://www.deewr.gov.au/highereducation/review/pages/reviewofaustralianhighereducationreport.aspx

Ehlers, U. D. (2009). Understanding quality culture. *Quality Assurance in Education, 17*(4), 343-363.

EFPI. (2011). *Standards for professional and practice-based education.* Sydney: The Education For Practice Institute, Charles Sturt University.

Ewell, P. (2010). Twenty years of quality assurance in higher education: What's happened and what's different? *Quality in Higher Education, 16*(2), 173-175.

Gvaramadze, I. (2008). From quality assurance to quality enhancement in the European Higher Education Area. *European Journal of Education, 43*(4), 443-455.

Huisman, I., & Westerheijden, D. F. (2010). Bologna and quality assurance: Progress made or pulling the wrong cart? *Quality in Higher Education, 16*(1), 63-66.

Stensaker, B., Langfeldt, L., Harvey, L., Huismann, J., & Westerheijden, D. (2010). An in-depth study on the impact of external quality assurance. *Assessment & Evaluation in Higher Education, 36*(4), 465-478.

Westerheijden, D. F., Hulpiau, V., & Waeytens, K. (2007). From design and implementation to impact of quality assurance: An overview of some studies into what impacts improvements. *Tertiary Education and Management, 13*, 295-312.

Joy Higgs AM PhD
The Education For Practice Institute
Charles Sturt University, Australia

Edwina Adams BAppSc, MAppSc, PhD
The Education For Practice Institute
Charles Sturt University, Australia

MARCIA DEVLIN AND HELEN LARKIN

13. THE STUDENT EXPERIENCE

Interest in the university student experience is a relatively recent phenomenon. As a health professional, depending on your specific profession, on when you were educated into your profession, and on whether you took a vocational or university route into your profession, the notion of "the student experience" may be new to you or something about which you might not have heard a great deal.

The student experience can be understood as the totality of what happens to, around, and with, students while they are undertaking their course of study. The academic, cognitive, affective, social, emotional and psychological dimensions of students' experience are all encapsulated under this notion. Interest in the notion has grown alongside a move from an elite system of higher education to one that has opened up to a larger number and wider range of students. In this more recent "massified" system, it is now well recognised that there is no such thing as a "typical" student or a homogeneous student population, and that no assumptions about students as a homogeneous group can be made. Where it was once the case that only males from white, upper-class and privileged backgrounds who had graduated from private schools could go to university, it is now the case that males and females from all races and strata of society, with a wide range of schooling and educational backgrounds, can and do attend university.

As these huge shifts have taken place, not all students have had the same sorts of experiences at university. For example, initially taught by white, upper-class males from privileged backgrounds who made up the teaching staff of universities, and surrounded by the male students outlined above, many of the small number of early women to go to university felt ostracised, isolated and out of place. As female students have become part of the higher education landscape, members of later minority cohorts have similarly felt the effects of being different from the dominant group(s). The importance of understanding the impact of such experiences and feelings on learning and academic performance has grown as university student populations have diversified further over time.

The notion of the student experience has matured into recognition of the complex interplay of factors that contribute to an individual's education and learning outcomes. With that recognition has come the development of a parallel understanding that, in relation to teaching a diverse student population, one size does not fit all, if indeed it ever did. With the massification of higher education, we now have "the brightest and most committed students … but they sit alongside students of rather different academic bent" (Biggs & Tang, 2007, p. 2). University educators need to ensure that all students have a positive experience and, in particular, the opportunity, support and guidance to achieve academically at similar

S. Loftus et al. (Eds.), Educating Health Professionals:
Becoming a University Teacher, 145–158.
© 2013 Sense Publishers. All rights reserved.

levels to those at which students who are more naturally academically inclined achieve. This is one of the key modern-day challenges of university teaching.

If you are new to the field of academic work, you are likely to have a wide range of discipline-specific and other clinical skills. Even though you might have undertaken postgraduate study or professional development activities, your knowledge of what it is like to be a university student may be based predominantly on your own experiences, that may have been some time ago. Modern universities and the students who attend them are very different from those of previous generations. Stepping into an academic role can, therefore, require some adjustment.

In exploring the student experience, this chapter draws on both relevant research and literature, as well as the combined experience of the authors. The chapter first examines the complex lives of current university students, including their several roles and paid work commitments. Some of the generational differences between current students and those in the past are also discussed, and the first year student experience is explored. These sections provide a background and contextual information for the more detailed sections that follow. The chapter then explores the student experience through the lenses of academic literacy, the academic program, and the quality of both the teaching and related support offered to students while they are at university.

THE COMPLEX LIVES OF STUDENTS

Multiple Roles

Modern university students often have a number of roles besides that of student. Many students juggle roles as parents, carers, partners, employees, members of families and so on. As much as university teachers might wish it to be and it once was perceived to be, the student role is not always a student's primary role. This is sometimes a choice for students, but in many cases, responsibilities related to family or to an employer must take a higher priority than those related to study. University students typically have several competing demands on their time and on what should be prioritised. Some students also manage physical, sensory and/or mental health conditions, and these may or may not be disclosed to university teachers. An awareness of the realities of students' lives can assist you as an educator to design learning environments, activities and assessment tasks that accommodate and take advantage of the complexity in which students live.

Finances and Paid Work

Australian students spend more time in paid work on average now than ever before. A 2006 national study of student finances (James, Bexley, Devlin, & Marginson, 2007) found that more than seventy percent of full-time undergraduate students worked an average of over 14 hours per week, the equivalent of almost two days per week during semester. One in six of those students worked more than

20 hours per week – around the equivalent of 3 days per week. This research also found that, contrary to popular beliefs about students working to fund a lifestyle filled with drinking, partying and fun, the 19,000 students surveyed reported that they worked primarily to fund their study. This included paying for travel costs to and from university, textbooks, stationery and fees, either through the Higher Education Contributions Scheme, through loan repayments or, if they were international students, through full fees. One in eight students surveyed said they regularly went without food or other necessities because they could not afford them.

In the same study, students living away from home and supporting themselves also reported using income from paid work to pay their rent and bills as well as food, clothes and essentials such as computer and Internet costs, the latter being a requirement for any student enrolled in university study. The research also showed that it was not unusual for students to miss classes to meet paid work requirements and for their paid work requirements to interfere with their ability to study outside of class (James et al., 2007).

Student Contact Hours

In previous generations, student face-to-face teaching hours in many health professional courses were often equivalent to full days, 5 days per week. Some educators new to their role may be surprised at an apparently lower number of student contact hours in some instances than may have been their experience as a student. That does not mean, however, that student learning outcomes and requirements have necessarily been reduced. Today's university students undertake a range of teaching and learning activities through blended learning approaches, that is, a "blend" of face-to-face, online and other strategies, and may be engaged in learning in which you are not directly involved and about which you are not aware. However, students might not be engaging in such self-directed learning, and the issue of where your responsibilities start and stop is one that engages academic and support staff across not only health but all disciplines in universities.

Generational Differences

Although we are wary of making sweeping generalisations about what is a sizeable proportion of the current generation of university students, "Generation Y" students do appear to bring a particular approach to their learning that is different from the general approach of previous generations. Considered to be those born between 1982 and 2002 (Prensky, 2001), Generation Y seem to learn differently from previous generations and communicate in a fundamentally different way (Nimon, 2007; Pardue & Morgan, 2008; Larkin & Hamilton, 2010). Given their several priorities, they are often strategic in their learning and may elevate study to a higher priority only when absolutely necessary, for example, when there are impending exams or assessment tasks to complete. This creates challenges for teaching staff in engaging students consistently over the course of a semester's study or indeed over several years of a program of study.

Generation Y students also often have a belief that aspects of their experience can be negotiated. For example, it is not uncommon for students to advise that they are going on holiday during semester and to seek to negotiate alternative examination or assignment arrangements. This can take some adjustment for those new to higher education. It can be challenging to find the balance between making clear what is expected of students and modelling appropriate professional behaviours, while at the same time recognising the changing face of society, generations and education. We explore this notion further, later in the chapter.

The Ubiquity of Technology

One of the most visible and undeniable changes in higher education in recent years has been the expansion in the use of teaching and learning technologies and the blurring of boundaries between traditional on-campus and off-campus or "distance" enrolment and study. These changes are often seen to be a response to a generation of students who are perceived as "digital natives" (Prensky, 2001, p. 1), who learn and communicate in fundamentally different ways (Arhin & Cormier, 2007; Nimon, 2007), although this notion is also contested (see e.g. Kennedy et al., 2008). That said, in their day-to-day life outside of university, Generation Y and other students often expect rapid responses to their electronic communication and these expectations can flow over into the university environment. They may expect instant answers to their study-related questions and, being used to dealing with information presented in short, "bite-sized" chunks (Gresty, Skirton, & Evenden, 2007; de Leeuw, 2012), they can expect particular sorts of responses from teaching staff. The ubiquitous nature of online learning, and the sometimes unrealistic expectations of students in terms of response times and the nature of responses given by academic staff, can lead to tensions.

One of the challenges for educators is to have realistic expectations with regard to response to students' online queries and requests. Answers from teachers in the bite-sized chunks that they might expect are not always appropriate. Students often need to be challenged to find their own solutions; to seek the support of their online colleagues; to realise that solutions are often not simply right or wrong; to recognise that there may be several solutions; and to reflect on and further research what they are seeking to understand. Setting realistic expectations also involves creating boundaries around the times you will be online and answering queries.

In an attempt to engage as many students as possible with the curriculum and learning outcomes, it is now an expectation in most universities that teachers will use blended learning environments and approaches to accommodate the range of student needs and learning styles (Bodie, Powers, & Fitch-Hauser, 2006; Blake, 2009). Blended learning includes not only traditional face-to-face teaching but also a range of e-learning approaches. Online material may include lecture notes, lecture recordings, teaching resources and materials, multimedia resources, library access, peer and teacher discussion sites, and synchronous "virtual" classrooms; as well as email access to teaching staff. Thus the focus has shifted away from what the teacher does and a dependence on face-to-face teaching, to facilitating students' access to a range of methods to engage with the academic curriculum, teaching staff and their peers. When faced with the realities of technology, multiple modes of study and the new generation of students and the ways in which they choose to study and learn, it can be difficult for many new academics to adjust.

Student learning now often occurs in a place and space far removed from the university campus, and at a pace dictated by the student rather than the teacher. However, regardless of the range of teaching technologies available, there is evidence to support that students still value face-to-face teaching and will attend class if they perceive it to be of value (Copley, 2007; Gosper et al., 2008; Larkin, 2010). Students are strategic about how they engage with the curriculum and academic staff and, as Larkin suggests, "if you could be replaced by a recorded lecture then why wouldn't you be?" (p. 248).

THE FIRST YEAR EXPERIENCE

One aspect of the university student experience that receives particular attention is the first year of study and attendance at university, known as "the first year experience". There are several reasons for the focus on first year. One of these is that students in their first year of study at university are at the greatest risk of dropping out. This is often because of the magnitude of adjustment that first year students must make when they move into university study. This occurs regardless of whether students move straight from high school to university, come through Vocational Educational and Training (VET) pathways, return to study as mature age students after a break, or come to higher education as international students from another country.

All first year students experience what has become known as "transition" to university. But not all first year university students are transitioning into the first year of their course. For example, students who come through "articulated pathways", where, for example, part of their nursing studies are completed in VET, often enter university at second year and experience their transition to university later in their course. Research in the area of the first year experience and transition shows that the more connected students can become with their academic work, their teachers, their fellow students and the institution at which they are studying, the more likely they are to have a smooth transition into university and to be more successful as students.

An important role for the teacher of first year health students is ensuring that students gain insight into the nature of their future profession. Students need to start to develop a sense of professional identity in the first year of their course so that they have information upon which to base decisions about the suitability of the profession for them. Without such early exposure, some students will live with doubts about the choice they have made until later in their course when they are assured of its validity, or when they realise they have made a poor choice.

ELEMENTS OF THE STUDENT EXPERIENCE

As mentioned in the introduction, the student experience comprises many dimensions including the academic, cognitive, affective, social, emotional and psychological experiences that students have at university. In this section, we examine in detail four aspects of experience that cut across these dimensions. These are the development of academic literacy; the content and foci of academic programs; the quality of teaching and learning; and the support provided to students within and outside the formal learning environment. Each is explored in turn.

THE DEVELOPMENT OF ACADEMIC LITERACY

In a massified system, students can find themselves entering higher education without the requisite skills and understanding to study appropriately and perform in ways that are expected. That is, their academic literacy can be at lower levels than is ideal. Some students arriving at university have what Margolis, Soldatenko, Acker, and Gair (2001) called a reservoir of cultural and social resources and familiarity with "particular types of knowledge, ways of speaking, styles, meanings, dispositions and worldviews" (p. 8), which allow them to feel comfortable in the university environment and give them decoding skills. Devlin (2010) highlighted that some students do not have such a reservoir and that successful university study can be difficult for them. Many students without a family history of university study can find navigating the discourses and norms of academia challenging. There are many such "first in the family" students who now attend university.

Researchers Collier and Morgan (2008) referred to the "implicit expectations" (p. 426) of students by staff and the "tacit understandings" (p. 426) that students need in order to be successful at university. Many "non-traditional" students without parents, family members or friends who are familiar with university study may not know that these unspoken requirements exist, never mind that they must understand and then respond appropriately to them (Devlin, 2010).

One Australian study of the first year experience of 2,422 students found that students from a low socioeconomic background were more likely than their higher socioeconomic peers to say that they have difficulty comprehending material and adjusting to teaching styles within the university environment (James, Krause, & Jenkins, 2010). Part of this difficulty in comprehension and adjustment might be due to the discourses of university, with which students with no family history of university study may not be familiar or comfortable.

As an academic, teaching either small or large groups of health students, it is important to consider what your role is with regard to the academic literacy of your students. Universities now invest considerable resources in student support programs, including student academic services. Students have access to language and academic skills advisors who are specifically skilled in assisting students to upgrade and improve their skills in this area. You can do much to contribute to improving the academic literacy skills of students in collaboration with institutional colleagues. Academic literacy programs can be more effective when embedded within the specific academic subjects being taught, in a "just-in-time" way. For example, there is little benefit to students being taught how to do an online literature search using multiple databases in the first week of the first year of study, if this skill is not going to be required by students until second year.

Much anecdotal discussion takes place between academic staff in universities about the role of feedback and the benefit that students may or may not derive from teaching staff providing, for example, written feedback on assignments. With current academic workloads, it can be a challenge to provide good quality feedback and corrections on assignments as part of the marking process. However, feedback is an important mechanism by which students can improve their academic literacy skills as well as consolidate their learning. You need to work towards providing this in a way that is both beneficial to students and sustainable for yourself as an educator in an increasingly busy academic environment.

Collegiality, Collaboration and Academic Standards

One area in which students can struggle in particular in relation to academic literacy is the area of plagiarism and collusion. Health practitioners need to share experiences and knowledge and work in a collegial and collaborative manner to achieve the best outcomes for clients. Such collegiality and collaboration should be a focus in any health professional education program. Indeed, in such programs, students often undertake interprofessional learning and work in problem-based learning groups and other shared and collaborative learning experiences. However, academics need to understand that in their quest for developing these attributes in students, they can run the risk of students becoming confused about where the line is drawn between collaboration and contravening the important academic standards of collusion or plagiarism. Specific attention needs to be paid, therefore, to explaining university requirements and "rules" in this area so that students are clear about what the relevant requirements are and are not at risk of being asked to answer charges of academic misconduct. You can work with language and academic skills advisors to help students understand these requirements.

THE ACADEMIC PROGRAM

In terms of the content and foci of the academic program, we have chosen to explore three areas – lifelong learning, the development of professional attributes and the development of professional competence through work integrated learning. Each of these is discussed in turn.

A Focus on Lifelong Learning

One central purpose of a modern university education is the development in students of lifelong learning attributes. In the past, learning at university has sometimes focused on surface approaches to learning (Biggs & Tang, 2007) and on students learning large amounts of facts and figures. Such approaches relied to a large extent on rote learning and on the reproduction of memorised material, often under exam conditions. Over the years, understanding about how students learn and how they translate what they have learned in formal settings to their professional and wider roles later on has become more sophisticated. Rote learning and exams are still in evidence in many disciplines, but they are widely understood to be limited to ensuring that students reproduce facts and have limited usefulness in assessing students' understanding at deeper levels, which is required to ensure high-quality learning outcomes.

As educators we need to focus on ensuring that part of students' academic experience involves developing the skills and abilities to critically reflect on practice, to be informed by evidence using sound research skills and to approach their future professional practice with an emphasis on the importance of lifelong learning. It is becomingly increasingly recognised in many disciplines, including health, that the rapid and exponential growth in knowledge and technology means that much of what is learned today becomes obsolete in a few years (Grubb & Lazerson, 2005; Boud & Falchikov, 2006; Walsh, 2007). In a sense we are preparing graduates for jobs in the future that don't exist today. It is no longer sufficient, therefore, for students as future practitioners to "know things". They must be able to reflectively apply their knowledge in changing clinical, technological and broader contexts. With so much knowledge available at the click of a button, particularly in health, a central aspect of teaching is for students to know how to select information that is authoritative and how to critique, analyse and apply it, and for educators to evaluate students' effectiveness in having done all of the above. The role of health educators, therefore, is not to transmit facts, but to facilitate the learning of our students.

Yet students can be resistant to a broadening of their academic activities to encompass teaching activities and assessments that don't necessarily have a clear right or wrong answer. Indeed, de Leeuw (2012, p. 59) has warned us that in relation to medical education "thinking about options, considering one's own stance on globalisation and other challenging issues, reflecting on matters of life and death, seems beyond many medical students in a universe where clinicians tell them that they can and need to rely on the facts, and only the facts". One challenge for you as an educator is to help students to understand that their current course and experience is just the start, or some point on a continuum, of learning over their lifespan, and that learning continues long past the point at which they graduate.

The Development of Professional Attributes

As health educators, we have a responsibility not only to prepare students with the relevant discipline-specific skills and attributes, but to also ensure that they leave university with an understanding of what constitutes professional behaviour in a more generic sense. As a health educator, you will have a personal interest in graduating students that you can confidently and proudly welcome as future colleagues. It is important, therefore, to embed into your teaching, from an early stage, appropriate expectations and standards with regard to professional practice and behaviour. As well as reflecting on your own behaviour in the classroom, online and in personal communication, you may also need to provide advice and feedback to students about personal presentation, communication and behaviour, at various points in their progression through the course. This may be either on a group or an individual basis, particularly as it applies to the undertaking of fieldwork practicums. Students are often unaware that they need to apply different standards of communication and behaviour while on fieldwork to those that may be acceptable in other university learning environments. Students can behave in a way that they would not think of behaving in their paid job and sometimes struggle to elevate their commitment and professionalism to an appropriate level for fieldwork practicums. As an educator, it is your role to make clear to students the expectations of them and their responsibilities while undertaking practicum.

The Development of Professional Competence

Clinical fieldwork and student practicums have long been a mandated component of most, if not all, health education programs. These programs now have to be considered in a wider context of what is generally referred to in higher education as "work integrated learning". Many academic programs now aspire to include some experience out in the field for students where previously none existed. The health disciplines, which have traditionally been doing this for many years, have much to offer in terms of leadership within universities around such programs. However, the context in which work integrated learning currently takes place in higher education means that consideration needs to be given to factors that might not previously have been of significant concern to health educators.

A recent national study (Patrick et al., 2008) reinforced the need for program co-ordinators to take account of some of the ways that work integrated learning programs can disadvantage students. Traditional "block" placements, where students undertake full-time fieldwork practicums, can seriously disadvantage students who depend on paid work to support their basic living requirements. Many students need to take time off work to complete their fieldwork placements or need to make alternative arrangements in relation to family responsibilities such as caring for family members. Additional travel costs associated with attending fieldwork also need to be considered, and as discussed earlier in this chapter, as a group representative of the general community, students bring to fieldwork a range of health, disability and personal concerns. It is important, therefore, for fieldwork co-ordinators and others responsible for managing work integrated learning programs to be sensitive to these issues and not only plan these programs in collaboration with health settings and agencies, but also do this in collaboration with students and endeavour to accommodate to some extent the difficulties and disadvantages they experience.

Although finding sufficient clinical placement opportunities remains one of the biggest challenges in health education programs, this can no longer be undertaken in isolation from or at the expense of individual student circumstances. Mechanisms need to be in place that give students prior opportunity to seek accommodations that can provide some flexibility regarding place, time, hours, and the like. At the same time, however, students need to take responsibility for alerting academic staff in advance to any specific circumstances that could impact on work integrated learning programs. If students and academics thus work together they can significantly increase the likelihood of positive and successful student experiences in work integrated learning programs.

THE QUALITY OF TEACHING AND LEARNING

The third critically important aspect of the student experience we address is the quality of teaching and learning. This section explores the notion of effective, high-quality teaching and the need to focus on learning rather than just teaching.

Effective, High-Quality Teaching

There is much research about being an effective teacher (Ramsden, 2003; Biggs & Tang, 2007) and no shortage of academic material and professional development opportunities for new academics. It may also come as a surprise to those new to academia that there is a large body of knowledge in relation to the scholarship of teaching and learning that sits separate from your discipline or area of clinical expertise. When you commence in higher education this body of knowledge might not be immediately obvious to you, or, when you find it, it can feel overwhelming in its scope. When starting to teach, new academics instead often revert to doing what "seems right" or what appears to make sense from their own past experiences or personal preferences.

One model that might be useful to consider is that of the development and understanding of teaching excellence in higher education, by Kane, Sandretto and Heath (2004). In this model, the authors proposed that the characteristics of excellent teachers are subject knowledge, teaching skills, interpersonal relationships, personality attributes, and a connection between teaching and research. This model is well suited to health practitioners who choose an academic career. Kane et al. emphasise the importance of teaching staff having strong discipline-specific knowledge and skills that they bring to the learning environment, which enhance their credibility in students' eyes. As a recent, and perhaps continuing practitioner, you will have much depth in this dimension of teaching. Teaching skills cover a range of attributes and include but are not limited to the ability to bring real-life examples to the classroom (online or physical) to illustrate teaching. Making real-world connections for students and bridging the gap between theory and practice is a highly regarded attribute of excellent teachers by students. Teaching skills also refers to your ability to communicate information in a way that engages students. Again, from your experience as a practitioner, you will have much to contribute to this dimension of excellent teaching.

In their model, Kane et al. (2004) also emphasise the need for good relationships with students, a willingness to bring characteristics of your own personality to your teaching, having a sense of humour, and showing that you enjoy your work. Finally, the research/teaching nexus is important so that you can demonstrate that your teaching is informed by evidence. This model may assist in increasing your confidence about what you can do to promote positive learning experiences and environments for your students.

Focusing on Learning

Fundamental to a consideration of what constitutes effective, high-quality teaching is that the focus needs to be on learning and not just on teaching. Such a focus is the basis of a student-centred approach to education. In the past, the role of the academic was conceived as merely "transmitting information, usually by lecturing" (Biggs & Tang, 2007, p. 16) and the lecturer stood in front of the class as "the sage on the stage" (p. 17) imparting his/her wisdom and experience. Students' minds were considered to be "empty vessels" into which knowledge was poured. Our understanding of teaching and learning has now shifted dramatically, in that not only is the teacher considered to be the "guide on the side", but more importantly the focus is on what students need to do and their need to be active in constructing their knowledge and understanding (Biggs & Tang, 2007). although Kane et al. (2004) acknowledged the importance of what the teacher does and the teaching strategies that they use, Biggs and Tang argue that this is merely "a means of setting the stage on which good learning occurs, not […] an end in itself" (p. 18).

Many health practitioners are comfortable with concepts of person- or client-centred practice. Yet when you start in an educational role it might not be immediately obvious to consider using a similar approach with students. However, students often see the irony of a lecturer who purports to be committed to the principles of person-centred clinical practice but does not treat students according to similar standards. Reflecting on the principles you hold strongly when you work with clients in a clinical setting and considering how you might apply these same principles to your students can be a fruitful exercise. This does not mean that you should become indulgent or accept lower academic standards. Instead, it goes to the heart of thinking about teaching as (a) providing students with as many opportunities as possible to engage with the learning material to accommodate their learning styles and needs, (b) demonstrating a willingness to be flexible and take account of personal circumstances where appropriate, and (c) treating students with respect so that their learning is maximised.

THE SUPPORT PROVIDED TO STUDENTS

A fourth and final important aspect of the student experience is the support provided by their teachers and more broadly by the institution. Health and other educators can provide support to students through their careful and professional approach to preparing for and engaging in teaching and learning activities.

Teachers who provide clear, organised, coherent classes that integrate authentic and realistic examples and provide opportunities for students to become engaged with the content can promote and support students' learning and positive student experiences. It is also important in a general sense to communicate clearly with students about your availability, preferred methods for communicating with you depending on the context or presenting issue, and your willingness to assist with student queries. Assistance may be in the capacity of timely responses to questions raised on online discussion sites, email contact, or meeting with students on a one-to-one basis when circumstances require it.

As discussed earlier in this chapter, students are representative of the population in general and as such can present with substantial personal, social, economic and health issues. It might be a one-off situation for some students, or the problem could be pervasive throughout their university enrolment. It is not necessarily your role as their teacher to address these concerns or to provide solutions. But it is important to understand how these issues are affecting their experience as students and their ability to engage with and to complete their studies. Part of your responsibility is to ensure that students have information about the full range of special consideration and extension processes available for the subjects they are studying. Your role is also to refer or direct students to the relevant student services where they can seek more direct and specialised assistance. Such services include student counselling, medical, accommodation, financial, disability-related, study skills, career and other services. It is important to familiarise yourself with the range of services available to support students. You should also find it helpful to seek advice from senior colleagues such as subject co-ordinators, course co-ordinators and other school or faculty representatives to ensure that the support and assistance that you provide is at an appropriate level and is in line with faculty and university policy and processes.

Supporting Students in Placements

In fieldwork education it is important that you work closely with your clinical colleagues in agencies that offer student placements. Unlike you, they might not be aware of the major changes in higher education in recent years. You could be liaising with fieldwork educators who expect universities and the students who attend them to be the same as they were 20 to 30 years ago. An important part of your role is to work with fieldwork educators to ensure that they are up-to-date with what is happening in higher education and the way that academic programs are organised. As an educator, you also need to be concerned and interested in preparing students for those positions and for roles that are newer and emerging or might not yet have been created. This approach is not always recognised by those already working in the field who are supervising students and who might prefer to focus on what might be considered "traditional" roles, skills and placements. You may need to champion the cause of current students who, as a whole, can and do contribute much to their communities, studies and their future profession.

156

CONCLUSION

In this chapter we have outlined the current experience of university students, including their multiple roles, paid work and other commitments, and generational features. Issues related to students' experience of transition to university, the development of academic literacy, the academic program they undertake, and the quality of both the teaching and the related student supports have been examined. Consideration of the student experience is a critical aspect of what it means to be a teacher in higher education and, more importantly, how to be effective in that role. With the massification of higher education and the marketing of university education as a commodity for sale, the quality of the student experience comes under the spotlight. Students are increasingly considered as, and consider themselves to be, "consumers" within this market. Regardless of whether you agree with this notion or oppose it, the quality of their experience is important. We hope that this chapter contributes to the conversation about how best to maximise the quality of the higher education student experience.

REFERENCES

Arhin, A. O., & Cormier, E. (2007). Using deconstruction to educate Generation Y nursing students. *Journal of Nursing Education, 46*(12), 562-567.

Biggs, J., & Tang, C. (2007). *Teaching for quality learning at university* (3rd ed.). Berkshire: McGraw-Hill, Society for Research into Higher Education & Open University Press.

Blake, H. (2009). Staff perceptions of e-learning for teaching delivery in health-care. *Learning in Health and Social Care, 8*(3), 223-234.

Bodie, G. D., Powers, W. G., & Fitch-Hauser, M. (2006). Chunking, priming and active learning: Toward an innovative and blended approach to teaching communication-related skills. *Interactive Learning Environments, 14*(2), 119-135.

Boud, D., & Falchikov, N. (2006). Aligning assessment with long-term learning. *Assessment & Evaluation in Higher Education, 31*(4), 399-413.

Collier, P. J., & Morgan, D. L. (2008). "Is that paper really due today?" Differences in first-generation and traditional college students' understandings of faculty expectations. *Higher Education, 55*(4), 425-446.

Copley, J. (2007). Audio and video podcasts of lectures for campus-based students: Production and evaluation of student use. *Innovations in Education and Teaching International, 36*(3), 501-512.

de Leeuw, E. (2012). The politics of medical curriculum accreditation: Thoughts, not facts? *International Journal of User-Driven Health Care, 2*(1), 53-69.

Devlin, M. (2010). *Non-traditional student achievement: Theory, policy and practice in Australian higher education.* Keynote address, First Year in Higher Education (FYHE) international conference, Adelaide, June 27-30.

Gosper, M., Green, D., McNeill, M., Phillips, R., Preston, G., & Woo, K. (2008). *The impact of web-based lecture technologies on current and future practices in learning and teaching.* Australian Learning and Teaching Council. Retrieved from https://www.mq.edu.au/ltc/altc/wblt/dissemination.htm

Gresty, K., Skirton, H., & Evenden, A. (2007). Addressing the issue of e-learning and online genetics for health professionals. *Nursing and Health Sciences, 9,* 14-22.

Grubb, W. N., & Lazerson, M. (2005). Vocationalism in higher education: The triumph of the education gospel. *The Journal of Higher Education, 76*(1), 1-25.

James, R., Bexley, E., Devlin, M., & Marginson, S. (2007). *Australian university student finances 2006: Final report of a national survey of students in public universities.* Canberra: Universities Australia.

157

James, R., Krause, K., & Jenkins, C. (2010). *The first year experience in Australian universities: Findings from 1994 to 2009*. Canberra: Department of Education, Employment and Workplace Relations.

Kane, R., Sandretto, S., & Heath, C. (2004). An investigation into excellent tertiary teaching. *Higher Education, 47*(3), 283-310.

Kennedy, G., Judd, T. S., Churchward, A., Gray, K., & Krause, K. (2008). First year students' experiences with technology: Are they really digital natives? *Australasian Journal of Educational Technology, 24*(1), 108-122.

Larkin, H. (2010). "But they won't come to lectures." The impact of audio recorded lectures on student experience and attendance. *Australasian Journal of Educational Technology, 26*(2), 238-249.

Larkin, H., & Hamilton, A. (2010). Making the most of your fieldwork learning opportunity. In K. Stagnitti, A. Schoo, & D. Welch (Eds.), *Clinical and fieldwork placement in the health professions* (pp. 159-170). Melbourne: Oxford.

Margolis, E., Soldatenko, M., Acker, S., & Gair, M. (2001). Peekaboo. In E. Margolis (Ed.), *The hidden curriculum in higher education* (pp. 1-20). New York: Routledge.

Nimon, S. (2007). Generation Y and higher education: The other Y2K. *Journal of Institutional Research, 13*(1), 24-41.

Pardue, K. T., & Morgan, P. (2008). Millenials considered: A new generation, new approaches and implications for nursing education. *Nursing Education Perspectives, 29*(2), 74-79

Patrick, C., Peach, D., Pocknee, C., Webb, F., Fletcher, M., & Pretto, G. (2008). *TheWIL [Work Integrated Learning] report: A national scoping study [Australian Learning and Teaching Council (ALTC) Final report]*. Brisbane: Queensland University of Technology. Retrieved from http://www.altc.edu.au and http://www.acen.edu.au

Prensky, M. (2001). Digital natives, digital immigrants, Part 1. *On the Horizon, 9*(5), 1-6.

Ramsden, P. (2003). *Learning to teach in higher education*. London: RoutledgeFalmer.

Walsh, A. (2007). An exploration of Biggs' constructive alignment in the context of work-based learning. *Assessment & Evaluation in Higher Education, 32*(1), 79-87.

Marcia Devlin BA, DipEd, Grad Dip Appld. Psych, MEd, PhD
Executive Director of Academic Products & Services
Open Universities Australia

Helen Larkin BApp Sc (OT), MAppSc, Grad Dip Health Admin, Grad Cert Higher Ed
School of Health and Social Development
Faculty of Health
Deakin University, Australia

CHRIS ROBERTS AND STEPHEN LOFTUS

14. THE DEVELOPMENT OF HEALTHCARE RESEARCHERS

This chapter focuses on the journeys of healthcare practitioners who want to or are required to undertake research in academia. We have used a case-based approach in an effort to integrate some of the scholarship published in this area with the stories of the many practitioners with whom we have had the privilege of sharing personal research journeys. These cases are fictionalised to protect the identity of colleagues. We examine some of the personal and other factors that might influence all healthcare practitioners in making a constructive career choice to engage in research, navigate academia, and perhaps become research practitioners. Consideration is given to some of the contextual factors that facilitate healthcare practitioner research as well as those that are barriers to its conduct. Although the utilisation of healthcare research is the business of all practitioners, we focus on the experiences of those who seek to produce research and the processes of the research education that they might undertake to qualify them to do good research. Finally, this chapter briefly considers some of the theoretical frameworks that have been used to provide a scholarly perspective on the experience of making the transition between healthcare practice and research.

In an academic context, research has traditionally been thought of as the province of the higher education sector, and in particular the university. For example, academic medicine has been defined as "the discovery and development of basic principles, effective policies, and best practices that advance research and education in the health sciences, ultimately to improve the health and wellbeing of individuals and populations" (Kanter, 2008, p. 205). It is founded on the three pillars of clinical service, research and teaching, and the interrelationships between them (International Working Party, 2004). Kumar, Roberts, and Thistlethwaite (2011) have suggested a helpful typology for academic medicine which attempts to broadly define the types of career that doctors undertake, based on whether their main focus is clinical service, research or teaching. We have adapted this typology in Figure 14.1 for healthcare practitioners with the authors' permission. In this chapter we consider the challenges of the research journey for all four groups in Figure 14.1, but focus on the intersection of research practice and the university. The main distinction between the categories that some are principally salaried through the university and others principally through healthcare providers.

S. Loftus et al. (Eds.), Educating Health Professionals:
Becoming a University Teacher, 159–172.

Academic practitioner-scientists: university-salaried healthcare practitioners who are primarily engaged in biomedical clinical sciences or health services research, maintain some clinical practice, and have variable involvement in teaching.

Practitioner-researchers: healthcare practitioners who are employed by health service providers, are primarily engaged in clinical practice, regularly undertake research, and have some or little involvement in teaching.

Academic practitioner-educators: university-salaried healthcare professionals who are primarily engaged in teaching and learning, maintain some clinical practice, and have variable degrees of involvement in research.

Practitioner-educators: healthcare practitioners who are employed by health service providers, are primarily engaged in clinical practice, regularly teach, and have some or little involvement in research.

Figure 14.1. Definitions of four subgroups of clinicians engaged in teaching and research (after Kumar et al.)

PERSONAL FACTORS

Health-related research encompasses a large number of themes related to achieving the health and wellbeing of individuals and the communities they live in. Health researchers pursue research questions using a full range of research methodologies from the laboratory to the bedside, through to the community level. With such a varied range of research careers available for healthcare practitioners, it is unsurprising that there are many pathways into research careers.

ACADEMIC PRACTITIONER-SCIENTISTS

Bazeley (2003) emphasised the wide differences between, on the one hand, pure "scientists" who complete doctoral studies, gain postdoctoral research experience as a member of a team, and then step onto the ladder of an academic career, and on the other hand, academic practitioner-scientists in a health professional context, who complete their doctoral studies early following a healthcare professional degree. The postdoctoral journey of the latter will include publications, but will be dependent on a successful track record of gaining national competitive research grants. There is considerable variation among healthcare disciplines as to whether such academic practitioner-scientists maintain a clinical commitment or not. This career pathway for academic practitioner-scientists is not without its challenges. O'Sullivan, Niehaus, Lockspeiser, and Irby (2009), in a study of academic doctors, for example, identified elements that enhanced participants' interest in becoming medical academics, including early exposure to research, interaction with role models and mentors, visibility of career pathways, career support for junior staff, and a complex interplay between their personal and social factors. We meet an academic clinician scientist in one of the cases studies (Susan) later in this chapter.

This traditional "scientific" pathway can be contrasted with professionals such as the physiotherapist or the general practitioner with many years of professional experience, who then undertakes a doctoral candidature and endeavours to build a research profile while still in practice. Within this cohort of practitioner-researchers, some may have approached academia through the teaching route as a practitioner-educator, for example providing supervision around clinical placements. Others will have become involved in research activities through an association with research units (Kumar et al., 2011), which might be in the health service sector or through a university academic unit. Many practitioner-researchers do not ultimately gain a salaried position within a university, but continue principally in their clinical service role. Such practitioner-researchers offer a basis for collaborative partnership with university-based academics to create a research base within the profession (McCrystal, 2000). We emphasise that the quotation marks around the word *scientific* above are deliberate. It is more appropriate to talk of rigorous and scholarly inquiry. This may engender qualitative or quantitative or mixed techniques depending on the research question (Roberts & Conn, 2009). However, in many research-led universities there is a perception that "scientific" research means laboratory-based pure basic health science research or clinical randomised controlled trials of new healthcare initiatives. We discuss later, when considering contextual issues, what kind of "science" funding bodies and increasingly universities themselves are prepared to fund, an important concern for any would-be healthcare researcher. For now, we consider the stories of the many healthcare practitioners who have not followed a traditional "scientific" route and have transitioned from full-time clinical practice into research. There are two broad categories, the academic practitioner-educator and the practitioner-researcher. We begin with an academic practitioner-educator who is salaried by a university and whose job is principally teaching focused.

THE ACADEMIC PRACTITIONER-EDUCATOR

Vijay's story (see Case Study 14.1) illustrates the opportunities and challenges for the academic practitioner-educator. At first Vijay wanted to argue that the university should value academic practitioner-educators. He wished to emphasise that he had left full-time clinical practice because he wanted to teach, and considered teaching a vital component of the university's mission. He felt it unfair that he should feel a lack of credibility and even a sense of marginalisation because he favoured teaching over research. Perhaps, he thought, there was a way that academic practitioner-educators could be better supported in developing a professional identity commensurate with an expanded notion of academic scholarship (Kumar et al., 2011). For example, Trigwell, Martin, Benjamin, and Prosser (2000), have provided a useful model for academic scholarship that includes constructing an argument to demonstrate the scholarly nature of practice, assembling the evidence to support the argument, and presenting this evidence as a teaching portfolio. The scholarship of teaching and learning includes being scholarly and evidence-based as well as conducting original educational research. For Vijay, however, it seemed that although a promotion system for educators had been proposed in his university, it was a long way off widespread acceptance and implementation. His job, he perceived, was on the line.

Vijay is a speech pathologist who has been in the university for 4 years. He has a heavy teaching load and is active on a number of committees. His role includes co-ordination of clinical placements, tutor professional development, and clinical supervision. His only publications have been as fourth author on a couple of papers with one of his senior colleagues. At his recent performance management review he was advised that the university required all incumbents in academic posts to be research active, or to have their role re-designated as a teaching focused post. Vijay left the meeting realising that he would probably need to do a doctorate in order to give him the skills and knowledge he would need to have any credibility as a researcher. He has a particular interest in student support and decided that this could be a suitable topic for a research project. As this would be research on his professional practice, Vijay has to decide between doing a conventional PhD or a professional doctorate.

Case Study 14.1. Vijay's research journey

Vijay recognised that in the modern university, becoming involved in research as an "academic practitioner-educator" would mean having to acquire the credentials to be a researcher. In most cases, this means that the long-established academic clinician-educator like himself must acquire a doctoral level qualification. Although he perceived that advancement in his university would be more dependent on publications and grants, he could see that the doctorate would be an essential first step along the road. The doctorate allows academics to claim the credibility to be accepted as independent researchers in their own right, with the ability to conduct research projects with all that this entails, such as the ability to think and write critically, to devise appropriate research questions and to design and conduct projects that can provide answers to those questions. It provides the opportunity to develop expertise in methodological skills as well as in-depth substantive content knowledge in a particular research area (Bazeley, 2003). Undertaking a PhD is a major commitment that takes 3 years if undertaken full-time, although Vijay realised that he would have to do it part-time while continuing to work (Phillips & Pugh, 2000).

With its focus on higher research training, the traditional doctorate by thesis is considered an important gateway into academe. The period of training typically also ensures socialisation into the academic research community and to the culture and style of the particular discipline (Becher & Trowler, 2001; Kumar et al., 2011), as well using the training period (doctoral and postdoctoral) to develop associations with distinguished researchers and to establish good scholarly habits (Bland & Schmitz, 1986). Nevertheless, Vijay recognised that the acquisition of a doctorate would not guarantee success or promotion in the highly competitive world of academe. He was aware of increasing casualisation of the research workforce in his own university.

Vijay asked himself whether he should do a traditional thesis or a thesis by publication. Both the traditional PhD by thesis and the PhD by publication require a thorough grounding in research methodology. Many universities now insist that the would-be doctoral student has done some kind of research training at Masters level. From the university perspective, doctoral attrition rates average from 30% to 50% depending on the subject field. The factors influencing attrition and retention are complex and relate to a dynamic intersection between student and supervisor, involving also societal, institutional, departmental and disciplinary factors (McAlpine & Norton, 2006). In a PhD by publication, students are expected to produce a series of peer-reviewed papers that have been published or accepted for publication. The series of papers must represent the equivalent of 3 years' full-time study. Vijay certainly did not feel he had the necessary grounding in methodology to realise his very early thoughts on researching student support.

A major review of doctoral education was conducted by the Carnegie Institute, and an attempt was made to reframe the purpose of doctoral education within the contemporary research environment (Golde, Walker, & associates, 2006). The authors particularly challenged the traditional apprenticeship model of doctoral study that is inherent in the supervised thesis approach, which they considered largely ineffective and inefficient. From a series of disciplinary studies, the authors examined practices and elements of doctoral programs and showed how they could be made more powerful by relying on principles of progressive development, integration and collaboration. They offered an alternative model of doctoral programs in which students learn while being apprenticed with several faculty members. In this model, high-quality graduate education is dependent on each department within an institution creating or being part of a vibrant and forward-looking intellectual community. Such knowledge-centred, multi-generational communities foster the development of new ideas and encourage intellectual risk-taking (Golde et al., 2006). Professional doctorates have become widely available in recent decades, and have also been reviewed by the Carnegie Institute (Jean-Marie & Normore, 2010).

Professional doctorates designed to meet the needs of particular groups have been established in health, for example in nursing, psychology, pharmacy and health sciences, and the doctorate now encompasses a wide range of academic pursuits (Boud & Tennant, 2006). Professional doctorates involve "a program of research and advanced study, which enables the candidate to make a significant contribution to knowledge and practice in their professional context, in which the candidate may also contribute more generally to scholarship within a discipline or field of study" (Kemp, 2004). Typically a professional doctorate will enable "candidates to become leaders in areas such as practice, research, management and education in [their] respective discipline and thereby shape professional knowledge and practice" (Doctorate in Pharmacy, Kings College London, http://www.professionaldoctorates.com/search/CourseDetails.aspx?CID=13171).

All doctoral degrees have the commonality that students must engage in scholarship and research and generate new knowledge, which must be documented in some way. Traditionally, the PhD has been a qualification acquired by a new graduate at the start of an academic career (Bazeley, 2003), whereas the professional doctorate has been aimed at professional practitioners who are mid-career and who intend to stay within the world of professional practice. So whereas the PhD is seen as developing theory that might be applicable to practice, the professional doctorate is seen as research on practice, which might generate new theory. For some universities this reflects the aspiration for new relationships between industry, government and academe. For others it is maintaining the privileged position of the universities (Kemp, 2004). Particular target populations for new professionally-oriented doctorates have been postulated as "new knowledge workers" who operate in areas not covered by specialised doctorates and those who wish to negotiate transdisciplinary programs (Boud & Tennant, 2006). The professional doctorate is also seen as more experiential and encouraging more transdisciplinarity. This type of knowledge has sometimes been referred to as "Mode 2 knowledge" (Gibbons, 2000) whereas the traditional unidisciplinary knowledge of the PhD is referred to as "Mode 1 knowledge". The difference between them has been compared to the difference in the kinds of questions a physiologist and a surgeon might ask. A physiologist might ask timeless questions with answers that are always and everywhere true, whereas a surgeon might ask timely questions which need answers that can be applied more specifically and more immediately. As most professional doctorate candidates are often mid-career and frequently in senior management, they may well be in a position to apply the knowledge they develop within their professional practice.

There are also organisational differences, in that the professional doctorate usually begins with coursework and has a smaller research component. In Australia, for example, professional doctorates are expected to be two-thirds research and are regarded as fully equivalent to the PhD by thesis. The more modular approach is a distinctive attraction to many prospective doctoral students who want to be part of a cohort of other students who can, in theory, provide mutual support in a learning community. The modularity also enables students to take breaks. This can be essential for busy professionals with demanding jobs, who must study part-time and who often have families as well. In contrast, the PhD by thesis is often perceived as a monolithic undertaking requiring several years of sustained effort. In recent years, however, these differences have started to blur somewhat. More and more PhD programs are including formal coursework. A PhD can also be interdisciplinary and there is no good reason why a PhD project cannot have close involvement with the world of professional practice.

There is growing realisation that doctoral education is about achieving the formation of a particular kind of person (Golde et al., 2006). This raises the question of how the different doctoral programs impact on the development of the professional identity of a health professional academic. A doctoral graduate is someone who has learned how to *know* and *be* differently; someone who can take a critical look at the field and distinguish between the established knowledge that needs to be preserved and what needs to be discarded, as well as having the ability to contribute effectively to that body of knowledge, or that professional practice. This ability can be summarised under the notion of stewardship. PhD graduates have been described as people who can become stewards of their discipline and professional doctorate graduates as people who can become stewards of their professional practice. This stewardship requires not just the ability to conduct research and critique knowledge and practice but other abilities, such as being able to communicate with the wider society so that everyone can understand the role of one's discipline or one's profession in society. The development of criticality also raises other issues. For example, the professional doctorate has often been seen as a means to train people to solve work-related issues. However, the development of criticality can educate people to take a deeper look at what constitutes a work-related issue. In other words, doctoral education enables people to be more reflexive, to take a step back and ask, "What's really going on here?" So, whereas a simplistic, or training, view of doctoral education might assume that graduates are equipped to deal with and solve complex problems, a more realistic, educational view sees graduates as having the ability to open up the complexity of problems and explore underlying issues. This latter view is more in keeping with the notion of stewardship.

One of the critiques of professional doctorates asks whether they will produce independent researchers in the same manner as the traditional doctorate. An additional concern is the quality and relevance of the taught components. In Vijay's case, he has significant prior experience of research, and it would be fair for him to question the relevance of a degree for future leadership, when his specific requirements are to develop associations with distinguished researchers and to establish good scholarly habits (Bland & Schmitz, 1986). Vijay's initial thoughts were to go back to his supervisor to see what support would be given to him to undertake a professional doctorate in health science studies offered at his university.

PRACTITIONER-RESEARCHERS

Many healthcare practitioners develop their interest in research while doing clinical practice. Let us now reflect on Rachel's story, which is given in Case Study 14.2, as an example of someone who transferred successfully into full-time academe, by a different route to Vijay. In helping to understand the richness of health practitioner research careers we then consider Jacinta, who is happy to remain in practice but with strong university links (Case Study 14.3).

Rachel is now in her late forties with two adult children, 18 and 23. She was a frontline nurse for many years, including a spell within hospital management. She undertook a Masters in Primary and Community Care in her 30s, on a scholarship over a year, and then returned to practice for several years. She then completed a PhD by thesis in qualitative health services research, part-time over 5 years, while continuing in part-time clinical work. On completion of her PhD, she took up a post as a university lecturer and left clinical practice. Her doctoral thesis provided the intellectual basis for her subsequent research output, research funding applications, teaching and consultancy.

Case Study 14.2. Rachel's research journey

There are many considerations that established healthcare practitioners, such as Rachel, need to reflect upon in deciding if research is the right career choice for them. Even if it is the right personal choice, a major consideration is the likelihood of making research a significant part of their future careers. Issues to be considered might include personal motivation, resilience, prior experience, intellectual passion, and self-efficacy. This last concept describes belief in one's capability to organise and execute various courses of action. The strength of such belief determines whether an action will be pursued, the level of effort expended, persistence in the face of obstacles, and subsequent performance (Lent, Brown, & Hackett, 1994). Self-efficacy in research was the strongest predictor of intention to do research in the future among trainee clinical psychologists (Wright & Holttum, 2012). Rachel needed to have a long-term belief that after expending considerable effort over a sustained period of time, at some financial loss to herself, she will become an independent and salaried researcher. In her case the motivation was to make a difference to the health and wellbeing of the community she had served as a clinician. She wanted to have a voice that was respected around the table when decisions affecting members of the public about whom she was passionate were made. The research journey was not easy, requiring personal sacrifice in lost evenings and weekend study, lost earnings in being able to work only part-time, and an impact on her family life. Careful consideration was needed around her financial situation and the need for considerable flexibility. Her research journey also impacted on her work. The isolation of pursuing an intellectual quest, which few around her were able to understand, was at times overwhelming. Personal sacrifices in the workplace in order to undertake research are a common theme for many. For example Woodward, Webb, and Prowse (2007) found that nurses felt that these sacrifices were not recognised by their managers. Health professional researchers needed more structured support systems and recognition of the value of their research, as well as mentorship from more experienced researchers. Others are motivated in different ways to become a research-practitioner. Woodward and colleagues (2007) suggested that the challenges of becoming a practitioner-researcher need to be set against the lack of challenge, boredom, and burnout with workload in highly service-driven clinical roles in the modern health service.

Rachel recalls many of her early difficulties in making the transition, such as learning to write academically, and she has become a strong supporter in her mentoring role to aspiring researchers, for example helping them develop academic writing skills. Shah, Shah, and Pietrobon (2009) provided a number of insights into the challenges faced by novice researchers in their early attempts at academic writing, noting that significant educational intervention is required to substantially improve this particular skill. Rachel also tried to encourage her colleagues to view the world in ways that were different from the conventional views of clinicians. She encouraged them to be more critical, more questioning. In other words, Rachel was promoting a change of identity, a change that would make them more like the stewards mentioned above. To some extent what Rachel is trying to promote through an apprenticeship model resonates with what Vijay is trying to achieve through a professional doctorate. Jacinta's story (Case Study 14.3) suggests an alternative path for practitioners engaged in research.

Jacinta is a physiotherapist working part-time in a community-based rehabilitation service. She has two children aged 9 and 13. She has had a part-time job over several years as a research fellow within the regional campus of a metropolitan university. She has been funded through various collaborative research grants obtained by the Director (Susan) of the university department, who has an interest in community care and has published several papers with Jacinta as an author. As Director, Susan has encouraged Jacinta to undertake a PhD to help her gain a more secure academic post. Jacinta suggests that it will be some time before she and her partner would have the time and the financial security for her to commence such an enterprise. There were few new posts at the regional campus and Jacinta didn't particularly want to move nearer the main campus.

Case Study 14.3. Jacinta's research journey

In this case, Susan, who is Director and an established academic practitioner-scientist, is maintaining a research team within a university departmental setting. Like Rachel in the previous case, Susan often finds herself counselling clinicians about the opportunities and challenges in becoming a researcher. Research supervisors spend considerable effort in supporting novice researchers and helping them develop necessary research skills, as well as supporting professional development activities. She has to take a long-term view of maintaining the research capacity of her team, and to consider the long-term personal development plans of those she identifies as motivated, productive, and good team players. In supporting healthcare practitioners such as Jacinta to advance their research ambitions, Susan has encouraged Jacinta's engagement with research mentors and potential doctoral supervisors, liaising with staff from local health provider research-focused departments and the local research network co-ordinators.

The challenges for Jacinta entering academia have been well described. The deterrents to her pursuit of an academic career in relation to research echo those found by the Walport Report (UK Clinical Research Collaboration, 2005). They include lack of a clear entry route, a transparent career pathway, an available post near where she lives, an achievable balance of work between service, academia and her private life, and the availability of a funded post on completion of her research training. Jacinta's research journey was serendipitous. She had enjoyed the opportunity to work with one of the other healthcare practitioners who had a substantive university position in the regional campus. Jacinta had undertaken some interviewing and qualitative data analysis. She had found the work stimulating and taken some research methods courses, developing her skills as she worked on particular projects. Accordingly, she had developed into a reasonably competent research fellow, but she needed to work clinically as funding for her research skills was limited. She was comfortable with this arrangement. Jacinta was also aware of colleagues who had completed a PhD but who did not remain active researchers (Bazeley, 2003). As in many areas of clinical practice, a role model or mentor can be inspirational in providing the impetus to take up research. However, she was not going to do that PhD!

CONTEXTUAL

Having considered becoming a researcher from a personal healthcare practitioner viewpoint, we now consider how the university and health research systems view career pathways into research. Scientific evidence is increasingly seen as the key driver of policy and practice. For example, in Australia, as elsewhere, decision makers are keen to receive rational and disciplined evidence provided by science in a context where democratic accountability demands that public money be wisely spent (Roberts & Conn, 2009). One benchmark for the quality of scientific research in the university sector to guide allocation of government funding is provided by the *Excellence in Research for Australia* initiative. Consequently, most universities are only likely to support individuals or groups in fields where the research will be recognised internationally, the evidence being a track record of publication in peer-reviewed journals with high impact factors. Such exercises in assessing research quality emphasise that the challenge of improving the reputation and the scientific quality of research lies squarely in the hands of the researchers themselves. One can perhaps understand now why Vijay (Case Study 14.1) was being directed to engage in research, and why the universities were keen to recruit established researchers such as Rachel (Study 14.2) and Jacinta (Study 14.3) and retain Susan (Study 14.3). Equally, one can understand the pressure that all individual researchers are under to perform according to the new metrics of research success. Potentially such metrics would not drive Vijay's wish to grow as a professional practitioner through a professional doctorate. Is the scholarship of teaching and learning likely to be a recognised research grouping in university health discipline settings?

The dominant message from contemporary research is that the production of a successful academic researcher is linked to the creative intersection of person, department and institution, where a motivated individual interacts with a supportive, stable and adequately resourced environment, with accessible skill development opportunities and the prospects for collaborative research (Grbich,

1998; Walker, Golde, Conklin Beuschel, & Hutching, 2008). Although this statement will resonate with many in the research community, the achievement of such a culture is problematic. To what extent can an individual department like Susan's address these questions? The universities themselves need to develop new academic cultural practices to meet the needs of new populations of doctoral candidates (Boud & Tennant, 2006) as would-be researchers.

CONTEXTUAL BARRIERS

In the highly competitive funding environment of the last decade, a new generation of academic researchers has found it difficult to compete with those who have long since established their credentials, and who are well known to those assessing, advising or making funding decisions (Bazeley, 2003). Those not already in academic employment typically seek an ongoing research position following their doctoral studies. This has been seen as more difficult than obtaining funding for research, as opportunities to access research funding often accompany a position (Bazeley, 2003). Researchers who succeed in gaining academic employment face the further problem that, even though they are highly trained in research, once hired as academics, in entry-level academic posts they spend only a small amount of time in research and do not receive supervisory support (Bland & Schmitz, 1986). Laudel and Gläser (2008) suggested that the two major factors affecting the transition into an academic career are a successful PhD and a research-intensive phase prior to academic employment. This implies that the new researcher must think about self-funding not only the preparation time for the PhD proposal but also the PhD itself and the immediate postdoctoral period before gaining an academic position. Some of the factors which deter doctors, for example, from pursuing any type of academic career were summarised by the Walport Report (UK Clinical Research Collaboration, 2005) and include the lack of clear entry routes and transparent career tracks; poor flexibility in terms of the geography of available places; difficulty in balancing work between service, academia and a personal life; and poor availability of properly structured and funded posts on completion of training. Also within the academic medicine context, Bakken, Byars-Winston, and Wang (2006) found that the development of a clinical research pathway entailed many challenges. These included low self-efficacy beliefs, negative outcome expectations, ill-defined personal goals, over-commitment, lack of early and continuous learning opportunities, and conflicting demands and expectations of the multiple environments an individual may inhabit.

There have been a number of calls for structural reforms to support capacity building in healthcare professional research, for example in medicine (UK Clinical Research Collaboration, 2005) and allied health (Pickstone et al., 2008). In the UK, the Clinical Research Collaboration's (UKCRC) (Latter, Clark, Geddes, & Kitsell, 2009) made recommendations about establishing career pathways for nurses and allied health professionals that would enable them to combine a focus on both clinical and academic roles. However, implementation has been complex due to the ongoing need to establish joint university–health service employment contracts, harmonising clinical and research roles and ensuring sustainability of funding for clinical academic posts (Latter et al., 2009). Others have developed and evaluated research networks and proposed their utility for developing and supporting beginning researchers (Perreault et al., 2009). Some researchers have reminded us that the problem of research capacity, in this case among nurses, is amplified in lower- and middle-income countries (Edwards, Webber, Mill, Kahwa, & Roelofs, 2009).

RESEARCH PERSPECTIVES

Understanding the journeys of healthcare practitioners who undertake research is a dynamic and rapidly evolving area for scholarship. The personal issues of career choice, values, motivation, and capabilities are enmeshed within the socialising influences of becoming a health professional, working in the health service, and entering and successfully navigating academia. In reflecting on the material we have appraised in writing this chapter, we suggest that there are three broad theoretical perspectives that have potential to illuminate this area to advance scholarship. First is the theoretical framework provided by socio-cognitive career theory (Lent et al., 1994), which is in the early stages of adoption by healthcare researchers (Bakken et al., 2006; O'Sullivan et al., 2009; Kumar et al., 2011). Secondly, there is the notion of the development of a professional identity as practitioner-researcher and considering the socialising influences that impact upon this identity formation (Grbich, 1998; Golde et al., 2006; Kumar et al., 2011). Finally there is the notion of developing communities of practice in which the development of healthcare practitioner-researchers takes place largely in the situated learning environment of the workplace, where the learner participates and is socialised in multiple communities of practice (Lave & Wenger, 1991). Integration of theoretical perspectives is needed, derived from theories that emphasise individual choice, motivation and competence and theories that emphasise the powerful socialising influences in the health and academic workplace, in order to understand the rise of the healthcare practitioner academic.

CONCLUSIONS AND RECOMMENDATIONS

This chapter has highlighted a number of factors that should help guide healthcare practitioners and their junior colleagues to understand the issues in becoming a healthcare practitioner-researcher. Although this involves a complex interplay between, personal, social and contextual factors, a number of broad themes arise. Those in the health service who wish to become academics need to ensure that as well as being good teachers they acquire the skills to do independent good quality research. In planning to acquire these skills, academics need to focus on what kind of professional identity they aspire to, always of course taking account of the institutional context. Do they see themselves as a professional researcher who teaches, or as a professional educator who collaborates on research projects? It then becomes an easier matter of aligning, in conjunction with a good mentor, the kind of training program required. A professional doctorate provides a broader reflection on practice, which can include leadership, teaching, research and community engagement. A more self-directed doctorate by thesis or publications is for those becoming professional researchers. Those who remain in the health service can focus on either teaching or research, but are advised to consider appropriate professional development opportunities.

Universities, in partnership with communities of health service providers, need to make changes to the culture if they wish to assure the rise of the healthcare practitioner-researcher and to maintain the credibility of the healthcare practitioner-educator. The practice of research in the health professions and the education of researchers are both areas ripe for further scholarship.

REFERENCES

Bakken, L., Byars-Winston, A., & Wang, M. F. (2006). Viewing clinical research career development through the lens of social cognitive career theory. *Advances in Health Sciences Education, 11*(1), 91-110.

Bazeley, P. (2003). Defining "early career" in research. *Higher Education, 45*(3), 257-279.

Becher, T., & Trowler, P. (2001). *Academic tribes and territories: Intellectual enquiry and the culture of disciplines* (2nd ed.). Buckingham: The Society for Research into Higher Education & Open University Press. Retrieved from http://ceps.pef.uni-lj.si/knjiznica/izbirni/D.c.%202001%20Becher%20and%20Towler_Academic%20Tribes%20and%20Teritories.pdf

Bland, C. J., & Schmitz, C. C. (1986). Characteristics of the successful researcher and implications for faculty development. *Journal of Medical Education, 61*(1), 22-31.

Boud, D., & Tennant, M. (2006). Putting doctoral education to work: Challenges to academic practice. *Higher Education Research & Development, 25*(3), 293-306.

Edwards, N., Webber, J., Mill, J., Kahwa, E., & Roelofs, S. (2009). Building capacity for nurse-led research. *International Nursing Review, 56*(1), 88-94.

Gibbons, M. (2000). Mode 2 society and the emergence of context-sensitive science. *Science and Public Policy, 27*(3), 159-163.

Golde, C. M., Walker, G. E., & Associates (Eds.). (2006). *Envisioning the future of doctoral education: Preparing stewards of the discipline. Carnegie Essays on the Doctorate.* San Francisco: Jossey-Bass.

Grbich, C. (1998). The academic researcher: Socialisation in settings previously dominated by teaching. *Higher Education, 36*(1), 67-85.

International Working Party to Promote and Revitalise Academic Medicine. (2004). ICRAM (the International Campaign to Revitalise Academic Medicine): Agenda setting. *British Medical Journal, 329*(7469), 787-789.

Jean-Marie, G., & Normore, A. H. (Eds.). (2010). *Educational leadership preparation: Innovation and interdisciplinary approaches to the Ed.D and graduate education.* New York: Palgrave Macmillan.

Kanter, S. L. (2008). What is academic medicine? *Academic Medicine, 83*(3), 205-206.

Kemp, S. (2004). Professional doctorates and doctoral education. *International Journal of Organisational Behaviour, 7*(4), 401-408.

Kumar, K., Roberts, C., & Thistlethwaite, J. (2011). Entering and navigating academic medicine: Academic clinician-educators' experiences. *Medical Education, 45*(5), 497-503.

Latter, S., Clark, J. M., Geddes, C., & Kitsell, F. (2009). Implementing a clinical academic career pathway in nursing: Criteria for success and challenges ahead. *Journal of Research in Nursing, 14*(2), 137-148.

Laudel, G., & Gläser, J. (2008). From apprentice to colleague: The metamorphosis of early career researchers. *Higher Education, 55*(3), 387-406.

Lave, J., & Wenger, E. (1991). *Situated learning: Legitimate peripheral participation.* Cambridge: Cambridge University Press.

Lent, R. W., Brown, S. D., & Hackett, G. (1994). Toward a unifying social cognitive theory of career and academic interest, choice and performance. *Journal of Vocational Behavior, 45*(1), 79-122.

McAlpine, L., & Norton, J. (2006). Reframing our approach to doctoral programs: An integrative framework for action and research. *Higher Education Research & Development, 25*(1), 3-17.

McCrystal, P. (2000). Developing the social work researcher through a practitioner research training programme. *Social Work Education, 19*(4), 359-373.

O'Sullivan, P. S., Niehaus, B., Lockspeiser, T. M., & Irby, D. M. (2009). Becoming an academic doctor: Perceptions of scholarly careers. *Medical Education, 43*(4), 335-341.

Perreault, K., Boivin, A., Pauzé, E., Terry, A. L., Newton, C., Dawkins, S. et al. (2009). Interdisciplinary primary health care research training through TUTOR-PHC: The insiders' view. *Journal of Interprofessional Care, 23*(4), 414-416.

Phillips, E. M., & Pugh, D. S. (2000). *How to get a PhD: A handbook for supervisors and their students.* Philadelphia, PA: Open University Press.

Pickstone, C., Nancarrow, S., Cooke, J., Vernon, W., Mountain, G., Boyce, R. A. et al. (2008). Building research capacity in the allied health professions. *Evidence & Policy: A Journal of Research, Debate and Practice, 4*(1), 53-68.

Roberts, C., & Conn, J. (2009). Building capacity in medical education research. *Medical Journal of Australia, 191*(1), 33-34.

Shah, J., Shah, A., & Pietrobon, R. (2009). Scientific writing of novice researchers: What difficulties and encouragements do they encounter? *Academic Medicine, 84*(4), 511-516.

Trigwell, K., Martin, E., Benjamin, J., & Prosser, M. (2000). Scholarship of teaching: A model. *Higher Education Research & Development, 19*(2), 155-168.

UK Clinical Research Collaboration, M.M.C. (2005). *Medically and dentally-qualified academic staff: Recommendations for training the researchers and educators of the future.* London: Report of the Academic Careers Subcommittee of the Modernising Medical Careers and the UK Clinical Research Collaboration: UK Clinical Research Collaboration, Modernising Medical Careers.

Walker, G., Golde, C. M., Conklin Beuschel, A., & Hutching, P. (2008). *The formation of scholars: Rethinking doctoral education for the twenty first century.* San Francisco: Jossey-Bass.

Woodward, V., Webb, C., & Prowse, M. (2007). The perceptions and experiences of nurses undertaking research in the clinical setting. *Journal of Research in Nursing, 12*(3), 227-244.

Wright, A. B., & Holttum, S. (2012). Gender identity, research self-efficacy and research intention in trainee clinical psychologists in the UK. *Clinical Psychology & Psychotherapy, 19*(1), 46-56.

Chris Roberts MBChB MRCGP MMedSci PhD
Charles Perkins Centre
The University of Sydney, Australia

Stephen Loftus PhD
The Education For Practice Institute
Charles Sturt University, Australia

ELAINE DUFFY AND WAYNE (COLIN) RIGBY

15. INDIGENOUS ISSUES IN HEALTH PROFESSIONAL EDUCATION

Indigenous peoples around the world have experienced historic injustices as a result of colonisation and dispossession of their lands, territories and resources. These injustices are acknowledged in the *United Nations Declaration on the Rights of Indigenous Peoples* (United Nations, 2008, Article 14, p. 7), which mandates:

> Indigenous peoples have the right to establish and control their educational systems and institutions providing education in their own languages, in a manner appropriate to their cultural methods of teaching and learning.

Furthermore, the Declaration advocates that Indigenous peoples have the right to the dignity and diversity of their cultures, traditions, histories and aspirations, which shall be appropriately reflected in education. Through Indigenous leadership and academic pursuits, countries such as Australia, the USA, Canada and New Zealand have explored and continue to explore ways of dealing with the effects of colonisation by actively pursuing decolonising strategies in both education and research.

The provision of a well-educated and culturally competent health workforce is critical to the alleviation of health inequities and the achievement of optimal health outcomes for Indigenous peoples throughout the world, not just in Australia (West, Usher & Foster, 2010). Marked improvements in Indigenous health can be achieved by increasing the participation of Indigenous people in the health fields.

This chapter explores Indigenous issues in health professional education from several perspectives, including issues for Indigenous students in mainstream health programs and those dedicated to Indigenous populations, Indigenous academics new to the academy, and Indigenous pedagogy. We debate these issues from a critical stance and hope that our debates stimulate your thinking and reflecting as a newcomer to the world of teaching and learning in the academy. We aim also to assist your understanding of the complex nature of Indigenous issues, particularly in the context of health and health professional education. We adopt an Australian perspective, but the issues raised are relevant in many countries.

Indigenous Students

Many Indigenous students who come to university, often academically under-prepared, are motivated to improve Indigenous futures through their choice of profession (Nakata, Nakata, & Chin, 2008) and many choose health professions because of the appalling health of their own people. There is a concern, however,

S. Loftus et al. (Eds.), Educating Health Professionals:
Becoming a University Teacher, 173–184.
© 2013 Sense Publishers. All rights reserved.

that education takes Aboriginal people away from country and family and they might never come back. Despite this concern, Main, Nichol, and Fennell (2000) claimed that education can be seen as a resource for community development in health by maintaining cultural identity while developing professional and leadership skills. Thus, graduates can return to their communities with their Aboriginality intact, together with skills, knowledge and established networks to help improve their people's health. Yet on entering the academy, Indigenous students often struggle with a confronting alien environment.

Indigenous students and Indigenous academics in the higher education sector enter a world that is dominated by Western theories, pedagogies and pedagogical spaces. The why and the how of the learning process is equally dominated by Western knowledges, concepts, theories and traditions. Indigenous students bring with them important knowledges and experiences that are not well represented in Western disciplinary knowledges or course content. Thus, Indigenous students are often left to negotiate and navigate on their own across a "conceptual chasm" (Nakata et al., 2008). Indigenous students face extraordinary barriers when they enter the higher education sector, leading to high attrition rates.

In Australia in 2009 over 10,000 Indigenous students were enrolled in higher education, representing a 10% increase over 2008 (DEEWR, 2009). Yet Australian Indigenous students still represent less than 1% of all higher education students. This proportion is significantly short of the 2.5% of Indigenous people in the broader population (IHEAC, 2006). Attrition, retention and completion rates of Indigenous students are areas of concern. The attrition rate for first year Indigenous students is estimated to be between 35 and 39% (IHEAC, 2006). Overall completion rates for Indigenous students are less than 50%, compared with 72% among non-Indigenous Australian domestic students (Radloff & Coates, 2010).

Several authors report that although the participation rates of Indigenous students in higher education are increasing, attrition rates are significantly higher than that of the general student population and occur most commonly in the first year of study (e.g. West et al., 2010). There is growing recognition that universities, faculties and schools need to find ways to help Indigenous students to succeed in their programs, especially in the first year of study. There is plenty of research to show that when students do get through this first year of study they are more likely to continue and succeed (e.g. Rigby, Rosen, Berry, & Hart, 2011). On enrolment, Indigenous students have reported culture shock, racist attitudes, stereotyping and isolation from others of a similar culture as reasons for leaving (Usher et al., 2003; Usher, Lindsay, Miller, & Miller, 2005).

Some researchers (Rigney, 1999; Nakata et al., 2008) have called for the recognition of attrition rates as "rejection rates", that is, students' rejection of the very factors listed just above, and warned that unless the educational system reflects on its white Western knowledge base and begins to acknowledge other ways of knowing, Indigenous students will continue to reject the system. Authors suggest that there may be a need to better equip students to engage more meaningfully with Western knowledge. If Indigenous students are viewed as bringing assets in the form of Indigenous views and values to the learning interface, they can use their own knowledge and experiences to contest misrepresented or absent course content. Unless Indigenous views and values are seen as assets and used in a meaningful way, the university system is likely to be seen as nothing more than yet another assimilation strategy for Indigenous people and another reason for rejecting the system.

The pressure on universities to improve student retention and success has brought a focus on students' need to adapt to the demands of university expectations and has also brought increased pressure on universities to accommodate the broad needs of diverse student populations. This ongoing pressure has led universities to extend their focus, not only to academic skills support but also towards academic teaching and learning as an area of research and professional development (Bryant, Scoufis, & Cheers, 1999). Developments in teaching and learning are generally concerned with issues surrounding curricula and pedagogy – what and how course content is delivered and assessed – but less with student factors.

The range of factors that prevent students from completing higher education studies are well documented. Such factors may be personal, financial or cultural, and may relate to educational preparation and other social issues.

Researchers have investigated barriers faced by Indigenous students in their transition to university and their success at university (e.g. West, West, West, & Usher, 2011; Rigby, Duffy et al., 2011). Studies have been undertaken in a range of different contexts and different disciplines. Of particular note, West et al. (2011) studied Indigenous students' experiences in tertiary nursing education, and a recent study by one of the authors of this chapter (Rigby, Duffy et al., 2011) explored the experiences of Indigenous students in a university program dedicated to Indigenous Mental Health.

Rigby, Duffy et al. (2011) aimed to identify and address barriers to the retention of students, identify strategies that were especially helpful in sustaining students in the program, empower students to better prepare them for university, and inform academic staff about areas that could be improved to provide a culturally safer learning environment. This study was of a unique program offered exclusively to Aboriginal and Torres Strait Islander students in the field of mental health, with most of the teachers being of Aboriginal or Torres Strait Islander descent. The study highlighted key strengths of the program that were particularly relevant to this group, such as the learning journey of students, working together, mutual connection and growth, ownership of the program, and wellbeing.

Despite the plethora of research and reports, issues associated with academic content, writing and study skills, or teaching and learning methods are not considered to be critical determinants of Indigenous students' decisions to persist with or withdraw from courses (Nakata et al., 2008). Nonetheless, Nakata et al. (2008) acknowledge that the literature is consistent in identifying that academic issues can present particular difficulties for Indigenous students and that academic support initiatives are essential for the success of Indigenous students, especially for those who are under-prepared for university study. Unfortunately, the notion that Indigenous students are under-prepared for higher education study can be associated with cultural deficit theory, a by-product of assimilation legislation, which (in Australia) was adopted as an agreed government policy direction in 1937. Cultural deficit theory attributes students' lack of educational success to characteristics embedded in their cultures, traditions and communities. This leads to blaming the victim, negative stereotypes, and assertions about particular individuals, groups and communities. The endurance of cultural deficit theory is evidenced in a recent Australian education policy review suggesting that Indigenous peoples are disadvantaged, not because of inequity in society, but because of the "circumstances of their birth" (Bradley, Noonan, Nugent, & Scales, 2008, p. xi). This statement is characteristic of cultural deficit theory, in that circumstances of birth can be seen to represent cultural heritage. As Townsend-Cross (2011) has argued, there is need for a real shift away from "education as assimilation" to an understanding of the right to define and engage education that is founded on Indigenous objectives, philosophies, epistemologies, values and language literacy. There must be an acknowledgement that Indigenous objectives in education might have goals that include (but extend beyond) the dominant cultural objectives of English language literacy and employment outcomes. This is a key message of this chapter.

In comparison to non-Indigenous students, Indigenous students are more likely to be female, to be of lower socioeconomic status, to be of mature age, to be the first in their family to attend university, and to come from regional or remote Australia (Herbert, 2011). The student profile represented here may help us to understand the specific issues impacting on Indigenous students. For example, mature aged women may have families to care for, might need to move away from home, often have low income, and as well must deal with the unfamiliar academic environment.

Nakata et al. (2008) argued that, in the higher education context, the tensions between teaching and learning issues relating to curriculum content, pedagogy, and support measures for discrete academic skills need to be brought closer together. The authors suggest that "how Indigenous higher education students have been investigated in the literature both shapes and limits our understanding of them as learners in the academy" (p. 139). There is a need to understand Indigenous students as learners who are required to negotiate the complex junctures between their personal knowledge, perspective and experiences and the dominant disciplinary knowledges of the academy. One way to gain such understanding is to consider Indigenous pedagogy in the higher education context, which we address in the next section.

Indigenous Pedagogy

There is a need to develop a distinctive Indigenous pedagogy for learning in the health and human sciences. For this, a framework for appropriate knowledge and learning is required (Main et al., 2000). Importantly, education providers need to acknowledge the learner's personal agency in defining *success* within the parameters of the learner's values and belief systems. Herbert (2011, p. 5) questioned the capacity of (Australian) educational providers to:

accept the challenge of preparing the nation for its future as a culturally diverse nation. This is a vital issue for Indigenous education, for unless this nation can transition its peoples into a harmonious, democratic society where all people are treated with respect regardless of their cultural values and beliefs, then Aboriginal and Torres Strait Islander students will continue to struggle to achieve their rights and ensure that their success is a matter of choice – their own choice. This is a transition that has the power to change this nation's history.

There are complex relationships in the development of learning spaces, environments, models and enhanced literacy learning frameworks, with specific attention needed to participation, community and critical/quality engagement (Biermann, Garbutt, & Offord, 2010). Biermann et al. explicitly linked teaching with experience, in terms of engaging with the social, cultural and political realities of the world rather than in the form of more conventional professional placement (Couldry, 2000). The guiding principle of this methodological orientation comes from the renowned educationalist Paulo Freire, who explained, "studying is above all thinking about experience, and thinking about experience is the best way to think accurately" (1985, p. 3). A case study by Brown (2010), exemplifying this statement, focused on an *Indigenised space* at the intersection of Aboriginal pedagogy, philosophy and epistemology within a tertiary environment. The study focused specifically on relationships nurtured within a space created by Indigenous methods of teaching. Brown concluded that future research is vital in the theoretical implementation and description of this created space, as well as exploring the potential of pedagogies regarding the learning experience of both Indigenous and non-Indigenous students. Also important is the impact of the learning environment on the cultural competency and understanding of all students, and how this can be reflected in increasing the representation of Indigenous students through all levels of education (Brown, 2010, p. 15).

As Nakata (2004, p. 9) suggested:

To defend Indigenous peoples, Indigenous students require understanding of the concepts and methodologies of both systems of knowledge. That is, one can't do battle with Western systems of thought without understanding it, likewise, its inconsistencies cannot be turned around and an Indigenous perspective substituted without rigorous understanding of Indigenous concepts.

Clearly there is a need for reconciliation of both systems of knowledge, i.e. Indigenous and Western knowledges. Brown (2010) considered Indigenisation of the academy to be important in changing mainstream attitudes and creating learning environments where Indigenous peoples and knowledges are valued and equal. However, as highlighted by Townsend-Cross (2011), "Indigenous knowledges have been disembodied, dismembered and synthesised through dominant culture conceptual, ideological and theoretical assumptions and appropriated by the disciplines of the Academy" (p. 10). Furthermore, Nakata et al. (2008) noted that the literature on Indigenous student performance consistently confirms that changes to curricula and pedagogy remain negligible in the disciplines and in mainstream courses and programs. Changes are most evident in dedicated Indigenous programs run by or in conjunction with Indigenous departments and academic staff. Many universities now have Indigenous education strategy documents; some professional accreditation authorities, such as nursing and medical programs in Australia, require Indigenous content as part of curriculum content.

The proportion of Indigenous academics in the Australian university system is miniscule and is on a par with the proportion of Indigenous students at less than 1% (IHEAC, 2008). In response to the challenges faced by Aboriginal and Torres Strait Islander people in the higher education sector, and to increase the number of Indigenous academics in the higher education sector, a *National Indigenous Higher Education Workforce Strategy* (2011) was developed. In committing to the strategy, universities are urged to undertake capacity building; prioritise academic over non-academic appointments; and make efforts for faculties to actively recruit, develop and offer a career path for Indigenous employees at a level that reflects population parity. In the next section Wayne (Colin) Rigby shares his reflections about his experiences of becoming an Indigenous academic.

Becoming an Indigenous Academic: A Personal Reflection by Wayne (Colin) Rigby

This section is written particularly for Indigenous people starting off their career as University academics, based on reflections upon my experiences as a teacher in the higher education sector, especially teaching on courses dedicated to Indigenous students. Many issues, such as different interpretations of knowledge and the learning challenges discussed above, will confront Indigenous academics. How each of these issues is addressed and dealt with will depend on an individual's life experiences, academic knowledge, resilience and personality. The academic's attitude and commitment makes a significant difference for the student experience and the student's learning journey. As an Indigenous academic you are faced with social justice issues and the recognition that Australian Aboriginal people are the most educationally disadvantaged group within the country (Dodson, 1993). According to Dodson, education brings the prospect of genuine employment and good health, a life of choices and opportunity, and freedom from discrimination. In addition, Indigenous academics can take on a strong leadership role in the wider institution in advising on curriculum development, Indigenous issues and perspectives, teaching and learning, policy development and representation on various committees. Most importantly, Indigenous academics can advocate culturally appropriate practices in learning, teaching and assessment, as recognised in the following quotes:

You can only be a proud Aboriginal person if you carry your own learning and cultural lifestyle with you. (Galarrwuy Yunupingu, Chairman Yothu Yindi Foundation)

To me, Aboriginality is about that shared experience, that shared culture and that shared pride. (Amy McQuire, Aboriginal journalist, Koori Mail)

(Read more: http://www.creativespirits.info/aboriginalculture/people/aboriginal-identity.html#ixzz1t0avS1Gm)

A key to surviving as an academic in the higher education sector is to be adaptable, respectful and able to relate real-life experiences to academia. A cliché I have often used is that "if you haven't lived it you should not be teaching it". Relating personal experiences in teaching and facilitating the sharing of experiences from students can make learning and teaching more meaningful, and in professional health programs helps the teacher to maintain credibility. Furthermore, listening genuinely and sensitively to students' stories and experiences can generate learning that respects different cultures, values and diversity:

> ... a very special kind of listening, listening that requires not only open eyes and ears, but open hearts and minds. We do not really see through our eyes or hear through our ears, but through our beliefs ... we must learn to be vulnerable enough to allow our world to turn upside down in order to allow the realities of others to edge themselves into our consciousness. In other words, we must become ethnographers in the true sense. (Delpit, 1988, p. 297)

This method of two-way or dialogical learning can be the start of an academic adventure for both the student and the academic. Storytelling is an integral part of Aboriginal oral cultures and this can include stories from our experiences as a teacher, and stories from our own individual life, family and community. Storytelling is a means of passing on beliefs and social, spiritual, cultural and economic practices to the younger generations. This oral culture enabled a learning process commonly known as the Dreamtime, by which survival stories were passed on to the succeeding generations over many thousands of years. Shared stories and experiences allow connections with family and land which are important in the Australian Indigenous context. These kinds of interactions will assist in connecting with the Indigenous student, improving relationships and engaging the student, which in turn leads to a positive learning experience.

Some pedagogic methods and styles, such as didactic teaching and delivering information without interaction, can be alien to many Indigenous students who may feel that their own knowledges and experiences are therefore not valued. But there are many useful methods of teaching that can enhance learning within an Aboriginal pedagogy framework (Yunkaporta, 2007-2009). Visualised learning and the use of symbols is a core cultural learning technique and includes at times a hands-on approach closely related to what is now known as work-integrated learning. Reflective techniques can be especially useful to ensure that students are grasping what is taught. The use of land-based learning is equally crucial in establishing connection to land and family. This is because Australian Indigenous peoples have developed systems of knowledge and understanding in terms of a living symbiotic relationship with the land and waters of their traditional origins. This understanding of land is at the basis of all Aboriginal relationships, economies, identities, cultural practices, health and social and emotional wellbeing (Rigby, Rosen et al., 2011).

Through mentoring and role modelling the teacher facilitates teaching and learning processes and practices that can engender enthusiasm and motivation. This close support is a form of scaffolding (Rose, Lui-Chivizhe, McKnight, & Smith, 2003). A key strategy of such scaffolding when teaching unfamiliar content is to utilise information that the student is already familiar with and work from the familiar to the unfamiliar.

It is important to recognise that local Indigenous community engagement is integral to teaching Indigenous students and for university education and research. Engagement and involvement of the local Indigenous community is vital to the success of any university program that aspires to appeal to Indigenous students. An underlying aim is to enable students to bring new knowledge home to help "our mob", i.e. Indigenous communities. This requires a holistic approach to curriculum development and a pedagogy that involves strong family and community partnerships.

The learning environment for Indigenous students and for all students requires a focus on cultural competency, which is crucial in enhancing meaningful pathways for self-determination for students. For example, Indigenous cultures have a great wealth of knowledge to share about sustainability that are seen in terms of spiritual relationships to "Mother Earth". This is closely related to the belief that those who understand their culture can understand their past (Treuquil & Lem Masc, 2010). In recent years we have begun to realise that there is a need for the wider population to understand these issues; this has driven the move to develop cultural competency as a requirement of all university graduates in countries like Australia and New Zealand.

Cultural competence, which is different from cultural competency (see below), requires a strong awareness of how one's own culture shapes attitudes, perceptions and behaviours. It also requires recognition of the importance of diversity, willingness to learn about other people's cultures, language, customs and values, and the ability to feel comfortable and communicate effectively with people from diverse cultural backgrounds. A position paper developed by the Diversity Health Institute succinctly captures the meaning of cultural competence at the individual level:

> The ability to identify and challenge one's own cultural assumptions, one's values and beliefs. It is about developing empathy and connected knowledge, the ability to see the world through another's eyes, or at the very least, to recognise that others may view the world through different cultural lenses. (Fitzgerald, 2000, cited by Stewart, 2006, p. 3)

The term *competence* here describes a broader outcome to be achieved, whereas *competency* refers to a narrower concept that is used to label specific skills and abilities that are observable and assessable. At the broader university level, cultural competence involves integrating respect for diversity in education programs, teaching guidelines and policies, which need to be transparent and practised in the teaching environment. Cultural competence requires:

that organisations have a clearly defined, congruent set of values and principles, and demonstrate behaviours, attitudes, policies, structures and practices that enable them to work effectively cross-culturally. (NCCC, 2006)

Cultural competence is best viewed as an ongoing process and an ideal to strive towards and, as (Diller, 2004) argued, rather than simply complying with legislation, meeting minimum standards of practice, or having a fixed end-point, cultural competence is a continually evolving process.

In recognition of the importance of cultural competence and competency, Universities Australia (2011b, p. 175) developed a national best-practice framework for Indigenous cultural competency in Australian universities, which is based on an extensive literature review, the evaluation of practice both in Australia and overseas, and four pilot projects. These data have informed the creation of a set of five guiding principles for Indigenous cultural competency:

- Indigenous people should be actively involved in university governance and management.
- All graduates of Australian universities should be culturally competent.
- University research should be conducted in a culturally competent way that empowers Indigenous participants and encourages collaborations with Indigenous communities.
- Indigenous staffing will be increased at all appointment levels and, for academic staff, across a wider variety of academic fields.
- Universities will operate in partnership with their Indigenous communities and will help disseminate culturally competent practices to the wider community.

Going beyond this, however, Universities Australia (2011a) also developed "Guiding principles for developing Indigenous cultural competency in Australian universities" in the area of learning and teaching, stating that all graduates of Australian universities should be culturally competent. The following recommendations and examples can assist Australian universities in learning and teaching development:

a) Embed Indigenous knowledges and perspectives in all university curricula to provide students with the knowledge, skills and understandings which form the foundations of Indigenous cultural competency.

b) Include Indigenous cultural competency as a formal graduate attribute or quality.

181

c) Incorporate Indigenous Australian knowledges and perspectives into programs according to a culturally competent pedagogical framework.

d) Train teaching staff in Indigenous pedagogy for teaching Indigenous studies and students effectively, including developing appropriate content and learning resources, teaching strategies and assessment methods.

e) Create reporting mechanisms and standards which provide quality assurance and accountability of Indigenous studies curricula. (2011a, p. 9)

These guiding principles provide the higher education sector with a framework for embedding Indigenous cultural competencies within and across institutions in sustainable ways that engender reconciliation and social justice by supporting the factors that contribute to social, economic and political change.

SUMMARY

In this chapter we have explored Indigenous issues in health professional education from several perspectives: Indigenous students in mainstream and dedicated health programs, Indigenous academics new to the academy, and Indigenous pedagogy. We have presented these issues from a critical stance that will stimulate further inquiry for new academics entering the world of teaching, learning and research in the academy. We hope this chapter helps your understanding of the complex nature of Indigenous issues, particularly in the context of health and health professional education.

REFERENCES

Biermann, S., Garbutt, R. G., & Offord, B. (2010). Cultural studies in action: Principled socially inclusive pedagogy and higher education equity projects. In N. Riseman, S. Rechter & E. Warne (Eds.), *Learning, teaching and social justice in higher education* (pp. 85-99). Melbourne, VIC: Electronic Scholarly Publishing.

Bradley, D., Noonan, P., Nugent, H., & Scales, B. (2008). *Review of Australian higher education: Final report.* Canberra: Commonwealth of Australia.

Brown, L. (2010). Nurturing relationships within a space created by 'Indigenous ways of knowing': A case study [online]. *Australian Journal of Indigenous Education, 39*(Suppl.), 15-22. Retrieved from http://www.uwa.edu.au/_data/assets/rtf_file/0009/.../Brown_Abstract.rtf

Bryant, M., Scoufis, M., & Cheers, M. (1999). The transformation of higher education in Australia: University teaching is at a crossroad. *Proceedings of the Higher Education Research Development Society of Australasia Annual International Conference.* Retrieved from http://www.herdsa.org.au/?page_id=182

Couldry, N. (2000). *Inside culture: Re-imagining the method of cultural studies.* London: Sage.

Delpit, L. D. (1988). The silenced dialogue: Power and pedagogy in educating other people's children. *Harvard Educational Review, 58*(3), 280-298.

Department of Education, Employment and Workplace Relations (DEEWR). (2009). *Selected higher education statistics 2008.*

Diller, J. V. (2004). *Cultural diversity: A primer for the human services* (2nd ed.). Belmont. CA: Brooks/Cole.

Dodson, M. (1993). *Annual report of the Aboriginal and Torres Strait Islander Social Justice Commissioner.* Canberra: Australian Government.

Freire, P. (1985). *The politics of education: Culture, power and liberation.* New York: Bergin and Garvey.

Herbert, J. (2011). *Educational success: A sustainable outcome for all Indigenous students when teachers understand where the learning journey begins.* Australian Council for Educational Research Conference. Indigenous Education: Pathways to success. Keynote address, 7-9 August 2011.

Indigenous Higher Education Advisory Council (IHEAC). (2006). *Improving Indigenous outcomes and enhancing Indigenous culture and knowledge in Australian higher education.* Canberra: Department of Education, Science and Training.

Indigenous Higher Education Advisory Council (IHEAC). (2008). *Supplementary submission to the review of Australian higher education.* Retrieved from http://foi.deewr.gov.au/documents/indigenous-higher-education-advisory-council-supplementary-submission-review-australian

Main, D., Nichol, R., & Fennell, R. (2000). Reconciling pedagogy and health sciences to promote Indigenous health. *Australian and New Zealand Journal of Public Health, 24*(2), 211-213.

National Centre for Cultural Competence (NCCC). (2006). *Conceptual frameworks/models, guiding values and principles.* Washington DC: Georgetown University Child Development Centre.

Nakata, M. (2004). *Indigenous Australian studies and higher education.* Paper presented at the Wentworth Lectures, Canberra.

Nakata, M., Nakata, V., & Chin, M. (2008). Approaches to the academic preparation and support of Australian Indigenous students for tertiary studies. *The Australian Journal of Indigenous Education, 37*, 137-145.

National Indigenous Higher Education Workforce Strategy (NIHEWS). (2011). Retrieved from http://foi.deewr.gov.au/documents/national-indigenous-higher-education-workforce-strategy

Radloff, A., & Coates, H. (2010). *Doing more for learning: Enhancing engagement and outcomes. Australasian student engagement report.* Camberwell: ACER.

Rigby, C. W., Rosen, A., Berry, H. L., & Hart, C. R. (2011). If the land's sick, we're sick: The impact of prolonged drought on the social and emotional well-being of Aboriginal communities in rural NSW. *Australian Journal of Rural Health, 19*, 249-254.

Rigby, W., Duffy, E., Manners, J., Latham, H., Lyons, L., Crawford, L. et al. (2011). Closing the gap: Cultural safety in Indigenous health education. *Contemporary Nurse, 37*(1), 21-30.

Rigney, L. I. (1999). The first perspective: On or with Indigenous peoples. *1999 Chacmool Conference Proceedings, University of Calgary, Alberta, Canada.* Internationalisation of an Indigenous anti-colonial cultural critique of research methodologies: A guide to Indigenist research methodology and its principles. *Higher Education Research and Development in Higher Education (HERDHE), 20*, 629-636.

Rose, D., Lui-Chivizhe, L., McKnight, A., & Smith, A. (2003), Scaffolding academic reading and writing at the Koori Centre. *The Australian Journal of Indigenous Education, 32*, 41-49.

Stewart, S. (2006). *Cultural competence in health care.* Sydney West Area Health Service: Diversity Health Institute Position Paper.

Townsend-Cross, M. (2011). Indigenous education and Indigenous studies in the Australian academy – assimilationism, critical pedagogy, dominant culture learners and Indigenous knowledges. In G. Dei (Ed.), *Indigenous philosophies and critical education* (pp. 2-23). New York: Peter Lang.

Treuquil, F., & Lem Masc, V. (2010). The wisdom of Indigenous cultures. Retrieved from http://www.celsias.com/article/wisdom-indigenous-cultures/

United Nations. (2008). *Declaration on the rights of Indigenous peoples.* Geneva, UN.

Universities Australia. (2011a). *Guiding principles for developing Indigenous cultural competency in Australian universities.* Canberra: Universities Australia. Retrieved from http://www.universitiesaustralia.edu.au/lightbox/1312

Universities Australia. (2011b). *National best practice framework for Indigenous cultural competency in Australian universities.* Canberra: Universities Australia. Retrieved from http://www.universitiesaustralia.edu.au/lightbox/13123

Usher, K., Miller, A., Lindsay, D., Miller, M., O'Connor, T., Turale, S. et al. (2003). *Successful strategies for the retention of Indigenous students in nursing courses*. Unpublished report to the Queensland Nursing Council Research Committee, School of Nursing Sciences, James Cook University, Queensland.

Usher, K., Lindsay, D., Miller, M., & Miller, A. (2005). Challenges faced by Indigenous nursing students and strategies that aided their progress in the course: A descriptive study. *Contemporary Nurse, 19*(1-2), 17-31.

West, R., Usher, K., & Foster, K. (2010). Increased numbers of Australian Indigenous nurses would make a significant contribution to 'closing the gap' in Indigenous health: What is getting in the way? *Contemporary Nurse, 36*(1-2), 121-130.

West, R., West, L., West, K., & Usher, K. (2011). Tjirtamai – 'To care for': A nursing education model designed to increase the number of Aboriginal nurses in a rural and remote Queensland community. *Contemporary Nurse, 37*(1), 39-48.

Yunkaporta, T. (2009). *Draft report for DET on Indigenous research project: Aboriginal pedagogies at the cultural interface* (pp. 1-43). Aboriginal Education Consultant in Western NSW Region Schools.

Elaine Duffy RN, RM, DipAppSc(CHN),BAppSc(AdvNsg),MN, PhD, FRCNA
School of Nursing and Midwifery
Griffith University, Australia

Wayne (Colin) Rigby RN, BSW, MHSc(PHC)
Mental Health
Murrumbidgee Central, Australia

HUGH BARR AND JULIA COYLE

16. INTRODUCING INTERPROFESSIONAL EDUCATION

Health professionals everywhere are working with a more damaged, more dependent and more demanding clientele than in the past: in wealthier countries resulting most obviously from the number of older people living longer with chronic, complex and multiple problems; in poorer countries from the number of families at the mercy of infant mortality, malnutrition, the killer childhood diseases and the HIV pandemic (WHO, 2009). Professionals under pressure to respond to these situations have three choices: to set aside those problems for which they have neither authorisation nor training; to go beyond their roles at risk of stress and overload for themselves and less than adequate care for their patients; or to work more closely with other professions to spread the load and respond more fully to the range of needs (Barr & Gray, forthcoming). The third option may seem self-evident, but as the interprofessional literature confirms (Meads, Ashcroft, Barr, Scott, & Wild, 2005), it is easier said than done. How then can professional education best prepare the entry-level practitioner?

SURMOUNTING THE BARRIERS

The barriers to closer collaboration erected during pre-licensure courses are formidable. Each profession engages in a process of "closure" through its own educational system with its own regulations, governance, corpus of knowledge and field of practice (Freidson, 1993). Students are socialised into the values of their newfound profession, each with its different culture and its unique ways of thinking and acting (Clarke, 1995, 1997; Hall, 2005). Distinctive semantics and discourses, modes of dress, demeanour and norms of behaviour associated with a profession perpetuate professional mores and beliefs.

There is much in the professionalisation process that is precious and worthy of preservation, but that same process comes with a downside in need of remedy before tomorrow's workers will be ready for the demands of collaborative practice. Courses for the various professions may be scattered across schools, campuses and universities. Often, neither students nor teachers from the different professions interact, rendering opportunities to learn with, from and about each other well nigh impossible. Small wonder that students identify with their intended profession to the exclusion of others if reciprocal perceptions are, at best, ill-informed and, at worst, stereotypical. Yet in spite of this progress is being made.

Barriers are being lowered as educational institutions amalgamate and modular courses are introduced. Learning is being liberated by technology as advances in

S. Loftus et al. (Eds.), Educating Health Professionals:
Becoming a University Teacher, 185–196.

informatics and communication pave the way for the professions to learn together. Common studies are being included in curricula, and extended over time. Educators are identifying overlaps in curricula in their professional courses, learning to trust each other with their students as they respond to pressures to effect economies of scale, but these are not enough without also including interprofessional education (IPE) (Barr, 2002).

This chapter:

- distinguishes between multiprofessional and interprofessional education
- describes interprofessional teaching and learning and its theoretical underpinnings
- focuses on the teacher's facilitation role
- reviews the evidence for the efficacy of IPE.

MULTIPROFESSIONAL AND INTERPROFESSIONAL EDUCATION

Learning shared between professions may comprise *multiprofessional* education, as with core subjects that span professional curricula such as physiology or psychology, or *interprofessional* education, as in collaborative learning for collaborative practice. The multiprofessional learning may be part of common curricula delivered in large groups by didactic teaching. The interprofessional learning is interactive between the professions, in small groups typically comprising 8–12 students from different professional courses drawn from the hundreds or even thousands in the interprofessional cohort. Understanding the difference in outcomes, content, learning methods and teaching roles between multiprofessional and interprofessional learning is critical. Each complements the other operationally, provided that they are distinguished conceptually.

INTEPROFESSIONAL EDUCATION IN ESSENCE

IPE occurs where two or more professions learn with, from and about each other to improve collaboration and the quality of care. (CAIPE, 2002)

IPE is outcome- and competency-based, enshrined in Canadian, UK and U.S. statements that promote models of good collaborative practice (Canadian Interprofessional Health Collaborative, 2010; Combined Universities Interprofessional Learning Unit, 2010; Interprofessional Education Collaborative, 2011, respectively) and formulated sufficiently broadly to be adapted in other countries such as Australia (Brewer & Jones, 2011). IPE strives to promote flexible, mutually supportive and cost-effective collaborative practice in interprofessional teams as students explore ways in which their professions can work better together, to respond more fully to compound and complex needs of individuals, families and communities within a policy-aware understanding of organisational relationships. It is dedicated to holistic care and the improvement of services, within a transcending socially accountable concept of professionalism.

Central to the achievement of those outcomes is the need to be responsive to patient and public expectations, while preserving and protecting the identity and integrity of each profession (Barr & Low, 2012). Thus, IPE is characterised by experiences that explore not only similarities between the professions but also differences, which range from the more tangible such as roles, responsibilities, knowledge and skills to the less tangible such as attitudes, perceptions and values. Facilitating this exploration requires a repertoire of interactive learning methods (such as those included below) that educators "mix and match" in response to different learning needs, to ring the changes, and to hold students' interest (Barr & Gray, forthcoming).

Examples of teaching approaches supportive of interprofessional learning

---

Case-based learning

Presents multiple and progressively more complex problems for the students to assess, focused towards developing a holistic understanding beyond that which any one profession may identify alone, opening the way to explore how each profession can best exercise its role and deploy its expertise to complement that of the others within the team (Higgs & Jones, 2000).

Observation-based learning

Enables groups of students from different professions to compare their perspectives, for example, when following patients throughout their treatment experience (D'Avray, Gill, & Coster, 2007) or making joint visits by invitation to patients in their homes (Lennox & Anderson, 2007).

Appreciative inquiry

Enables students to exchange their experiences of good practice and explore ways to disseminate it (Cooperrider & Whitney, 2005).

Problem-based learning

Enables students to learn how to work together, focusing on the resolution of problems (Barrows, 1996).

Continuous quality improvement

Derived from "total quality management", is a cyclical process to engage practising professionals in improving systems and services from the bottom up, with interprofessional learning as a by-product (Walton, 1988, citing Deming).

Collaborative inquiry
Involves the interested parties in a similar investigative process (Heron & Reason, 2008).
Simulation-based learning
Has referred for many years in IPE to exercises such as role-play, but increasingly includes also the creation of virtual learning environments (Walsh & van Soeren, 2012) and the adoption of laboratory-based simulated learning on manikins in IPE. For example, students from, medicine, nursing and physiotherapy practise their respective interventions as members of an interprofessional team observed by their fellows, followed by debriefing (Freeth, Ayida, Berridge, Sadler, & Strachen, 2006; Mikkelsen Krykjebo, Brattebo, & Smith-Strom, 2006).

Educators tend to prefer methods commonly employed in their field of professional education, but opting for only one method is needlessly constraining, inhibiting opportunities to respond to the range and diversity of students' needs and learning styles. Experienced teachers ring the changes to hold the interest of their students and to match the content.

Interprofessional learning methods such as these may be introduced from the beginning of students' pre-licensure[i] courses or later when they have had time to identify with their respective professions and have some experience to share. The learning may be discrete, as in dedicated modules or sequences, or permeate the professional curricula in the classroom and clinical settings. It may be mediated by technology, including simulated learning, reusable objects and virtual environments adapted from professional learning, or originate in interprofessional learning (Barr, Helme, & D'Avray, 2011). It may put the emphasis on improving mutual understanding, countering ignorance and resolving misconceptions between the professional groups, with the expectation that closer collaboration will follow, although that can overplay the negatives in interprofessional relations, driving students into a downward spiral where the positives (from which interprofessional learning draws its examples) are obscured. Inducing guilt is counterproductive. A culture of blame has no place in interprofessional learning.

Students feel less threatened when educators help them to understand how rivalries and misunderstandings between professions can result from differing structures, boundaries, cultures, priorities and policies between organisations. Introducing such explanations does not detract from interpersonal and interprofessional responsibilities; it does, however, keep them in proportion. Official inquiries, such as into child abuse or medical error, bring these issues into sharp relief, attributing as they do adverse events to lapses in communication and trust between professions (see e.g. Institute of Medicine, 2000; Kennedy, 2001; Laming, 2003, 2009). Their reports provide powerful learning material, but students encountering a critical report for the first time can be disconcerted, dispirited or even debilitated, more so if it is accompanied by damning coverage in the media. Such reports are nevertheless a compelling source of learning, driving home "the collaborative imperative" as they forewarn and forearm students for the rough ride that may lie ahead.

Interprofessional teaching is more effective when it values the positive which each profession brings to collaborative practice, harnessing energy and expertise across professions to improve services and to provide more rounded care in response to the complex needs of individuals, families and communities. Problems that impede collaborative practice can be dealt with if and when they arise.

Teaching which is outward and forward looking encourages and enables students to establish mutually supportive relationships as they discover how their respective expertise, albeit in its formative stages, complements and reinforces each other towards shared goals. Trust and mutual respect may be cultivated over time as they learn from each other, grounded in mutual understanding of their abilities, experiences and perspectives (McCallin, 1999; Blue & Fitzgerald, 2002).

All placements can provide interprofessional learning opportunities such as shadowing members of another profession or observing team meetings. They may be linked to create opportunities for students from different professional courses to get acquainted, compare experiences, discuss cases and perhaps engage in joint activities such as service audits and surveys. Some may be lucky enough to be placed in an interprofessional student team, such as on an interprofessional training ward (Jacobsen, Fink, Marcussen, Larsen, & Hansen, 2009). Barr and Brewer (2012) have made the case for greater investment in interprofessional student team placements in community and hospital settings, to build on interprofessional learning during uniprofessional placements.

Learning methods introduced into IPE apply and extend the principles of adult learning, where students are responsible for managing their own learning not only individually but also collectively and collaboratively (Barr et al., 2011). The students construct their learning experientially (Kolb, 1984) and reflectively (Schön, 1987) within a community of practice (Lave & Wenger, 1991). Schön's distinction between reflecting in practice (at the time) and on practice (after the event, with benefit of hindsight) is critical in interprofessional learning, where the significance of the complex interactions observed in practice may be overwhelming but can be made clearer during debriefing. So is Wackerhausen's (2009) distinction between first order reflection, which is confirmatory, and second order reflection, which casts experiences in a fresh light. Students may co-reflect from their different professional perspectives, testing and sometimes challenging others' attitudes and assumptions, perceptions and prejudices.

Those from the humanistic professions may be more accustomed to such constructivist learning than those from the positivist science-based professions in which more emphasis is placed on didactic teaching that hands down evidence-based knowledge (Barr et al., 2011). Evidence nevertheless must be applied in different settings by different professions, calling for discussion between the parties. Didactic teaching needs therefore to be complemented by constructivist learning between the professions for it to be applied in collaborative practice.

IPE is grounded not only in the principles of adult learning, but also in a coherent and consistent theoretical rationale which the educators distil as they compare and contrast anthropological, educational, psycho-dynamic, socio-psychological or sociological perspectives which they introduce from their academic disciplines and practice professions (Barr, Koppel, Reeves, Hammick, & Freeth, 2005; Colyer, Helme, & Jones, 2005; Hean, Craddock, & O'Halloran, 2009; Barr, 2013).

The assessment of IPE may be formative or summative. Formative assessment is preferable in the early stages of developing such learning and for group assignments where it is difficult to isolate the contribution of each student. However, students may value interprofessional learning more when assessment is summative and counts towards their professional qualifications. For example, demonstrating what they have gained from interprofessional learning experiences can be incorporated into profession-specific assignments. Peer appraisals may be better confined to formative assessment where they feed back into ongoing learning not only for the individual being assessed but also for the group. A practice teacher should be designated to work with each ad hoc interprofessional student group co-located in the same placement setting, at the same time, working in partnership with their uniprofessional practice teachers.

Arrangements are often made to combine professions from different schools, faculties and even universities to obtain the preferred student mix. However, balancing numbers can remain less than ideal, given the markedly different size of the student populations in the professional courses. Nurses invariably comprise the largest single group, with the smaller professions, including those from allied health, thinly spread. This imbalance may hamper students' capacity to voice a professional opinion if they find themselves in the minority. It is critical in this respect for educators to consider at the outset the implications of the group's composition for its culture and dynamics, especially where one or more much-needed party to collaborative practice, such as medicine or social work, is missing.

There is a case for including as many of the practice-related health and social care professions as possible in pre-licensure IPE, but the wider the spread the greater the challenge for students and educators. A large group comprising many professions may be better subdivided for part of the interprofessional experience, bringing together students from no more than two or three professions for learning designed to focus on cases and situations where they are likely to collaborate in working life. Adverse experiences resulting from teachers' inability to facilitate large, diverse groups effectively can impact negatively on students' perceptions of IPE and, by association, interprofessional practice.

TEACHING AND FACILITATING

Facilitating interprofessional learning requires insights and skills additional to those needed when facilitating professional learning. It entails working with students, teachers and practitioners from other professions in unfamiliar fields. The facilitator enables the student group to optimise its learning by calling on resources in, through and beyond its members and their respective professions, sensitive to the perspectives and perceptions of each, above all enabling the group to translate problems into opportunities (Rees & Johnson, 2007; Howkins & Bray, 2008; Anderson, Cox, & Thorpe, 2009; Freeman, Wright, & Lindqvist, 2010; Barr et al., 2011).

The facilitator resists pressure to assume the didactic role unless and until the group has exhausted its own learning capacity. He or she encourages the students to view the group as a microcosm of collaboration in working life, as a test-bed under safe and controlled conditions to develop their collaborative skills, as an opportunity to review what can get in the way and to explore more productive ways of working together. Co-facilitating enables colleagues from different professions to complement each other's insights and interventions.

Experienced facilitators understand how students behave in an interprofessional group, the roles that each may play in leading or obstructing its work, assisting or impeding the learning of others, and the conflicts and rivalries that can intrude, overlaid by power and status differentials. Some students are less accustomed than others to learning in small groups or feel at a disadvantage by virtue of their social or educational backgrounds. Others may be more forthcoming, more confident in taking the lead, in ways that fellow students may welcome or resist.

Facilitation entails briefing students for an interprofessional assignment, identifying with them during the learning process and helping them to compare and contrast what they experienced or observed from their different professional perspectives. It relates back to earlier learning, applying theory to practice as students come to understand their own and fellow group members' feelings, responses and behaviour, reinforcing positive examples of collaborative practice and remedying weaknesses. Much the same process applies for educators as they plan the interprofessional learning experience, review its progress and evaluate its outcomes, taking into account their own effectiveness in exercising their roles and managing their relationships with each other.

The facilitation process applies critically before, during, and after practice placements and is shared between the university and the practice educator. Responsibility for the briefing rests, in the first instance, with the university educator, then with the practice educator when the student(s) arrive in the placement setting. On-hand facilitation during the placement clearly rests with the practice educator, but may be complemented by the university educator during one or more visit during the placement. Responsibility for debriefing rests in the first instance with the practice educator followed by further debriefing with the university educator when the student(s) return. A fuller exploration of the roles of these two facilitators would extend beyond the scope of this chapter. Suffice it to say that the learning for the student(s) depends critically on the rapport and mutual understanding between them.

ESTABLISHING THE EVIDENCE

IPE is frequently included in validation for pre-licensure courses, less often for post-licensure courses, except when they are university-based within approved programs. Furthermore, interprofessional inputs may be subject to evaluation to elicit student feedback to inform revision of content and learning methods for subsequent intakes. These evaluations typically use questionnaires administered post-hoc focusing on students' satisfaction. More rigorous evaluations comprise before-and-after studies using questionnaires, validated instruments and sometimes interviews or focus groups, which can provide evidence of changes of attitude or behaviour during the interprofessional learning period; yet others intervene measures during the learning and sometime afterwards. Data generated are illuminating, provided that they are accompanied by evaluations of process (Freeth, Hammick, Reeves, Koppel, & Barr, 2005a; Freeth, Reeves, Koppel, Hammick, & Barr, 2005b).

Evidence regarding the efficacy of IPE has been assembled in successive systematic reviews of international databases (see Reeves, Goldman, Burton, & Sawatzky-Girling, 2010, for a review of reviews). Two employed criteria agreed with the Cochrane Collaboration (Zwarenstein et al., 2001; Reeves et al., 2008). A less restrictive review (Barr et al., 2005, refined subsequently by Hammick, Freeth, Reeves, Koppel, & Barr, 2007) focused on 107 rigorous evaluations, of which half came from the U.S. and a quarter from the UK, with the remainder thinly spread. Four-fifths were post-licensure. Outcomes classified on a scale adapted from Kirkpatrick (1967) indicated that pre-licensure IPE established foundations for collaborative practice. They also found that IPE modified reciprocal attitudes and perceptions between the professional groups, laying the foundations for the post-licensure IPE which could change practice.

INTERPROFESSIONAL NETWORKING

Progress made in promoting and developing IPE as described in this chapter would have been inconceivable had it not been for the readiness of IPE teachers to share their experience locally, nationally and internationally through conferences and peer-reviewed articles and reports in the *Journal of Interprofessional Care* dedicated to the promotion of collaboration in education, practice and research (http://www.informaworld.com/jic).

"Collaboratives" and "networks" have been launched in those world regions where IPE is firmly established, to facilitate the exchange of information, mount conferences and respond to enquiries.

- The American Interprofessional Health Collaborative (AIHC)
  http://www.aihc-us.org/
- The Australasian Interprofessional Practice and Education Network (AIPPEN)
  http://www.aippen.net/

- The UK-based Centre for the Advancement of Interprofessional Education (CAIPE)
  http://www.caipe.org.uk
- The Canadian Interprofessional Health Collaborative (CIHC)
  http://www.cihc.ac.
- The European Interprofessional Education Network (EIPEN)
  http://www.eipen.org/
- The Japan Association for Interprofessional Education (JAIPE)
  http://www.jaipe.jp/
- The Nordic Interprofessional Education Network (NIPNET)
  http://www.nipnet.org

These organisations support a rolling program of global biennial *All Together Better Health* conferences (http://www.k-co.co.jp/atbh6.html) and are working towards establishing an effective international and interprofessional "umbrella" body.

CONCLUDING THOUGHTS

IPE is taking root in a growing number of countries, enjoying various degrees of backing and endorsement from government and professional institutions, but underscored in reports commissioned by the World Health Organization (WHO, 1988, 2010) and forming a central plank in the strategy to promote global health (Frenk et al., 2010). It is constantly adapting and evolving as it extends into wider fields in response to the changing demands of practice in countries with different approaches to the organisation and delivery of health and social care. Progress has nevertheless been made in defining terms and in formulating principles and methodology which enjoy widespread and consistent currency, which we have tried to capture in this chapter.

NOTES

[i] Licensure is defined as "the granting of a licence, especially to carry out a trade or profession" (Oxford Dictionary, 2011). Thus, pre-licensure refers to all health courses that graduate students at an entry level to their professions.

REFERENCES

Anderson, E. S., Cox, D., & Thorpe, L. N. (2009). Preparation of educators involved in interprofessional education. *Journal of Interprofessional Care, 23*(1), 81-94.

Barr, H. (2013). Towards a theoretical framework for interprofessional education. *Journal of Interprofessional Care, 27*(1), 4-9. doi:10.3109/13561820.2012.698328

Barr, H. (2002). *Interprofessional education: Today, yesterday and tomorrow.* London: LTSN Health Sciences and Practice.

Barr, H., Helme, M., & D'Avray, L. (2011). *Developing interprofessional education in health and social care courses in the United Kingdom.* Higher Education Academy: Health Sciences and Practice, Occasional Paper 12. Retrieved from http://www.health.heacademy.ac.uk

Barr, H., & Brewer, M. (2012). Interprofessional practice-based education. In J. Higgs, J.R. Barnett, S. Billett, M. Hutchings, & F. Trede (Eds.), *Practice-based education: Perspectives and strategies* (pp. 199-212). Rotterdam: Sense.

Barr, H., & Gray, R. (forthcoming). Interprofessional education: Learning together in health and social care. In K. Walsh (Ed.), *The Oxford textbook of medical education.* Oxford: Oxford University Press.

Barr, H., Koppel, I., Reeves, S., Hammick, M., & Freeth, D. (2005). *Effective interprofessional education: Argument, assumption and evidence.* Oxford: Blackwell.

Barr, H. & Low, H. (2012). *Interprofessional education in pre-registration courses: A CAIPE guide for commissioners and regulators of education.* London: CAIPE.

Barrows, H. S. (1996). Problem-based learning in medicine and beyond: A brief overview. In L. Wilkerson & W. H. Gijselaers (Eds.), *Bringing problem-based learning to higher education: New directions for teaching and learning* (pp. 3-12). San Francisco: Jossey-Bass.

Blue, I., & Fitzgerald, M. (2002). Interprofessional relations: Case studies of working relationships between registered nurses and general practitioners in rural Australia. *Journal of Clinical Nursing, 11*, 314-321.

Brewer, M., & Jones, S. (2011). *Client centred care: The foundation for an interprofessional capability framework.* European Interprofessional Education Conference, 14-16 September, Ghent, Belgium.

CAIPE. (2002). Interprofessional education – A definition. Retrieved from http://www.caipe.org.uk

Canadian Interprofessional Health Collaborative. (2010). *A national interprofessional competency framework.* Retrieved from http://www.cihc.ca/files/CIHC_IPCompetencies_Feb1210.pdf

Clarke, P. (1995). Quality of life, values and teamwork in geriatric care. Do we communicate what we mean? *The Gerontologist, 35*(3), 402-411.

Clarke, P. (1997). Values in healthcare professional socialisation: Implications for geriatric education in interprofessional teamwork. *The Gerontologist, 37*(4), 441-451.

Colyer, H., Helme, M., & Jones, I. (2005). *The theory–practice relationship in interprofessional education.* London: Higher Education Academy Health Sciences & Practice, Occasional Paper No. 7.

Combined Universities Interprofessional Learning Unit. (2010). *Interprofessional capability framework 2010 mini-guide.* London: Higher Education Academy Subject Centre for Health Sciences and Practice.

Cooperrider, D. L., & Whitney, D. (2005). *Appreciate inquiry: A positive revolution in change.* San Francisco: Berrett-Koehler.

D'Avray, L., Gill, E., & Coster, S. (2007). Interprofessional learning in practice in South East London. In H. Barr (Ed.), *Piloting interprofessional education: Four English case studies*, Occasional paper no. 8 (pp. 30-42). Higher Education Academy: Health Sciences and Practice. Retrieved from http://repos.hsap.kcl.ac.uk/content/m10208/latest/occp8.pdf

Freeman, S., Wright, A., & Lindqvist, S. (2010). Training for educators involved in interprofessional learning. *Journal of Interprofessional Care, 24*(4), 375-385.

Freeth, D., Ayida, G., Berridge, E., Sadler, C., & Strachen, A. (2006). MOSES: Multidisciplinary Obstetric Simulated Emergency Scenarios. *Journal of Interprofessional Care, 20*(5), 552-554.

Freeth, D., Hammick, M., Reeves, S., Koppel, I., & Barr, H. (2005a). *Effective interprofessional education: Development, delivery and evaluation.* Oxford: Blackwell with CAIPE.

Freeth, D., Reeves, S., Koppel, I., Hammick, M., & Barr, H. (2005b). *Evaluating interprofessional education: A self-help guide.* Higher Education Academy, Health Sciences and Practice. Retrieved from http://repos.hsap.kcl.ac.uk/content/m10250/latest/occp5.pdf

Freidson, E. (1993). How dominant are the professions? In F. W. Hafferty & J. B. McKinlay (Eds.), *The changing medical profession: An international perspective* (pp. 54-66). New York: Oxford University Press.

Frenk, J., Chen, L., Bhutta, Z. A., Cohen, J., Crisp, N., Evans, T., et al. (2010). Health professionals for a new century: Transforming education to strengthen health systems in an interdependent world. A Global Independent Commission. *The Lancet, 376*(9756), 1923-1958. doi:10.1016/50140-6736(10)61854-5

Hall, P. (2005). Interprofessional teamwork: Professional cultures as barriers. *Journal of Interprofessional Care, 19*(Suppl. 1), 186-196.

Hammick, M., Freeth, D., Koppel, I., Reeves, S., & Barr, H. (2007). A best evidence systematic review of interprofessional education: BEME Guide No. 9. *Medical Teacher, 29*(8), 735-751. doi:10.1080/01421590701682576

Hean, S., Craddock, D., & O'Halloran, C. (2009). Learning theories and interprofessional education. *Learning in Health and Social Care, 8*(4), 250-262.

Heron, J., & Reason, P. (2008). Extending epistemology within a cooperative inquiry. In P. Reason & H. Bradbury (Eds.), *Handbook of action research* (2nd ed., pp. 367-380). London: Sage.

Higgs, J., & Jones, M. A. (2000). Clinical reasoning in health professions. In J. Higgs & M. A. Jones (Eds.), *Clinical reasoning in the health professions* (pp. 3-14). London: Butterworth-Heinemann Medical.

Howkins, E., & Bray, J. (2008). *Preparing for interprofessional teaching: Theory and practice.* Oxford: Radcliffe Publishing. Retrieved from http//www2.Cochrane.org/reviews/en/ab000072.html

Institute of Medicine. (2000). *To err is human: Building a safer health system.* Washington, DC: National Academy Press.

Interprofessional Education Collaborative Expert Panel. (2011). *Core competencies for interprofessional collaborative practice: Report of an expert panel.* Washington, D.C: Interprofessional Education Collaborative. Retrieved from https://www.aamc.org/download/186750/data/core_competencies.pdf

Jacobsen, F., Fink, A. M., Marcussen, V., Larsen, K., & Hansen, T. B. (2009). Interprofessional undergraduate clinical learning: Results from a three year project in a Danish interprofessional training unit. *Journal of Interprofessional Care, 23*, 30-40.

Kennedy, I. (2001). *The report of the public inquiry into children's heart surgery at the Bristol Royal Infirmary, 1984-1995.* London: The Stationery Office.

Kirkpatrick, D. L. (1967). Evaluation of training. In R. Craig & L. Bittel (Eds.), *Training and development handbook* (pp. 87-112). New York: McGraw-Hill.

Kolb, D. A. (1984). *Experiential learning: Experience as the source of learning and development.* Englewood Cliffs, NJ: Prentice Hall.

Laming, H. (2003). *The Victoria Climbie Inquiry: Report of an inquiry.* London: HMSO.

Laming, H. (2009). *The protection of children in England: A progress report.* London: The Stationery Office.

Lave, J., & Wenger, E. (1991). *Situated learning: Legitimate peripheral participation.* Cambridge: Cambridge University Press.

Lennox, A., & Anderson, E. (2007). *The Leicester model of interprofessional education: A practical guide for implementation in health and social care.* Special report 9. Newcastle: Higher Education Academy: Medicine, Dentistry and Veterinary Medicine.

McCallin, A. M. (1999). Pluralistic dialogue: A grounded theory of interdisciplinary practice. *Australian Journal of Rehabilitation Counselling, 5*(2), 78-85.

Meads, G., Ashcroft, J., Barr, H., Scott, R., & Wild, A. (2005). *The case for interprofessional collaboration in health and social care.* Oxford: Blackwell with CAIPE.

Mikkelsen Kyrkjebo, J., Brattebo, G., & Smith-Strom, H. (2006). Improving patient safety by using interprofessional training in health professional education. *Journal of Interprofessional Care, 20*(5), 507-516.

Rees, D., & Johnson, R. (2007). All together now? Staff views and experiences of a pre-qualifying interprofessional curriculum. *Journal of Interprofessional Care, 21*, 543-555.

Reeves, S., Goldman, J., Burton, A., & Sawatzky-Girling, B. (2010). Synthesis of systematic review Evidence of interprofessional education. *Journal of Allied Health, 39*(Suppl.1), 198-203.

Reeves, S., Zwarenstein, M., Goldman, J., Barr, H., Freeth, D., Hammick, M., & Koppel, I. (2008). *Interprofessional education: Effects on professional practice and health care outcomes* (Cochrane Review). Retrieved from http://www.nvmo.nl/resources/js/tinymce/plugins/imagemanager /files/20120926_Cochrane-20090121_Reeves-S-ea_.pdf

Schön, D. A. (1987). *Educating the reflective practitioner: Toward a new design for teaching and learning in the professions.* San Francisco, CA: Jossey-Bass.

Wackerhausen, S. (2009). Collaboration, professional identity and reflection across boundaries. *Journal of Interprofessional Care, 23*(5), 455-473.

Walsh, M., & van Soeren, M. (2012). Interprofessional learning and virtual communities: An opportunity for the future. *Journal of Interprofessional Care, 26*(1), 43-48.

Walton, M. (1988). *The Deming management method.* New York: Putnam.

WHO. (1988). *Learning together to work together for health.* Geneva: WHO.

WHO. (2009). *2008-2013 action plan for the global strategy for the prevention and control of non-communicable diseases.* WHO: Geneva.

WHO. (2010). *Framework for action on interprofessional education & collaborative practice.* Geneva: WHO. Retrieved from http://www.who.int/hrh/resources/framework_action/en/index.html

Zwarenstein, M., Reeves, S., Barr, H., Hammick, M., Koppel, I., & Atkins, J. (2001). *Interprofessional education: Effects on professional practice and health care outcomes.* (Cochrane Review).

Hugh Barr MPhil., PhD
Emeritus Professor, University of Westminster, UK
President, the UK Centre for the Advancement of Interprofessional Education

Julia Coyle MManipPhys., PhD
Head, School of Community Health
Charles Sturt University, Australia

SECTION 4: CASE STUDIES

MAREE DONNA SIMPSON AND NARELLE PATTON

17. MAKING THE MOST OF WORKPLACE LEARNING

LEARNING ANOTHER LANGUAGE AND DEVELOPING A NEW PROFESSIONAL IDENTITY

As an academic, you may have come to teaching directly from your profession, perhaps with experience as a clinical educator, or you may have arrived as an experienced academic but with no previous experience of workplace learning or possibly some previous experience of workplace learning in another course or at another university or campus. In each case, your success in workplace learning will depend to some extent on your ability to learn a new language – the language of workplace learning – and to develop a new identity as a workplace learning academic. This can be a challenging transition, as your focus and identity change from practitioner to educator for the profession.

A common truism today is that workplace learning is a key feature of the education of healthcare professionals. Yet in the education of healthcare professionals, the workplace is being re-discovered as a valid educational site for the development of skills, abilities, knowledge about the profession, professional practice and being a health practitioner (Brodie & Irving, 2007). Historically, many health professions were learned in an "apprenticeship" relationship in the workplace, with participation developing from observation, to assisting, to patient assessment, management and treatment. This method of training health practitioners has been largely replaced by education within a university setting. The current approach is not without its detractors, as some practitioners consider that current graduates may have good theoretical knowledge and may be able to articulate how to achieve certain patient-related treatment and management goals, but have fewer practice-ready skills and behaviours. Neither view is necessarily right or wrong. Today's graduates are expected upon graduation to demonstrate the skills and capacity of practitioners already in the workplace (Brodie & Irving, 2007). This attitude may reflect a greater sensitivity to these issues in recent years. The experience of this chapter's authors is that as new graduates they were expected to be competent but not experienced. Even with a university preparation there was a transition phase after graduation where a healthy apprenticeship with a more experienced practitioner was an important part of professional development.

This historical background may contribute to the view that simply adding workplace learning to a health professional course is sufficient to develop skills and professional socialisation. It is assumed that this exposure automatically allows students to apply their theoretical knowledge to a practice context. Learning and

S. Loftus et al. (Eds.), Educating Health Professionals:
Becoming a University Teacher, 199–210.

application, however, require more intentionality, structure and support to achieve desired learning and graduate outcomes, and the first approach that needs to be selected or confirmed is your teaching philosophy.

Identifying and Developing a Workplace Learning Teaching Philosophy

The academic literature, professional accreditation bodies and employers agree that work readiness is a key objective of professional education. Strategic incorporation of workplace learning within courses and subjects can help to achieve this. However, the workplace learning component requires articulation of specific learning outcomes and support prior to participation so that students have a clear understanding of the learning that is intended. The workplace learning also needs effective debriefing sessions. According to Brodie and Irving (2007), students need to be able to recognise and appreciate learning and knowledge presented in different ways in different venues. This means that students should not expect to learn in the same manner in a workplace as they do in a university lecture theatre or problem-based learning group. Further, students must appreciate that learning and knowledge imply change, which students need to be able to recognise in themselves and others. Therefore in your new role as a workplace learning academic you will need to expand your current teaching philosophy to include various learning approaches appropriate for facilitating student learning in the workplace.

Successful workplace learning needs to incorporate key essential elements. Williams (2010) identified three critical insights for workplace learning. The first is the appreciation that such learning is based in an authentic workplace during the normal practice of that workplace and is centred on a task that is student-led or related. Supervisors or clinical educators must navigate between responsibilities to patients and responsibilities to students who seek to learn. This can be a challenge in a busy health workplace. Moreover, goals for workplace learning may include skills acquisition, development or assessment alone, but may formally or informally include socialisation into professional practice. The second key element is the recognition that the creation and application of knowledge are shared activities and that workplace learning proceeds most successfully in workplaces with an organisation-wide learning philosophy and infrastructure (Williams, 2010). It has been established that organisational support across all levels is the key factor influencing whether students do well or poorly in their learning in health workplaces (Girot & Rickaby, 2008). Active support is required, since both non-responsive supervisors and uninterested and unengaged supervisors decrease the success of students' learning. Williams' (2010) final contention is that learners need to be self-directed and self-motivated. This last characteristic is crucial not only to success in workplace learning but also throughout future professional careers, as lifelong learning is now an expectation of all registered health professions.

Brodie and Irving (2007) advised that as academics we need to ensure that our students are prepared to engage effectively with workplace learning. We need to ensure that our students have a clear vision of what learning is, and that they understand learning theories to develop some knowledge of how they best learn. Hodge and colleagues (2011) proposed that, since workplace learning is so grounded in engaged practice, experiential and situated theories and perspectives offer the most useful insights into this form of learning. Apart from developing professional self-awareness, students also need to use workplace learning to identify areas in which they need to acquire further knowledge or skills. The ability to self-regulate, to critique skills and knowledge, and to commit to lifelong learning are valuable attitudes and behaviours that students should see in workplace learning.

It is helpful for the novice workplace learning academic to read the academic and vocational literature, exploring learning theories in general and in particular what has been learned from students' and educators' experiences of workplace learning. Other sources of useful information range from the formal to the informal, from meetings dedicated to workplace learning and from one's peers. An example of how both staff and students can learn from the workplace is the growing use of portfolios, especially electronic versions. Many students are expected to maintain portfolios of their experiences during workplace learning. There is now a trend for academics also to develop their own professional portfolios, based on their teaching and research. Such portfolios can be a useful way for academics to reach a deeper understanding of how they learn from their own workplace, and this can help them to understand how students learn from their workplace experiences.

Managing Workplace Learning

Developing your skills, capacities and philosophies is important, but it is necessary to actively manage workplace learning experiences so that students meet desired objectives. This requires pre-workplace learning preparation. It is important to have a clear understanding of what students must know or be able to do before they begin a workplace learning experience. This might include awareness of occupational health and safety or issues of ethics, privacy and confidentiality, apart from any disciplinary skills or knowledge considered important. Furthermore, it is necessary to ensure that students are attending the workplace and progressing satisfactorily through tasks and experiences. This requires some form of register, which could be quite unsophisticated or, with large groups, multiple sites and several cohorts, might require a customised database. In the case study that follows, we outline a solution developed by colleagues that incorporates workplace learning progression within the online subject presence.

CASE STUDY ONE

The setting: You are an academic responsible for a workplace learning subject with a compulsory 280 hours of placement. Your students are encouraged to select a community pharmacy in which to undertake their placement, to gain a broad range of experiences and to make valuable professional contacts in locations or areas of practice that they might wish to pursue as an early career practitioner.

The focus: You receive a somewhat terse phone call early on Tuesday morning of the first week of a planned 2-week clinical placement from Hasnaa, a pharmacy owner and clinical educator for your program. Hasnaa advises you that Justin, a third year student, has not attended the placement, and has not made any contact. Hasnaa therefore assumes that Justin had chosen another pharmacy site as she had not received a learning contract, assessment tasks or a placement site contract between the school and the pharmacy, as is your usual practice. Hasnaa is quite disappointed not to be advised of the change of plans by you or the university, as she has rostered extra staff for the next 2 weeks to cover the student's presence and learning.

You are surprised by this information, as you know that your placement administrative co-ordinator is usually very thorough in checking paperwork before booking a placement for any student. Furthermore, both you and the placement administrative co-ordinator present a briefing session in the first week of semester, and you also post the PowerPoint presentations to the subject online site for students to refer to if uncertain about any aspect of placement. You have also developed a workbook to support student learning on this 2-week placement, and your placement administrative co-ordinator has developed a placement manual which is essentially a handbook of expectations, information and forms.

The strategy: You walk to the office of your placement administrative co-ordinator to check where Justin is booked to go. Your placement administrative co-ordinator is also mystified; no student has formally booked a placement at Hasnaa's pharmacy and Justin is not booked to attend any pharmacy. In class, you have noticed that Justin seems distracted and lacking in motivation, has poor time-management skills with assignments, and demonstrates poor participation in tutorials. At this point, you decide to phone Justin to clarify the situation.

Justin tells you 4 weeks ago that he had phoned and spoken to Aimee, the front shop supervisor at Hasnaa's pharmacy, to see whether there was an opportunity for placement at this time. Aimee checked the pharmacy calendar and advised that no students were booked for either of Justin's two preferred weeks. Aimee advised that she had booked the placement for Justin in the pharmacy system and so Justin did nothing further. Justin tells you that he had been to a party on Sunday evening and so did not drive to the town where Hasnaa's pharmacy is located, as he knew it was likely that his blood alcohol level would be above the legal limit. Justin advises that he is planning to drive to Hasnaa's pharmacy today and will arrive about lunch time.

Challenges: You face two major issues – a student not following procedures adopted for risk management and governance and not demonstrating appropriate professional courtesies, and a clinical educator who is disappointed, has engaged additional staff specifically to be able to educate your student, and who may re-evaluate her commitment as a clinical educator.

You have a number of issues to consider:

1. Do you withdraw Justin from the placement due to inappropriate process which is not consistent with the legal and risk management strategies of your university?
2. Do you confirm with Hasnaa that she will still accept Justin and then allow him to undertake the placement but reiterate Hasnaa's feedback and check Justin's understanding of proposed strategies for improvement?
3. Do you schedule an immediate meeting with Justin to complete any legally required documentation and arrange feedback sessions with Justin and Hasnaa to monitor his progress for the remainder of the placement?
4. Do you explore with colleagues better strategies to identify and monitor all students on placement?

Reflections: While workplace learning does place students in an authentic work environment, with careful support and transparent processes it should entail no more risk than any other learning activity such as a practical laboratory session. It is essential that you, as the academic, are able to access information relevant to a placement about any student in your subject. Justin appears to have adopted a casual approach to placement, and the outcome could easily have been more serious.

This situation has provided you with an opportunity to review and redevelop your processes, and you seek strategies to identify potential solutions that track student progress in workplace learning preparation and participation. You had believed that your placement program was sound until this situation. Your placement administrative co-ordinator maintains a database within the student administration system at your university, and you know that a more comprehensive system is also being trialled. However, you need to ask the co-ordinator for access when required, as the database is password-protected for privacy.

Since placement supervisors often phone you if there are problems, it would be helpful if you could access key information while on the phone. You recall an innovation presented by two colleagues at staff educational sessions. You phone and speak to one of these colleagues, who confirms that they set up an online "site within a site" in their subject. The "placement site" is set up as a simple database of key milestones, and access is restricted to the teaching staff and students of that subject. Every student and member of the teaching team can see at a glance whether particular students are on placement, and if they are, at which site, the name and contact details of the workplace supervisor. Completion of prerequisite requirements and completion of reports or tasks can be confirmed. Your colleagues advise that their students find this approach convenient and enjoy being able to track their progress.

Critical Success Factors for Workplace Learning

Active participation by students has been established as central to successful student learning in a health workplace, and inclusion of tasks and assessment activities that encourage student participation will facilitate your development of successful workplace learning experiences. Various levels of participation may be more appropriate for students at different stages of their course and at different points through their workplace learning experience, and each level is associated with a different learning outcome (Dornan, Boshuizen, King, & Scherpbier, 2007). Observation might be an appropriate level of participation for a junior level student attending a workplace for the first time. It may also be appropriate for a more senior student entering a complex and new environment for the first time, such as an emergency department or the cytotoxic suite in a pharmacy. In these situations a higher level of risk applies and thus a more extended orientation may be needed. Participation might start in a passive manner, with the student watching how patients are managed and issues addressed, then transiting into more interactive participation by engaging in discussion with supervisors and other members of the patient care team.

Higher levels of participation include performing professional tasks such as taking a patient history and progressing to treatment, under supervision. As students need to interact with patients, supervisors can facilitate their transition by introducing them to patients and seeking the agreement of particular patients to be managed by the student.

Participation may be viewed as a relatively low risk, high gain learning activity, but actions of supervisors and practitioners can easily derail student learning and progress. As a workplace learning academic, it is helpful to engage with your profession and especially with your workplace learning supervisors. Student supervision adds to the workload of supervisors, and not all supervisors may be able or prepared to offer students the structure and support consistent with student workplace learning. At the beginning of the year or semester, you may choose to offer training in supervision, or an incentive such as subsidised continuing professional development, to indicate how valued supervisors are in the education of health practitioners. Further opportunities to engage with the university could include practitioner access to the library, opportunities to tutor on campus, opportunities to present workshops about health workplaces to prepare students to be more self-directed and self-sufficient during workplace learning.

Students, and the choices and behaviours they demonstrate, also significantly influence their own learning and success in health workplaces. Students were found to be more successful if they had a clear vision of what they wanted to achieve and could articulate that clearly with their supervisor, and were unafraid of asking questions (Dornan et al., 2007). However, a synergy resulted when both these characteristics were combined with good professional knowledge and competence appropriate to their level of study.

Supervisors were most likely to ask stage-appropriate questions and to have stage-appropriate expectations of students when they were familiar with the students' curriculum. Thus another strategy for making the most of workplace learning is to ensure that the supervisor receives an introductory letter, manual or supervisory pack a short time, perhaps 2-4 weeks, before the student's attendance at the workplace. If the supervisor is new to supervision or new to supervising a student from your course, it would be helpful to phone and address any uncertainties they might have. It is also often helpful to mention the small courtesies and considerations that can so affect a student's workplace learning experiences. These include being addressed by name and being introduced to others. They may also include interacting with students not just in a teaching role but perhaps in the staff room over lunch, having reasonable expectations of them, gently "grilling" them on clinical matters, and occasionally, but carefully, "throwing them in the deep end" in patient management (but having a life preserver handy) (Dornan et al., 2007).

Participation in a workplace may still not result in effective student learning without effective reflection. Critical reflection has been identified as crucial to effective student learning, as it develops students' ability to consider and evaluate information and knowledge, and to consider the validity, credibility and general or specific applicability of that knowledge (Brodie & Irving, 2007). The two case studies considered next illustrate two quite different approaches to encouraging critical reflection on workplace learning.

Case Study 2 outlines the use of a course-wide reflective professional portfolio which showcases students' capabilities to build confidence and serves as evidence for future job applications. This capacity to aid the development of self-monitoring skills and to signpost the achievement of learning goals is well recognised (Brodie & Irving, 2007).

CASE STUDY 2

The setting: You are an academic responsible for course co-ordination in a health program in a rurally sited university. You are part of a small team of academics and have come to academia after practice in your profession. Some of the team have decades of practice experience and others just a few years. Your course offers increasing time in the workplace from first through fourth year, and you teach the subject which contains workplace learning in third year.

The focus: In your role as course co-ordinator (oversight over the entire program, not just a subject) you note that student evaluations indicate that some students feel they do not learn significantly in workplace learning experiences. You believe that students are well supported by training or prerequisite requirements for workplace learning. Each subject includes a workbook to provide further structure for students' learning, including suggested activities for students to undertake when the workplace supervisor is unavailable, such as when in a meeting.

Over the last 2 years, you, your team leader and other colleagues have made changes to subject delivery and assessment modalities in an effort to showcase to students the learning opportunities they have enjoyed, and student evaluations have improved. However, there some of your students still fail to recognise what they have learned and how they changed as a result of being in the workplace

The strategy: In discussion with your team leader, you implement reflective professional portfolios starting in first year to support workplace learning and also to incorporate other learning from assessments in professional subjects. Reflective professional portfolios address subject needs and also address the requirement to be a reflective practitioner who develops and maintains competency applicable to current practice. These professional portfolios document not only skills and competencies for registration but dispositional skills relevant to practice, such as working effectively in a group to achieve patient education, and as such support students when they apply for intern year positions.

Challenges

- Although reflective professional portfolios appear to offer students significant advantages, such as preparation for their intern year and future professional practice, few studies document their effectiveness.
- This innovative practice offers not only a challenge but also an additional benefit, as research will be necessary to evaluate the impact of this activity.
- Your solution is to research the literature and you find sufficient support for portfolios as a learning tool, so you implement them and evaluate their impact. You do this with (a) a course-wide research project and (b) a research project with practitioners.

Reflections: Your challenge was to provide students with a "tool" with which to document and understand their learning in the workplace. In doing so you needed to identify factors that integrate workplace learning with future professional practice. The literature you consulted established that students consistently identified professionally relevant activities, assignments, and lectures or tutorials as highly desirable in courses and usually found them both useful and even enjoyable. Moreover, most if not all health professional students indicated that they chose a health profession to help patients, and the workplace provides opportunities to help patients in increasingly meaningful ways. However, the changes that the workplace facilitates within students might not be appreciated by them without critical reflection and incorporation of that learning.

Although students are not unanimous in their endorsement of them, professional reflective portfolios have been identified as another strategy to encourage and to facilitate student learning, with the additional benefit to the student of showcasing their skills and abilities to future employers, and to the registering authority as evidence of the development and maintenance of professional competence. Further, research arising from this initiative may help to clarify the role that reflective professional portfolios play in the professional lives of registered health practitioners, and could provide additional validation of their use in student learning.

Case Study 3 describes the use of photo-elicitation as a strategy to (a) assist identification of issues on placement, (b) debrief students, and (c) assist them to reflect on a workplace learning experience that can sometimes be emotionally overwhelming or indeed very negative for some. The photographs provide a means of initiating discussion about student experiences and their learning. In this case the academic (and co-author) restricted photographs to objects only, and to maintain privacy no people were allowed to be photographed. Nonetheless, objects such as coffee cups and place settings at a dinner table hinted at the person to whom they related and could provide a prompt to discussion.

CASE STUDY 3

The setting: You are an academic responsible for the co-ordination of workplace learning in an inland university physiotherapy program. You have practised for several years as a physiotherapist before choosing to develop an academic career, and have in recent years also become the program leader with oversight over the entire program which is offered over two geographically distant campuses.

The focus: In your workplace learning role you receive a phone call mid-way through a physiotherapy clinical placement from Susan, a supervisor, to discuss Mary's progress in her physiotherapy placement. Susan advises you that Mary is not progressing as would be expected for a final year student and has been identified as being at risk of failing the placement. You are surprised by this information as you regard Mary as an academically high-achieving student who has performed well on previous placements. Susan indicates that Mary lacks confidence and initiative, has poor time-management skills and has demonstrated poor clinical reasoning skills. Susan has discussed Mary's "at risk of fail" status with Mary and suggested several strategies to assist. Following this discussion, you phone Mary for additional information and clarification. Mary bursts into tears as soon as she recognises your voice, telling you that she hates the placement; it has been the worst experience of her life; the supervisor is intimidating and condescending. You are surprised by this feedback because previous students have enjoyed this placement and particularly noted the friendliness of the workplace supervisor. In your discussion with Susan you recall that she displayed concern for Mary, suggesting that external pressures might be interfering with Mary's ability to fully engage with the placement.

The strategies: This situation, where perceptions of the workplace supervisor and student are diametrically opposed, offers several challenges to you.

- Do you withdraw Mary from the placement due to conflict between her and Susan, which is causing considerable distress for Mary leading to decreased engagement with the placement?
- Do you allow Mary to continue but reiterate Susan's feedback and check Mary's understanding of proposed strategies for improvement?

- Do you, in addition, or perhaps instead, schedule regular feedback sessions with Mary to monitor her progress?
- Do you explore with Mary other factors that could be influencing her engagement with the placement, such as problems with accommodation, fatigue, health and wellbeing, or family and potential personal issues before you propose a strategy?
- Do you explore with Mary why she has gained the impression that Susan is intimidating and condescending; for example, is Susan asking questions that Mary can't answer, which might indicate poor background knowledge, or is Mary perceiving constructive feedback in a negative light, resulting in a loss of confidence?
- Do you explore with Mary why Susan has gained the impression that she has poor clinical reasoning skills; for example, is Mary providing justification for her treatment choices?

Challenges: Successful resolution of student issues requires an understanding that workplaces represent complex, multi-dimensional and often intimidating learning environments for students. As well as learning to apply theory to rapidly changing and uncertain practice situations, students must also learn to negotiate the unfamiliar terrain of a new workplace. This negotiation includes learning the physical layout of the workplace and understanding workplace cultures including power hierarchies (such as avoiding sitting in the consultant's chair at team meetings). Furthermore, individual student factors such as poor health, recent bereavement, or recent relationship difficulties contribute to the manner in which workplace factors influence students' learning. Therefore, an awareness of the numerous factors that influence students' workplace learning will increase your ability to maximise clinical learning opportunities.

You review ways to start a non-threatening discussion in a situation where students might be distressed and defensive, and recognise that photo-elicitation provides an immediate focus. You decide to adopt a policy that students may take photographs during workplace learning that do not include any humans, whether patients, staff, supervisor or casual passers-by. Your department purchases inexpensive, easily operated digital cameras which all students take on placement.

Reflections: This photo-elicitation activity offers an opportunity to start a conversation with a student about her or his workplace learning. When students return to university following workplace learning experiences, debriefing sessions are a useful vehicle for capturing students' experiences and the factors that shaped their learning experiences, positively or negatively. Images provide a link to past experiences and can be used as a stimulus for conversation – resurfacing memories that enrich clinical discussions individually or in the classroom to provide the student and you with deeper insight into a clinical placement from the student's perspective, and workplace factors that influenced the student's learning. You have found that digital photographs help students to talk about matters important to them and help you to identify potential causes of their problems. The benefits have been that fewer defensive conversations occur with students when problems have surfaced during their workplace learning.

Facilitating Positive Workplace Learning Experiences

A workplace learning academic fills an important and integral role in practice-based education which needs to be appreciated by all, most importantly by students, as workplace learning may be the prime source for students of new learning about their profession (Walkington & Vanderheide, 2008).

A workplace learning academic needs a broad skill set, including the skills of a diplomat, an auditor, an innovator, a counsellor and an architect, as well as the flexibility of a gymnast, to facilitate effective student learning in the workplace. Being and becoming a workplace learning academic is ongoing – always a work in progress as new situations arise with student desires and preferences, with changes in health organisation policies, with legislation such as that covering occupational health and safety. That sounds like hard work, and it is, but it is also very rewarding, very relevant, and can be greatly appreciated by students and practitioners alike. It takes only appropriate investment of time and energy on your part to become that competent, critically reflective, successful workplace academic.

ACKNOWLEDGEMENTS

Thanks to colleagues David Maxwell and Brett van Heekeren for permission and assistance to report their use of online management of workplace learning, to George John for permission and assistance to discuss his use of reflective professional portfolios, and to colleagues whose "corridor conversations" may have sparked a recollection of an example or an idea for an explanation of a concept.

REFERENCES

Brodie, P., & Irving, K. (2007). Assessment in work-based learning: Investigating a pedagogical approach to enhance student learning. *Assessment and Evaluation in Higher Education, 32*(1), 11-19.

Dornan, T., Boshuizen, H., King, N., & Scherpbier, A. (2007). Experience-based learning: A model linking the processes and outcomes of medical students' workplace learning. *Medical Education, 41*(1), 84-91.

Girot, E. A., & Rickaby, C. E. (2008). Education for new role development: The community matron in England. *Journal of Advanced Nursing, 64*(1), 38-48.

Hodge, P., Wright, S., Barraket, J., Scott, M., Melville, R., & Richardson, S. (2011). Revisiting how we learn in academia: Practice-based learning exchanges in three Australian universities. *Studies in Higher Education, 36*(2), 167-183.

Walkington, J., & Vanderheide, R. (2008). *Enhancing the pivotal roles in workplace learning and community engagement through transdisciplinary "cross talking"*. Paper presented at the HERDSA 2008 Conference, 1-4 July, Rotorua, New Zealand.

Williams, C. (2010). Understanding the essential elements of work-based learning and its relevance to everyday clinical practice. *Journal of Nursing Management, 18*(6), 624-632.

Maree Donna Simpson BPharm BSc (Hons) PhD
School of Biomedical Sciences
Charles Sturt University, Australia

Narelle Patton BAppSc(Phty), MHSc, PhD Candidate
School of Community Health
Charles Sturt University, Australia

MAREE DONNA SIMPSON, TERESA SWIRSKI,
NARELLE PATTON AND JOY HIGGS

18. WORKPLACE LEARNING IN RURAL AND REMOTE AREAS

Challenges and Innovative Strategies

Workplace learning (WPL) presents students with a range of opportunities and possibilities as they pursue their journey from student to novice practitioner. Simultaneously, staff involved in WPL, whether academics, general staff or practitioners who act as WPL educators, face many challenges in helping students to navigate these journeys. In this chapter we explore these challenges and consider innovative strategies with particular reference to rural and remote WPL settings. In our experience, such settings face specific organisational complexities that influence personal, social and professional learning experiences. There is a particular need in these challenging situations for innovative WPL strategies. We define WPL innovations as new and authentic strategies that add value to or enhance the way in which WPL is conducted.

We examine WPL from the context of Charles Sturt University in Australia, which has campuses across considerable distances within the state of New South Wales and is in a good position to reflect these emerging educational and partnership issues. Each year, CSU staff organise diverse WPL placements, visits and experiences for students across many different courses and disciplines. This is a demanding task. Some courses are dealing with diminished placement availability due to industry pressures and competition with an increasing number of course providers. Many courses need to deal with considerable distances between placements and campuses.

Moreover, the escalation of student technical communication capabilities has placed pressure on WPL course designers and educators to provide learning strategies that emphasise Web 2.0 assisted communication and learning approaches. We see these pressures as opportunities for both creativity and innovation.

To be effectively undertaken the task of designing and managing innovative WPL placements requires understanding of how WPL has been traditionally implemented in the course/profession, together with a vision for innovative practices that could be designed to address the unique disciplinary, student profile, learning opportunities and location challenges facing the course team. The two case studies described in this chapter highlight instances of WPL challenges and innovative strategies, to enhance understanding of these unique contexts.

S. Loftus et al. (Eds.), Educating Health Professionals:
Becoming a University Teacher, 211–222.

WPL IN RURAL AND REMOTE SETTINGS

Wakerman (2004, p. 213) highlighted that rural and remote definitions are "time and place sensitive" and should not be compartmentalised, suggesting alternatively that they be viewed as "something more complex which recognises the heterogeneity of non-metropolitan areas and the distinct features and similarities of different settings as reflected in various sociodemographic and health indicators". The rural and remote locations of WPL are similarly heterogeneous. For the purposes of this chapter, we have found the following definition to be useful: *rural* refers to non-urban; such locations oblige practitioners to acquire skills not usually required in urban practice. *Remote* rural practice is where the location is more than one hour by road transport from a specialist service (RACGP, 1997).

The implications of increasing understandings of rural and remote WPL challenges and innovations are manifold for higher education, the health professions and society. Foremost within the higher education context, understanding of the challenges and innovative strategies can enhance student learning, inform academic planning and facilitate administrative WPL tasks. More widespread is the impact upon a major issue facing the health professions – the shortage of graduates in rural areas – which affects the distribution of health services and wellbeing in Australian society (Barnett et al., 2011).

The strongest reason for identifying challenges and integrating rural and remote WPL innovations into curricula is that such changes may enhance students' learning experiences, academic approaches, WPL administrative planning and WPL partnerships. Secondly, improved engagement with both the place and the practice of the profession may positively influence graduates' choice to pursue work in rural locations upon graduation.

Killam and Carter (2010) noted the links between successful rural placements and subsequent recruitment in those areas. Johnson and Blinkhorn (2011) suggested the need for longitudinal studies to delve further into this perception. It is apparent that the immediate impact of identifying rural and remote WPL challenges and innovations may lie in enhancing students' experiences. The potential to foster graduates' capabilities and engagement with professional practice in rural and remote places is a longer-term outcome that can benefit multiple stakeholders: graduates, employers, co-workers, clients and communities.

To illustrate our discussion of challenges and innovative strategies of WPL we present two case studies. Within the literature, common issues identified across remote and rural placements include travel, time, isolation, the community, engagement as a community, and lack of support (Killam & Carter, 2010). The first case study highlights the personal and professional challenges of a student "going home" to a rural placement, as well as the subsequent issues which the academic WPL co-ordinator addressed in a variety of ways. The second case study, "going far away", illustrates the unique set-up of a placement in a remote Indigenous community. The ways in which innovative strategies address the associated complex challenges are discussed.

EXPLORING CHALLENGES IN RURAL AND REMOTE WPL STRATEGIES

Conducting WPL in remote and rural locations entails a range of challenging advantages and disadvantages. Students may gain greater skill development, social skills and independence; yet there are instances where students may wish to be (or may have to be) removed from their rural and remote placement as a matter of necessity and urgency. Costs, practical support, and a limited range of placement opportunities have been identified as prominent issues for students in regional and remote areas (Patrick et al., 2008). The first case study highlights the challenging personal and professional issues which can arise in such a situation.

Going Home

This case deals with a placement undertaken at a small rural hospital and the complex issues that can arise for both the student and WPL co-ordinator. In this instance, the role of the academic WPL co-ordinator involved co-ordination of physiotherapy student workplace learning placements across all four years of a physiotherapy program. The co-ordinator had worked consistently to establish strong relationships with WPL partners in metropolitan and rural areas, routinely contacting all sites while students were undertaking WPL experiences. The co-ordinator had processes in place to ensure that all students were prepared prior to undertaking placements and were debriefed following placements. She was therefore surprised when she received an email from "Sally", a fourth year physiotherapy student, requesting an appointment to discuss her fourth year clinical placement allocation.

The co-ordinator considered Sally to be a strong student; her last placement assessment reported that she had performed capably across all assessment items. The co-ordinator was astonished when Sally said that her previous placement had been difficult, since this placement in her home town should have provided a welcome opportunity for Sally to enjoy the company of family and friends before taking a staff position in a hospital the following year.

Sally arrived at the co-ordinator's office appearing agitated and distressed, requesting a change to her placement allocation. She burst into tears and disclosed that her last clinical placement, undertaken in a small rural hospital, had been extremely stressful, and she was consequently very anxious about undertaking another placement in a rural setting. Sally's previous clinical placement had been in her home town, where nearly every client she assessed greeted her with a warm hug and a variation of the greeting, "Little Sally, who would have imagined!" This familiarity challenged Sally's developing understanding of professional behaviour as she was unsure how to respond, which left her feeling awkward and uncomfortable.

Sally's discomfort was exacerbated when her supervisor behaved inappropriately during an overnight visit to an outreach centre. The supervisor appeared embarrassed for the remainder of Sally's placement, resulting in her spending less time supervising Sally, which left Sally feeling stressed by her increased sole responsibility for client care. Sally was reluctant to discuss the supervisor's unprofessional behaviour, as the supervisor's family was well known to Sally's family.

The WPL co-ordinator reminded Sally of the critical contribution WPL opportunities can make to the development of her professional practice capabilities and about the university's protocol for contacting an academic clinical co-ordinator immediately should problems arise while undertaking WPL. The co-ordinator discussed options that Sally could pursue to gain help in future placements, such as asking for supervision and guidance from a more experienced clinician. Following this, the co-ordinator helped Sally to identify other clinical staff (for example, doctors, nurses, and other allied health practitioners) who might be able to provide assistance and answer questions. Finally, they explored Sally's understanding of professional behaviour and why client familiarity challenged her confidence in her professional identity. At the end of the meeting Sally felt reassured and more positive about her upcoming rural placement.

Initially, Sally's WPL co-ordinator had focused on the positives of rural placements, particularly the wide range of opportunities that WPL partners and experiences in rural and remote settings can provide to students. Before their meeting, the co-ordinator had assumed that Sally would enjoy undertaking placements in her home town and had not fully appreciated the potential difficulties facing students working in small, close-knit communities in rural areas, particularly in their home town.

On reflection, the co-ordinator recognised the need for more targeted preparation and debriefing for Sally and other students attending rural and remote WPL placements. A clinical preparation session was developed for the physiotherapy students, to discuss specific characteristics of rural placements, highlighting rural practice opportunities as well as potential challenges involved in such placements. In the session, specific challenges faced by students undertaking rural placements were acknowledged (utilising stories shared from previous placements) and students were encouraged to brainstorm potential solutions.

A Case of Overlapping Personal and Professional Boundaries

Sally's dilemma highlights a number of key issues students may encounter when undertaking placements in rural or remote areas. In particular, Sally's case identifies the challenge of balancing personal and professional aspects of clinical placements. This situation was particularly difficult since the setting was a small country town where many people, including staff and clients in the hospital, knew each other well.

This was further exacerbated in Sally's placement as the workplace had only one physiotherapist, her supervisor, and Sally was the only student on the placement. She was therefore unable to seek advice or support from other physiotherapists or physiotherapy students while undertaking her placement. This lack of other discipline-specific support underlines the important contribution of interprofessional collaboration as a potential source of support for students undertaking rural placements.

Sally's experience highlights how students in rural placements can encounter isolation from professional support. These events prompted the WPL co-ordinator to work with clinical supervisors to discuss potential problems students could experience in rural placements and to ask targeted questions regarding students' progress (including social progress and performance) during placements. Given Sally's reluctance to contact the university while undertaking her placement, an automated mail merge system was implemented to establish initial contact with students on rural placements and to open a dialogue as a potential avenue for discussing any problems they might be experiencing.

"Going home" to a community where one is already known can raise key issues for students, supervisors and co-ordinators. The feelings of conflict between the student and the WPL supervisor were starkly apparent, with tensions further increasing when the student felt unsure about how to react. This is among the common issues faced by professionals in rural and remote places:

> Fitting into a rural community, being highly visible and therefore lacking anonymity and privacy, having unclear boundaries between personal and professional life, and being socially isolated [are] problems in remote and rural nursing today. (Wood, 2010, p. 57)

After communicating with the student, the WPL co-ordinator was able to identify and establish ways to enhance the placement experience. The more insights gained about our students the better our understanding of stressors and potential dislocations in their studies (Hemmings, Kay, & Kerr, 2011, pp. 106-107). The co-ordinator recognised the gap in social support that can occur in such rural placements; this was subsequently addressed in the design of the clinical preparation program to explore how such issues could be tackled. Social support is vital to rural and remote WPL. It can be a way of providing valuable information that can be significant for how students cope in rural and remote locations.

How students cope with social contingencies while on placement is often not explored unless a student submits a formal misadventure report and application for consideration in relation to grades, or is identified as being at risk of failing professional practice. A WPL co-ordinator's role is crucial to assist students to "deal with the ambiguity of their position in the community" (Wood, 2010, p. 56). This also relates to the relational and personal challenges highlighted by Killam and Carter (2010), who identified the importance of addressing potential conflicts of social participation in a new community or maintaining professional boundaries. Similarly, it is important to know how to foster students' motivation and self-directed learning.

While metropolitan and rural placements share many common challenges, rural placements present unique challenges for students during WPL. Distance is a particular problem, including distance to travel between campus and "home" during the placement, distance from support groups and, often, distance to travel during placements (e.g. visiting clients in remote areas). As has been highlighted in this case study, significant difficulties and adjustments can occur in such placements, even (or particularly) for students returning home to rural areas.

EXPLORING INNOVATIVE STRATEGIES IN RURAL AND REMOTE WPL

The diverse approaches to change and innovation can be broadly distinguished between "reform", a top-down approach, and bottom-up, grass-roots "innovation" (National Center for Postsecondary Improvement, n.d.). An example of top-down reform is an Australian government initiative which established the University Departments of Rural Health (UDRH) seeking to "increase rural academic input into all levels of nursing and allied health programs" (Playford, Wheatland, & Larson, 2010, p. 69).

The next case study focuses upon bottom-up or grass-roots innovation; that is, how all WPL stakeholders – students, academics, administrative staff and WPL partners – contribute to the arrangement and the implications of rural and remote WPL innovations.

Going Far Away

In this case study we explore a particular WPL program involving pharmacy students on a remote tropical island off the northern coast of Australia. Through this case study we challenge the notion that "rural and remote" settings are homogeneous and propose that a deep understanding is necessary of the unique opportunities and the scaffolding/support needs of students in any situation; particularly when setting up new placement programs that entail "going far away". This case study sets the scene for exploring innovative strategies in WPL practices.

Within a rurally-situated, multi-campus university, pharmacy students are offered placement opportunities in various remote locations. These locations may vary from year to year or remain available for several years, but are offered only to students who consider them as opportunities and are prepared to commit to long travel times, isolation, limited facilities and longer times being away from home and familiar environments than in placements in closer regional or metropolitan locations.

One such remote location is an island off the coast of the Northern Territory in Australia, which we here call "Northern Island". Students received information about the project and the project site during an information session in which previous program participants shared their first-hand perceptions and experiences of placements on the island. Afterwards, a number of students applied for the limited number of places in this program. Students were required to briefly outline their intended learning goals and to describe their particular interest in Indigenous health, tropical health and public health issues. This process identified students with a genuine interest in this healthcare field and population. This application process guided the academics and the community team in the selection of successful applicants.

For our students, access to this island requires permission from the Northern Land Council or the local community and a partnership with a health and research institute with offices in a number of states and in the Northern Territory. This institute has until recently conducted an eradication program for the medical conditions strongyloides and scabies, which affect the local population of Northern Island. The program operates in conjunction with local Aboriginal health workers and community elders and involves testing, explaining the eradication process, and administering either tablets or cream as appropriate. Our pharmacy students participated in this program.

The program provided many rich learning opportunities. This real-life project offered an authentic opportunity for students to participate in a direct healthcare program, to learn to engage with Indigenous Australians in a culturally sensitive manner, and to work to improve health outcomes for relatively neglected tropical diseases that increase the population's morbidity and mortality.

The program also generated a number of challenges around achieving learning outcomes and minimising risks. The first challenge for the university staff was to engage with health institute workers and researchers on the mainland and on site to verify that students' health, accommodation and facilities were consistent with their needs. It was necessary from a risk management perspective to ensure that any necessary vaccinations and prophylactic medications were obtained in advance, and that facilities were available should illness arise during the placement. Due to transport weight restrictions, students were permitted no more than nine kilograms of luggage; this allocation (including a towel) had to include sufficient clothes and essential belongings for a 6-12 week placement.

In advance of arrival, it was also necessary to discuss issues of access, participation, modest dress and behaviour. In essence, for the students to participate effectively, the community had to accept them as newcomers; the community became the students' family and they became the cousins of the community. It was also important that students were aware that some familiar items might not be the same as those they were used to, one example being the low-aromatic fuel, "Opal", in use. Similarly, seemingly common experiences such as going to school might well become vastly different experiences due to cultural, location and distance factors.

As well, it was important to ensure that students remained current with their studies during extended placements, as most who participated were final year students. This meant ensuring that they liaised with one another to take texts or resources between them, that they had on-line access to the university library and that they took sufficient of the resources that might be in short supply, such as USB drives. It also meant ensuring that an effective communication strategy was in place by obtaining mobile phone numbers in case of emergency.

The organisation of this "going far away" placement generally worked really well. Students were well supervised and greatly enjoyed their time at Northern Island. Some students found it more difficult than others to operate within the community, perhaps struggling with isolation and geographic distance, struggling with maintaining momentum with final year study, or finding it more challenging to operate as a healthcare provider in a more kin-based community. For such students it would be advantageous to identify some screening activity or shorter, more accessible workplace learning site in advance of the longer placement. This "trial run" would facilitate student reflection and identify necessary scaffolding and support. Another opportunity might be to send a small number of research and academic staff to the site with the students to facilitate student understanding and access at the site. This is such a rich learning environment that every opportunity needs to be considered to benefit all participants.

A Case of Slow Innovation

Although there are large inroads in the way digital technologies are transforming regional Australia (DBCDE, 2009), innovation does not always need to involve the quickest decision, latest gadget, or most expensive technology. An innovation can also be an idea, decision or activity that simply, effectively and authentically enhances practices within the student, academic, administrative and partnership arrangement. Within this context these are examples of "*slow* innovation in higher education" (Swirski & Simpson, 2012). Slow innovations are unique and are tailored to the specific and unique situations of rural and remote workplace learning. They are "an approach that provides room for exploration, reflection and learning, so that participants in an innovation process can constructively combine practice and theory and engage in joint learning and joint creation" (Steen & Dhondt, 2010, p. 2).

A better understanding of the significant relationship between enhancing WPL and slow innovation can foster creative ways of designing placements. For example, identifying and tailoring innovative strategies to specific rural and remote WPL contexts is key to enhancing student satisfaction and interrelationships among WPL stakeholders. Three innovative strategies identified from this case study were: *approaches, collaboration* and *communication*. Readers may be hesitant in thinking that these strategies should be described as innovative – especially if they have been applied in other contexts, or even within the same discipline. However, if these changes are tailored to the place, useful to practice, and add value to stakeholders within the specific and unique WPL situation, then they are certainly examples of slow innovation in action.

Thinking of different approaches to WPL in rural and remote settings can open up new ways of sustaining WPL, as well as maximising the wellbeing of stakeholders. In the case study "Going far away", approaching a remote Indigenous community and brokering discussions for establishing this location as a WPL setting was innovative. This brokering formed the basis of a partnership which sought to foster students' learning and the wellbeing of the island residents. Readers might wish to explore the potential for new WPL situations to emerge by asking: *What are the new and novel ways in which we can conceptualise and implement rural and remote WPL?* This exploration can open up novel possibilities for both the places and practices of WPL.

Thinking of new ways of collaboration can enhance WPL in rural and remote settings. This case study highlighted the collaboration that took place between the academic co-ordinators and the Indigenous health workers and elders of Northern Island in establishing the principles and strategies for organising WPL within this remote setting. Such building up of relationships is crucial to how students will be welcomed and integrated into the community. Readers seeking to innovate new forms of collaboration within WPL need to ask: *What are the new and novel ways in which we can collaborate with rural and remote WPL stakeholders?* Collaboration among partners, stakeholders, professions and universities is crucial to successful establishment and implementation of WPL in rural and remote places:

> Sharing student placement data, regular cross-disciplinary discussion about when, where and how students may be supervised and taught whilst on placement and actively looking for opportunities for them to participate in interprofessional learning and practice, is likely to contribute to expanding placement capacity and contribute to the development of a better prepared workforce. (Barnett et al., 2011, p. 4)

From this perspective, the community clerkship program designed by the University of Wollongong (Hudson, Weston, & Farmer, 2011) is another example of a novel way of collaborating with rural and remote placements. The introduction of a longitudinal, community-based arrangement within the Graduate School of Medicine has had reciprocal benefits, such as greater participation and engagement, for both students and supervisors. Influenced by international trends towards longer-term placements, a program was designed where third year medical students could experience continuity of learning and supervision by living and working in a regional or rural community for 12 months. An important aspect of this program was its focus upon placing students within a community-based general, or family practice. This provides diverse opportunities for students to increasingly participate within a healthcare team environment over the period of their placement. Through its longer-term community engagement and focus upon situated learning, this program offers an alternative approach to the traditional placement model of short-term clerkships.

Collaboration involves more than the "nuts and bolts" of how WPL is conducted. It also involves how we reflect upon and learn from prior WPL arrangements to inform future practices.

Being innovative about communication can also enhance WPL experiences in rural and remote settings. Experience with the placements on remote Northern Island identified that ensuring an effective communication strategy was vital to supporting final year students to remain on track with their learning in this crucial stage of their course. Enhancing communication among WPL stakeholders through innovative strategies is seen as key to enhancing students' experiences in remote and rural WPL.

This account may prompt readers to inquire (within your own contexts): *What are the new and novel ways in which we can communicate within rural and*

219

remote WPL? Clarity and ease of access need to be foremost in discussions about new ways of communicating among rural and remote WPL stakeholders. This focus upon communication can address some of the educational, political and environmental challenges highlighted by Killam and Carter (2010): orienting and supporting students in their learning, possible political impacts upon their placement, and potential transport and weather issues. Communication can enhance students' ability to deal with all of these complex situations.

In the case of Northern Island it was also made clear to students that the development of community connections could be facilitated through particular modes of dress, behaviour and modified expectations. This highlights how the cultural and communication aspects of rural and remote WPL can strongly affect students' experiences and learning. As illustrated in this case study, exploring new approaches, collaborations and ways of communicating can enhance the places, practices, experiences and potential of rural and remote WPL.

FINAL REFLECTIONS

WPL in rural and remote environments provides rich learning opportunities for students, and often, unexpectedly, for new WPL academics. These unexpected situations often provide opportunities for reflection and innovation which WPL academics can devise, perhaps inspired by some of the ideas discussed in this chapter.

The case studies described demonstrate that for students, academics and administrative staff there is a strong argument to recognise the heterogeneity of rural and remote places. Recognising the complex and unique practices which influence places "mitigates against treating rural as a natural and rooted identity" (Kelly, 2003, p. 2280). We need to acknowledge the diversity of rural and remote places, as de la Torre, Fickenscher, and Luft (1991) suggest. Such a perspective provides the foundation from which addressing challenges and integrating innovative strategies may emerge.

We also need to recognise the impact of scaffolding students' experiences to maximise their immediate learning as well as their longer-term positive disposition towards working in diverse community and workplace settings. WPL benefits not just the students and clients but also the evolving workforce and healthcare provision. The design and implementation of WPL is vital to how this continuum unfolds. It is important, therefore, to increase awareness of how understanding WPL challenges and innovative strategies can enhance and inform these processes.

ACKNOWLEDGEMENTS

Thanks to Ahmose Abrahim for his assistance in the preparation of case study 2. We appreciate the feedback from The Education For Practice Institute writing group, with special thanks to Celina McEwen for additional suggestions.

REFERENCES

Barnett, T., Walker, L. E., Jacob, E., Missen, K., Cross, M. D., & Shahwan-Aki, L. (2011). Expanding the clinical placement capacity of rural hospitals in Australia: Displacing Peta to place Paul? *Nurse Education Today*. Retrieved from http://www.nurseeducationtoday.com/article/S0260-6917(11)00212-7/abstract

de la Torre, A., Fickenscher, K., & Luft, H. (1991). The zip (postal) code difference: Methods to improve identification of rural subgroups. *Agricultural Economics, 5*, 253-262. Retrieved from http://www.sciencedirect.com/science/article/pii/0169515091900047O

Department of Broadband, Communications and the Digital Economy DBCDE. (2009). *Annual report*. Canberra: Australian Government.

Hemmings, B., Kay, R., & Kerr, R. (2011). The influence of social contingencies on teacher education students undertaking a rural internship. *Education in Rural Australia, 21*(1), 95-109.

Hudson, J. N., Weston, K. M, & Farmer, E. A. (2011). Engaging rural preceptors in new longitudinal community clerkships during workforce shortage: A qualitative study. *BMC Family Practice, 12*. doi:10.1186/1471-2296-12-103

Johnson, G. E., & Blinkhorn, A. S. (2011). Student opinions on a rural placement program in New South Wales, Australia. *Rural and Remote Health, 11*, 1703. Retrieved from http://www.rrh.org.au

Kelly, S. E. (2003). Bioethics and rural health: Theorizing place, space, and subjects. *Social Science & Medicine, 56*, 2277-2288. doi:10.1016/S0277-9536(02)00227-7

Killam, L. A., & Carter, L. M. (2010). Challenges to the student nurse on clinical placement in the rural setting: A review of the literature. *Rural and Remote Health, 10*, 1523. Retrieved from http://www.rrh.org.au

National Center for Postsecondary Improvement (n.d.). *Reform and innovation in higher education: A literature review*. Stanford University. Retrieved from http://www.stanford.edu/group/ncpi/unspecified/student_assess_toolkit/pdf/reforminnov_litrevie w.pdf

Patrick, C.-J., Peach, D., Pocknee, C., Webb, F., Fletcher, M., & Pretto, G. (2008). *The WIL [Work Integrated Learning] report: A national scoping study* [Australian Learning and Teaching Council (ALTC) Final report]. Brisbane: Queensland University of Technology. Retrieved from http://www.altc.edu.au and http://www.acen.edu.au

Playford, D., Wheatland, B., & Larson, A. (2010). Does teaching an entire nursing degree rurally have more workforce impact than rural placements? *Contemporary Nurse, 35*(1), 68-76.

Royal Australian College of General Practitioners [RACGP] (1997). *Advanced Rural Skills Curriculum Statement - RACGP Training Program*. Retrieved from http://www.wagpet.com.au/upload/child_health_curriculum.pdf

Steen, M., & Dhondt, S. (2010). Slow innovation. Paper presented at European Group for Organizational Studies Colloquium, Lisbon, 1-3 July, 2010.

Swirski, T., & Simpson, M. (2012). 'Slow innovation' in higher education: Re-imagining workplace learning. *Asia-Pacific Journal of Co-operative Education, 13*(4), 239-253. Retrieved from http://www.apjce.org/files/APJCE_13_4_239_253.pdf

Wakerman, J. (2004). Defining remote health. *Australian Journal of Rural Health, 12*, 210-214. doi:10.1111/j.1440-1854.2004.00607.x

Wood, P. J. (2010). Historical imagination and issues in rural and remote area nursing, *Australian Journal of Advanced Nursing, 27*(4), 54-61.

Maree Donna Simpson BPharm. BSc (Hons) PhD
School of Biomedical Sciences
Charles Sturt University, Australia

Teresa Swirski PhD
Postdoctoral Fellow (Practice-Based Education)
The Education For Practice Institute
Charles Sturt University, Australia

Narelle Patton BAppSc(Phty), MHSc, PhD Candidate
School of Community Health
Charles Sturt University, Australia

Joy Higgs AM PhD
The Education For Practice Institute
Charles Sturt University, Australia

NIGEL GRIBBLE AND ALMA DENDER

19. INTERNATIONALISATION AND HEALTH PROFESSIONAL EDUCATION

Excerpt from a student's Go Global reflective journal:
*"This trip has shaped me more than I can ever explain and possibly recognise –
not just as a therapist but as a human being."*

Annually, approximately 90 students from the occupational therapy, physiotherapy, pharmacy, nursing, dietetics, health promotion and speech therapy schools at Curtin University in Western Australia, participate in Go Global, an international interprofessional clinical placement delivering thousands of hours of service to patients and children in host sites in China, India, South Africa and Ukraine. This chapter describes the lessons the Go Global team have utilised to construct and grow this unique student mobility program.

The Go Global program is built around a series of strategically managed partnerships with Indian, Chinese, Ukrainian and South African healthcare providers, community-based organisations (government and non-government), industry and university partners. The program is ambitious. There is a collaborative approach to learning and teaching supporting the service learning and relationship marketing models used in the program. The program also aims to deliver services that contribute to the development of the host sites and their staff as well as providing a quality educational experience for students. The following quote is indicative of the recognition Go Global has received from employers of Curtin graduates:

> International interprofessional clinical education placements should become a part of health curricula to ensure students attain graduate attributes related to "cultural competence" and "global citizenship" critical to becoming an all-round health practitioner able to deal with the multifaceted cultural issues that are encountered in all health settings today … It encourages flexibility and creativity and skills to survive and add value to others in conditions that are not ideal. Basically it makes the students more worldly, and this in turn has a positive benefit on the person and the professional. (Senior Occupational Therapist reflecting on employing new graduate occupational therapists who had participated in Go Global, June 2010)

S. Loftus et al. (Eds.), Educating Health Professionals:
Becoming a University Teacher, 223–234.

THE SETTING

Go Global is an interprofessional program that offers students in a range of health professions an international fieldwork placement. Since 2001, exponential growth has seen over 500 students participate in the program, which currently is expanding to include sites in Malaysia and Cambodia.

A unique component of the Go Global program was the early adoption of a formal vision statement to:

Provide quality international opportunities for students to contribute to humanitarian based health services that can be sustained by those who follow.

A vision statement can empower the individuals in an organisation to perform above their expectation (Covey, Merrill, & Merrill, 1994). This is certainly the case for Go Global, where the vision statement has become a useful tool at the core of our communication and decision-making.

At the heart of the program's success is that, since its inception in 2001, students have only ever delivered services to the same health agency in the host country. Many international fieldwork placements utilise the "study tour" model whereby students visit a variety of sites. Go Global is different. Students in the program remain at the same one or two sites for the entire 4 or 5 weeks. Student cohorts in subsequent years continue the work of previous groups, building sustainability. A brief description of each host agency follows:

China: two placements per year at the Shanghai Boai Rehabilitation Centre, a centre where children with cerebral palsy receive therapy, and Hua Shan Hospital. The China program commenced in 2001.

India: two placements per year at Anandaniketan Society for Mental Health in West Bengal, 4 hours north of Kolkata. This program commenced in 2005, delivering services to the 400 children and adult residents.

South Africa: two placements per year in Uitenhage Provincial Hospital near Port Elizabeth. This program commenced in 2007 with a focus on children with HIV/AIDS and tuberculosis.

Ukraine: two placements per year in the Dzherelo Rehabilitation Centre, Lviv and Regional Children's Home, Novograd Volynski. This program commenced in 2008 and focuses on young children 5 years old and younger.

THE FOCUS

The program aims to graduate professionals who are highly employable global citizens with an education ranging beyond their first discipline. The program is worth credit points towards the completion of various Bachelor of Science degrees for health professionals. Only students in their final year are eligible to participate. Students who participate will enrol in the relevant discipline-specific fieldwork unit appropriate to their course. The learning outcomes, teaching strategies and assessment are specific to the Go Global fieldwork placement.

The current unit learning outcomes for the program are below. The majority of international fieldwork placements in Australian universities leverage off existing unit outlines. As a result, their learning outcomes focus on skills and knowledge related to the relevant healthcare discipline. In contrast, the learning outcomes for Go Global are focused on the international, interprofessional experience. The aims are to:

- Appraise personal and professional progression towards attaining cultural competence during an international fieldwork placement.
- Demonstrate and evaluate interprofessional practice in an international fieldwork placement.
- Differentiate and synthesise the current influences on the healthcare system of an international community.
- Select and apply interventions and programs that sustain a community-based rehabilitation program.
- Demonstrate culturally appropriate verbal, nonverbal and written communication.

The Go Global experience for any student ranges from 15 to 18 months from application to placement completion. Student cohorts travelling together undertake a comprehensive orientation program prior to departing Australia. The orientation program includes a comprehensive cultural and language orientation program specific to each host country prior to travelling; sessions on working in interprofessional teams and working in resource-poor environments; and theories related to the development of cultural competency.

Each student cohort uses the STEEP approach, requiring them to research the social, technological, and economic environment and political drivers of their host country, in order to produce a comprehensive environment analysis – and enabling the group to work together before travelling and the immersion experience.

Each cohort meets with the university Counselling Service prior to travelling to undertake team building exercises, engage in open discussion of any individual's anxieties and fears, and discuss team-based strategies to support each other. They meet again with the Counselling Service to debrief on their return.

The immersion component of the program requires the students to live and work for a period of 4 to 5 weeks in the host country, delivering allied health services in interprofessional teams to host site clients. Students experience learning 7 days a week, 24 hours a day, living and practising in the same environment as their clients. Action learning is generated from the interactions between the host facility staff, students and clients to resolve real issues with the ever-present cultural and language differences.

We realised there was no point coming in with fancy intervention ideas which were not going to be used once we left, thus awakening our notion of sustainable service delivery in the complexity of an often under-resourced environment. (Go Global student, reflective journal, 2011)

For the first 10 days of the immersion experience, the clinical supervisor orients, provides consultation for each of the client programs and guides the interprofessional practice. After 10 days of face-to-face supervision, the supervisor returns home, conducting remote supervision via email, phone and Skype™. The supervisor has usually been an occupational therapist, with some physiotherapists and nurse practitioners filling this role over the years.

Formal assessment is completed using the Interprofessional Competencies Assessment Tool (ICAT) developed by Curtin University (Brewer, Gribble, Lloyd, White, & Robinson, 2009). The ICAT tool focuses on students' interprofessional capabilities in the domains of communication, professionalism, collaborative practice and client-centred service. Student assessment is completed by the clinical supervisor, with staff of the host site providing input based on their observations of the students' programs and interactions with the children or adult patients. Students utilise the same tool to self-evaluate.

Reflective journals are mandatory and are updated daily. Journals are useful educational tools to increase students' understanding gained from clinical experience, to enhance their learning and to develop and guide their future practice (Jung & Tryssenaar, 1995). The journal, which is read by the supervisor before returning to Australia, allows insight to evaluate a student's progress and provide support in times of difficulty and transition (Landeen, Byrne, & Brown, 1998).

> Although the limited knowledge of the language did create some barriers, it made the whole experience much more of a challenge. At times I wish I was more fluent in Mandarin but then it wouldn't have been the same experience. It definitely increased our nonverbal skills and increased our knowledge of creative ways to communicate – definitely transferable skills. (Go Global student, reflective journal, 2009)

On completion of the placement, students hand over individual therapy programs to subsequent student cohorts via detailed Handover Reports and face-to-face meetings.

THE STRATEGY

Service Learning

The extraordinary growth and continuity of success of Go Global can be attributed to the utilisation of a service learning framework to guide decisions regarding the growth and pedagogy of the program. Service learning creates opportunities for students to integrate theory from the lecture theatre with real-world clients and organisations (Kenworthy-U'ren & Peterson, 2005). As such, service learning has a powerful impact on students' professional development by improving self-efficacy, self-esteem, and confidence in interpersonal skills in social and political arenas (Gitlow & Flecky, 2005). The "WE CARE" service learning model proposed by Kenworthy-U'ren and Peterson (2005) was selected to guide the program, underpinned by the principles of being *w*elcoming, *e*vidence-based, *c*omplementary, *a*ction-oriented, *r*eciprocal and *e*pistemic (and reflexive).

The program appoints a Country Co-ordinator to oversee the service learning for each host site. For example, the same staff member oversaw the China program for the first 7 years. Country Co-ordinators engage with host site staff in the creation of the student learning experiences, projects and goals.

In this international service learning model, the clinical supervisor's role is to step back from the placement, allowing students to assume responsibility for their learning while the clinical supervisor takes a subsidiary supportive role in the educational process. This is possibly due to the long-term trust-based partnerships developed with the host site, which have been achieved through participation in the problem-solving and decision-making processes with the host site staff. The action learning environment provides opportunity for problem solving and decision making to take on a life of their own as students see their ideas trialled and implemented. This teaching process questions students' knowledge, encouraging them to think outside their own assumptions, to collaborate with and be guided by the host site's needs before their personal learning needs.

Go Global demonstrates the true meaning of sustainable student learning partnerships for international health. (Director Goa Yali, Shanghai Boai Rehabilitation Centre, July 2006)

Relationship Marketing

Another influential factor in creating the successful infrastructure, capacity and growth in student academic mobility is the university's commitment to fostering relationships with key individuals in the partner organisations. A pivotal decision, made early in the program, was that only one site in each country was chosen, and through strategic interactions relationships were built with that one site so that the international service learning program could be sustained over many years. As such, a relationship marketing approach was implemented to foster these critical relationships.

Marketing professionals across a variety of industries have used relationship marketing strategies to transform potential customer leads into loyal customers (Morgan & Hunt, 1994; Berry, 1995; Payne, 2000). The underpinning concepts of relationship marketing transfer easily to the service industry and thus were appropriate for Go Global. Wong and Sohal (2001, p. 3) defined relationship marketing as a company's efforts oriented towards "attracting, maintaining and enhancing customer relationships"; Buttle (2000, p. 1) states that the objective of relationship marketing is "the development and maintenance of mutually beneficial long-term relationships with strategically significant customers". Of significant interest in maintaining the program's relationships across international borders is the claim by Peppers, Rogers, and Dorf (1999, p. 45) that relationship marketing is about "a firm being willing and (more importantly) able to alter their behaviour towards a specific customer, based on information gained directly from the customer or from external sources". The Country Co-ordinators pride themselves on actively listening to the key stakeholders in the host sites and being flexible in meeting their needs. An example has been the last-minute cancellations of two China trips, at the site's request, due to Severe Acute Respiratory Syndrome (SARS) in 2003 and swine flu in 2009.

Relationship development is a complex task requiring time, patience, determination and personal and team ability. The most significant challenge facing universities commencing an international service learning fieldwork program is the acquisition of partners or host sites with which to forge strong and sustainable relationships. The selected host countries and sites, in fact, become driving forces and foci for many subsequent decisions, including university staff recruitment, curriculum decisions, and the professional image and public perception of the university. Therefore, selection of a host site is a decision that should not be taken lightly.

The relationships between the Go Global host sites and Curtin University began as relationships between individual university faculty members and the host sites. These close personal connections were the starting point and have been a pivotal step in establishing the long-term sustainable institutional relationships between multiple partners that allow this program to grow. Integral to the enhancement of these relationships has been the personal and proactive commitment demonstrated by each pioneer Country Co-ordinator. The passion and determination of these staff members have become embedded in the culture of the program, with all staff members committed to the vision and values of the international fieldwork program.

For each of the four host countries, the university tapped into existing networks which facilitated an introduction to the host sites that might not have been possible on an individual basis. Many of these networks are with a non-government organisation (NGO) that has already built relationships with the host site; in fact, the NGO in many cases has been retained as a secondary stakeholder in the program, making valuable contributions to the operational nature of the program. In the case of China, a contact from within a World Health Organization Collaborating Centre was able to gain introduction to the host site in Shanghai through existing *guanxi* with the Director of the Boai centre. In India, initial contact with Anandaniketan occurred through Equal Health, a Perth-based NGO, which had been delivering medical and allied health services to Anandaniketan in India for 3 years. A fundraising organisation delivering essential food and clothing to the children in the centre in Ukraine provided an initial link. A faculty member who had previously lived and worked in Uienthage in South Africa gained access for the students to the Uitenhage Provincial Hospital through professional and personal affiliations that gave direct insight into the need for services in this area and the ability of the School to provide assistance.

The relationships between the university, the host sites and third party stakeholders have further strengthened the service delivery, ensuring continuity and consistency with the allied health program at the host sites. For example, the bond between Curtin, Equal Health and Anandaniketan in India ensures that the services delivered by the students in their July and December trips are continued by the Equal Health allied health team during their February visit. The provision of co-ordinated services between partners is critical to ensuring that the relationship with the manager and staff of the India site is sustained.

> These productive international partnerships enhance the study experience of students through a service learning partnerships model and contribute sustainable health services back to the partners in India and China. (Professor Kit Sinclair, President World Federation of Occupational Therapy, 2007)

In Payne's (2000) Ladder of Customer Loyalty, the first stage of the relationship between a company and customer is a "prospect". The higher on the ladder one moves, the less passive and the more active the relationship becomes. The task of relationship marketing is to focus on the cultivation of the relationship, in order that prospects progress up the rungs of the ladder through the customer, client and supporter phases until they attain the top levels of "partner" and "advocate". According to Buttle (2000 p. xi), "partners and advocates are so deeply enmeshed in the organization that they are not only very loyal long-term purchasers but they also influence others through positive word of mouth".

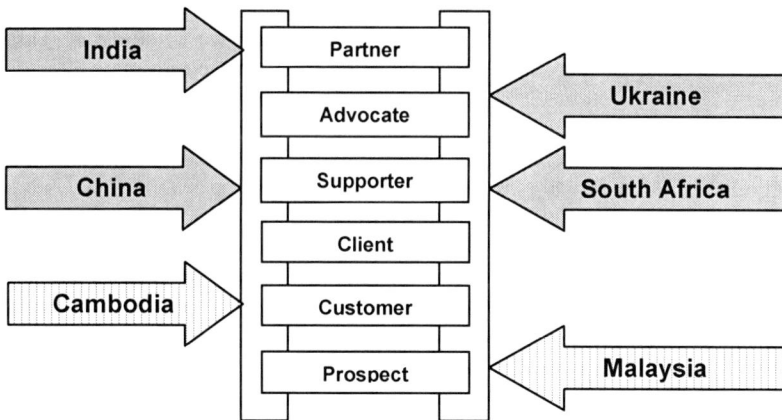

Figure 19.1. Ladder of customer loyalty and the Go Global partners (after Payne, 2000, p. 113)

Figure 19.1 depicts the status of the relationships between the Curtin and the Go Global host sites. Fluctuations in the relationships detail their dynamic and ever-changing scope. The India site has reached the highest rung on the ladder as a result of the mutual benefits each key party gains from the ongoing relationship. The India site actively greets each student cohort with a formal welcome ceremony. The Director has requested the inclusion of nursing students, a request that is now an ongoing part of the India program. The Director advocates for the program whenever asked. The Ukraine program, through the dedication and leadership of its Country Co-ordinator, has forged relationships with NGOs that are unparalleled in Eastern Europe. Staff of the host site have been flown to Perth to visit relevant centres.

At the time of writing, the relationships with China and South Africa are changing. The Boai Centre in Shanghai now has a competitor funded by the government and is struggling to maintain children and funds, and thus the resources to host the students have diminished slightly. The presence of Go Global students in the South African hospital acted as one of the catalysts for the hospital to commence employing therapy staff, and thus the need for the students is diminishing. The Malaysia program has been delayed but the first cohort of Go Global students will attend a Cambodian site in the near future.

The process of elevating a host site up the Ladder of Customer Loyalty towards "partner" is not simple. According to Payne (2000), organisations must develop explicit knowledge and in-depth understanding of a potential partner's needs – but most importantly, the university must deliver as promised. This is an important aspect of the sustainable nature of the relations that Curtin has built, making small but firm commitments to ensure that the promises made to a host site are deliverable. Payne (2000, p. 112) writes that customer satisfaction must be replaced with "customer delight, by offering a quality service that exceeds expectations". The Curtin program delivers this through the service component, by offering more to the host site than simply the presence of students. This is particular evident in Ukraine, where each year students co-ordinate donations from across the corporate sector of their home city, Perth, and take much-needed equipment to the host site.

There are significant challenges facing universities when implementing and co-ordinating a relationship marketing model to enhance international student mobility. Fournier, Dobscha, and Mick (1998, p. 85) warned managers of the difficulties in cultivating intimate relationships with customers as "it is alarming how quickly and thoughtlessly relationships can be destroyed through the muddled actions we often engage in … it is time to think about and act on what being a partner in a relationship really means". Understanding and demonstrating cultural sensitivities has been critical to climbing the Ladder of Customer Loyalty for the Go Global programs. For example, the presentation of a commemorative plaque to the Boai Centre in Shanghai, from Curtin University was a culturally appropriate method of expressing the gratitude the partnership has forged, and enabled the host site to promote itself locally as having a professional affiliation with an international academic institution. The level of trust that has developed allows problems to be resolved and the relationship to continue building.

Successful relationship marketing is interactive, rather than the arms-length approach more commonly associated with transactional marketing. Relationship marketing enhances mutual interdependence and co-operation, creating a win-win situation for both the host sites and the Curtin students. Sheth and Parvatiyar (2000) suggested that efficiencies and economies of scale are created from the interdependence between parties. The program has created synergies for students and the host site staff and clients whereby each key stakeholder is reliant on the other for the continuation of each program's excellence.

CHALLENGES FACED

Growth in operational costs and resources and the sustainability of the core values of service learning and relationship marketing have been the two primary challenges the Go Global team has faced.

The rapid growth from one host country with six participants to four host countries and 90 participants was an exciting yet challenging time. Go Global began in 2001 with only occupational therapy students. Four years later, other allied health students were invited to join as the international host sites requested an expansion in services. Until recently the School of Occupational Therapy operated all aspects of the program, from delivering the orientation program, booking flights and accommodation, to supervising students and marking all assessments, solely from the goodwill of the staff and without financial assistance from the faculty. It was eventually decided that the school must obtain financial support from the university. A proposal was presented to the Vice-Chancellor requesting more than $AUD500,000 over a 4-year period to fund a Director of Go Global, Country Co-ordinators and administrative staff, as well as provide 34 scholarships to students worth $2000 to each recipient. The central premise of the proposal was to assist Curtin University to achieve its internationalisation Key Performance Indicators which were central to its Strategic Plan. The Strategic Plan's fourth key strategy was to "drive international excellence". Go Global is now one of the flagship programs achieving this internationalisation goal. An important lesson for new academics everywhere is to align any initiatives in which you are involved with your institution's strategic plans wherever possible.

Since funding has been obtained, gaining and maintaining senior management support for resourcing the program has been relatively easy. Maintaining the core values of service learning and relationship marketing has not been so straightforward. The majority of international fieldwork programs are based on a "study tour" model which requires less effort and commitment to ensuring that partners are satisfied and their needs are being achieved. Being fully committed to these relationships takes time and resources. Thus, at times, there is a clash with the economic imperatives of university decision-making. We frequently return to the vision statement to ensure that decisions are made that align with the Go Global's direction.

Curtin's Faculty of Health Sciences prides itself on rapid uptake and integration of interprofessional education and practice for students (refer to http://healthsciences.curtin.edu.au/faculty/ipe.cfm). A few years ago, when we invited other disciplines to join the program at the request of the host sites, we were perhaps ahead of our time, as we immediately set up a Go Global Steering Committee made up of representatives from all seven schools within the Faulty of Health Sciences. Communication issues soon emerged, but were resolved through active listening and collaboration. Disagreements about learning outcomes and assessment procedures followed and were resolved in similar ways. At present, we are a cohesive group continuously working towards the betterment and expansion of the program. The passion of committee members, in particular the Country Co-ordinators and supervisors, has been another reason behind the continuation and growth of the program.

REFLECTIONS

What if we could go back and do one thing differently? We would have implemented a rigorous formal evaluation of all aspects of the program. However, research based on the program includes one completed Honours project. Currently two PhDs are under way and a master's study is in the planning stages. Only a few journal articles and conference presentations have transpired. The time required to operationalise the logistics often undermines the time available for research. Go Global may be one of the largest international interprofessional service learning programs in the world, and the lack of research output is an ongoing concern.

A major reason for the high student satisfaction is the interprofessional nature of the cohorts. Five disciplines are currently involved, and negotiations are under way with host sites to introduce health promotion, biomedical sciences, dietetics and social work students. Co-ordinating this number of disciplines, students, academic supervisors, fieldwork assessment processes and general logistics is complex. However, the interprofessional aspect of the program is crucial and very worthwhile:

> Having the opportunity to see first-hand the incredible benefits of multi-disciplinary intervention set me on my career path and gave me a deeper appreciation of the benefits of speech pathology. (Previous Go Global student reflecting on her involvement two years after returning from her India experience, 2010)

No structured evaluation of the host site experience has been developed, but it is planned. Most of the feedback at this point is anecdotal. Of most importance is that Curtin students are repeatedly invited to return each year to each host site. The Director of the Indian host site regularly requests more students and has specifically requested the inclusion of mental health nurse, dental hygiene and dietetics students.

> I have no language to express my gratitude. Your gift has uplifted our communication and work. I am not thanking you for the gift. I am thanking you for your great heart. (Director of Anandaniketan, Indian Go Global, 2009)

The benefit for Curtin University lies in the development of an interdisciplinary curriculum, and the increase in student global citizenship, student cultural awareness and increased global employability. Examples of the longer-term benefits for the university include the acknowledgement at a national level of the program through the recent granting of an Australian Learning and Teaching Council (ALTC) Award for Programs that Enhance Learning. Gaining national recognition such as this raises the university's profile internationally.

Since its inception Go Global has undergone many changes, except for the basic premise on which it was founded, that of service learning. It remains a matter of continual vigilance for the program to continue to function within this philosophy and to maintain the integrity of the uniqueness of the program.

This was definitely the BEST prac I have done. It was an honour and a privilege to come to AN [India]. I hope to come back in the future to visit or work. (Go Global student, reflective journal, 2010)

ACKNOWLEDGEMENTS

We are forever grateful for the passion and commitment of the inaugural Country Co-ordinators who have made Go Global what it is today.

REFERENCES

Berry, L. L. (1995). Relationship marketing of services: Growing interest, emerging perspectives. *Journal of the Academy of Marketing Science, 23*(6), 236-245.

Brewer, M., Gribble, N., Lloyd, A., White, S., & Robinson, P. (2009). *Interprofessional capability assessment tool (ICAT) 2009*. Retrieved from http://healthsciences.curtin.edu.au/local/docs/Interprofessional_Capability_Assessment_Tool.pdf

Buttle, F. B. (2000). The CRM value chain. Retrieved from http://suanpalm3.kmutnb.ac.th/teacher/FileDL/sakchai106255314285.pdf

Covey, S. R., Merrill, A. M., & Merrill, R. R. (1994). *First things first*. New York: Simon & Schuster.

Fournier, S., Dobscha, S., & Mick, D. G. (1998). Preventing the premature death of relationship marketing. *Harvard Business Review, 76*(1), 42-50.

Gitlow, L., & Flecky, K. (2005). Integrating disability studies concepts into occupational therapy using service learning. *The American Journal of Occupational Therapy, 59*(5), 546-553.

Jung, B., & Tryssenaar, J. (1998). Supervising students: Exploring the experience through reflective journals. *Occupational Therapy International, 5*(1), 35-48.

Kenworthy-U'ren, A. L., & Peterson, T. O. (2005). Service learning and management education: Introducing the "WE CARE" approach. *Academy of Management Learning and Education, 4*(3), 272-277.

Landeen, J., Byrne, C., & Browne, B. (1995). Exploring the lived experience of psychiatric nursing students through self-reflective journals. *Journal of Advanced Nursing, 21*, 878-885.

Morgan, R. M., & Hunt, S. D. (1994). The commitment-trust theory of relationship marketing. *Journal of Marketing, 58*(1), 20-38.

Payne, A. (2000). Relationship marketing: Managing multiple markets. In Cranfield School of Management (Ed.), *Marketing management: A relationship marketing perspective* (pp. 16-30). Great Britain: MacMillan Press Ltd.

Peppers, D., Rogers, M., & Dorf, R. (1999). The one-to-one fieldbook: The complete toolkit for implementing a 1 to 1 marketing programme. New York: Doubleday.

Sheth, J. N., & Parvatiyar, A. (2000). Relationship marketing in consumer markets: Antecedents and consequences. In J. N. Sheth & A. Parvatiyar (Eds.), *Handbook of relationship marketing* (pp. 171-208). Thousand Oaks, CA: Sage.

Wong, A., & Sohal, A. (2001). *Customer-salesperson relationships: The effects of trust and commitment on relationship quality.* Melbourne: Monash University.

Nigel Gribble MBA, B.Sc. (Occupational Therapy) (Hons)
School of Occupational Therapy and Social Work
Curtin University, Australia

Alma Dender PhD Candidate, DipEd, B.Sc. (Occupational Therapy)
School of Occupational Therapy and Social Work
Curtin University, Australia

MICHELLE LINCOLN AND SUE MCALLISTER

20. ASSESSMENT IN HEALTH PROFESSIONAL EDUCATION

THE SETTING

If effective teaching was a simple matter of filling student "cups" by pouring in enough knowledge from the teacher's "jug", then assessment would be a simple matter of measuring how much knowledge the students have managed to keep in their "cups" – and passing those who have "enough". However, over 20 years of teaching and assessment of clients and speech pathology students have taught us that the inter-relationship between learning and assessment is more dynamic, interesting and powerful than commonly assumed. Our learning about and use of quality assessment practices is founded in collaborative cross-institutional work in the assessment of clinical competency (McAllister, Lincoln, Ferguson, & McAllister, 2010) and ongoing engagement in curriculum revision.

In this chapter we aim to share what we have learned about assessment and its relationship to students' learning for clinical practice through presenting a case study of assessment in a case-based learning curriculum. Cased-based curricula have been adopted by our universities as a strategy to move from a focus on our students "knowing" to being able to "do" because of what they are learning. This makes intuitive sense to us as health professionals – we want our graduates to be able to use what they have learned in service of their future clients and communities. Students enter our programs as lay people and we are aiming for them to exit as competent health professionals.

THE FOCUS

Case-based curricula are informed by constructivist theories of learning and use inquiry-based approaches to learning, where students learn theory and skills for professional practice through active engagement with authentic case material (Kim et al., 2006; McCabe, Purcell, Baker, Madill, & Trembath, 2009). There are a number of ways of implementing a case-based curriculum but all approaches are underpinned by constructivist theories where learning is understood as a process that is actively constructed by the student rather than knowledge "poured in" by the teacher (Hager, 2004). Students' understanding of theory and related skills develops while using knowledge to intervene effectively in practical problems experienced by clients.

This change in teaching philosophy necessitates a change in assessment practices. If we are no longer "pouring in" theory and measuring how much the

S. Loftus et al. (Eds.), Educating Health Professionals:
Becoming a University Teacher, 235–244.

student has retained but are instead interested in whether the student can apply theory to practice, how can we assess "doing" instead of "knowing"? Tests of theoretical knowledge clearly are no longer relevant. Two overarching themes have informed our development of strategies to assess whether our students can apply knowledge to practice: assessment driving learning (Boud & Falchikov, 2006) and constructive alignment (Biggs, 1999).

Assessment Drives Learning

We have all heard the question "Will this be in the exam?" some time in our careers as learners or teachers. As learners we pay close attention to the answer; as teachers we may become exasperated because after all we wouldn't be teaching the material if we didn't think it was worth learning! It is easy to dismiss this question as a strategic "surface" or instrumental approach to learning where the student is only interested in learning enough to pass, as opposed to a "deep" approach that aims to build an understanding of the material and integrate it into future professional practice (Biggs, 1999).

However, assessment has many functions. We assess students to ensure that they possess the necessary foundational knowledge and skills to function competently in clinical practice and be certified as ready to enter our professions. We may also seek to judge clinical reasoning abilities and knowledge translation to individuals, organisations, communities and cultures. Our universities require that we also give consideration to whether our students are demonstrating graduate attributes such as lifelong learning, global citizenship and critical thinking. Our students understand this predominantly through the lens of the assessment task – the assessment defines for them what they are learning and why. For health professional students, each assessment task therefore defines the nature of professional practice in the future career they have chosen.

If we want students to be able to "do" or perform the tasks of our professions, we need to assess them in ways that require them to engage their knowledge and skills in the context of professional tasks. Professional practice is founded on the ability to take wise action on the basis of judgements informed by professional knowledge and skills. These skills include the ability to think critically about and use professional knowledge to inform our clinical reasoning and action (Higgs & Edwards, 1999). Assessing knowledge alone will not equip our students to undertake these important aspects of practice across their lifetime as health professionals.

Our students also need to be equipped with the skills and orientation required for successful lifelong learning post-graduation. It is critical that students be able to evaluate their own work, identify their learning needs and know how to acquire the knowledge and skills they require to continue to improve their practice, particularly as work environments are complex and changing, and unique clinical problems will inevitably be encountered (Boud & Falchikov, 2006). Explicitly aligning learning outcomes, activities and assessments is a strategy to support this process.

Constructive Alignment

Health professional students have chosen their programs based on the profession they would like to join in the future. Although they may not always have a full understanding of what this might entail, they are clear that they are at university to learn how to practise a particular health profession. Assessment that is obviously related to workplace requirements is therefore positively received by these students. This kind of assessment has authenticity – and indeed is often known as authentic assessment (Boud, 2007). Authentic assessment aligns well with the students' motivations, the needs of future clients, and the expectations of accreditation bodies and members of the students' future profession.

Constructive alignment also includes ensuring that assessment aligns with curriculum objectives and learning activities (Biggs, 1999). Ideally, assessment should align with the desired learning outcomes for a subject within a curriculum and should require integration of knowledge and skills across these learning outcomes. If these learning outcomes are expressed in specific terms requiring high-level thinking, such as "explain", "analyse" or "apply" rather than simply "identify", "list" or "understand", the assessment can be more easily and explicitly aligned with these expectations. The learning activities involved in a subject must closely link with both the learning outcomes and also the assessment activities. This may seem an obvious statement, but in our experience, assessments are sometimes designed that bear little relationship to what the students learn in a subject and do not provide evidence of learning across all aspects of the proposed outcomes.

We suggest that the best place to start when designing or reviewing a subject is to clearly identify what you expect students to be able to do by the end of the subject and how you will know that they can achieve this goal. Assessments should then be designed from this viewpoint. The learning outcomes should make the relevant components explicit for the students and it should be apparent how the learning activities will develop students' ability to successfully complete their assessments.

Another critical aspect of constructive alignment is to understand where the subject you are teaching sits within the overall course. This approach ensures that two important and related principles are embodied: developmental assessment and fairness. Assessments should be carefully located within the stage of the course. They should recruit and consolidate students' prior learning and prepare them for what they need to learn next – all with a view to what students need to be able to do to practise their profession on graduation. Moreover, assessment across a curriculum should integrate knowledge and skills at increasing levels of complexity. Hence a good piece of assessment is at the level appropriate to its location within the curriculum and requires students to extend their knowledge and skills but is not too easy or too hard.

Fair assessment makes clear to students that they have been enabled to perform to the best of their ability and their corresponding mark or grade accurately reflects their demonstrated ability. We conceptualise a fair assessment as one that is aligned with the desired learning outcomes of the subject. In other words, the assessment task samples the knowledge and skills that have been taught and learned in the subject. A fair assessment considers student workload, not just in the subject being assessed but across all the subjects in a semester. A fair assessment also has clearly communicated expectations and levels of performance. It is socially inclusive and does not advantage or disadvantage one group of students over another. As we discuss in this chapter, there is a significant challenge in designing case-based assessment where some student backgrounds, such as life experience, could advantage particular students over others. Finally, we argue that a fair assessment involves students having the opportunity to practise for the assessment task via formative assessment before they are required to complete a summative assessment.

Assessment in a Case-Based Curriculum: Doing, Not Just Knowing

As highlighted at the start of this section, a case-based curriculum brings to the fore the need to change from assessments of theoretical knowledge only to assessments that require the students to demonstrate the ability to apply that knowledge to practice in the context of real-life clinical problems. In the following section, an example of a case-based assessment within a speech pathology curriculum illustrates the themes and principles we have highlighted.

THE STRATEGY: DESIGNING A CASE-BASED EXAM IN A SPEECH PATHOLOGY CURRICULUM

One of the authors co-ordinates a discipline-specific subject called "Stuttering", which students complete in first semester of the second year of a 4-year undergraduate degree. In this subject, students learn important foundation knowledge about the cause, nature and epidemiology of stuttering. They also learn, within an evidence-based practice framework, how to assess and treat people of all ages who stutter. The entire undergraduate curriculum in this speech pathology program has been moving towards using cases to motivate and drive learning in all subjects.

Designing assessment for this subject has included balancing marking load for 80-90 students, ensuring a reasonable student workload, and constructively aligning subject learning outcomes and learning and teaching activities. Assessments include a written assignment, a case-based exam, participation in online case discussions and a skills-based viva assessment. This mix of assessment activities identifies for students the full range of professional skills required to competently provide assessment and intervention for people who stutter. The following example focuses on how the case-based exam was developed, contrasting it with a previous traditional exam format, and lessons learned as a result.

Assessment Drives Learning

Assessment supports learning with two main strategies:

– *Opportunities to practise the required performance:* Students practise case-based exam questions prior to the exam by interacting with six cases in an online learning environment during the semester. These cases present short scenarios and students post a response in an online discussion area to the problem posed at the end of the scenario. Each case is attempted in the week after relevant academic content has been presented in lectures (see Vignette 20.1 examples).

– *Formative feedback:* Formative feedback is provided to students on their online responses to the case. Formative feedback involves providing students with feedback on their ability to meet the learning outcomes for a subject – which in a constructively aligned course will align with the skills required to successfully complete the assessment tasks. Students are made aware that responses will be used as exemplars of different standards of performance and importantly that the questions are typical of what they could expect in the exam. The large class size is managed by providing feedback to the whole group on a selection of posts for each case rather than individually to every student. Online feedback and discussion are supplemented with some in-class discussions.

Vignette 20.1. Examples of formative cases

Case 1 – Marilyn: Videoed case history and questions
Marilyn is 60 years old and stutters. The speech pathologist takes a life history approach to the interview and elicits Marilyn's perspective on the cause and nature of her stuttering and how her stuttering has changed as she grows older. *Question*: Identify three pieces of information that Marilyn provides that are consistent with the theoretical and scientific information about stuttering and three pieces of information that are not consistent.

Case 2 – Lauren: Written case scenario and questions
You are a speech pathologist working in a private practice. You are referred a 4 year 3 month old girl, Lauren, who is stuttering. During your assessment you find out that Lauren lives with her mum and dad and younger brother and attends day care 3 days per week. Lauren is a quiet, shy girl who doesn't talk much at day care. She has been stuttering for approximately 8 months and her parents report that her stuttering has increased in severity over the past 3 months. During a speech sample collected while Lauren was playing with her brother you found she was stuttering on 11% of syllables and that fixed postures and repeated movements were present in her speech. *Questions:* What further assessment would you do? What further information would you collect from Lauren's parents? Considering the information available, what treatment approach would you commence with and why?

Constructive Alignment

Constructive alignment of the exam was attended to at several levels:

- *Locating the assessment within the context of the course:* The author reviewed students' formative and summative assessments prior to the stuttering topic (first year of their degree) and those they would be doing concurrently. The students had completed a case-based exam in the prior semester that assessed application of theory to case scenarios of children who have normal speech and language development. Hence the stuttering exam would be the first formal assessment under exam conditions applying theory to cases of children with communication impairment. In a concurrent subject, students interact with and complete short assignments on a longitudinal case with a different communication disorder. The author concluded that students had experienced previous exposure to case-based assessments but the requirements were at a low level. For example, the exam questions had asked students to "describe" and "explain" and the assignment had higher level expectations asking students to "plan", "justify" and "decide".
- *Building complexity across learning outcomes:* The author systematically increased the level of complexity of the cases and corresponding questions until they matched the level of the learning outcomes. For example, students moved from identifying theoretically consistent and inconsistent information to being required to integrate information about cases' stuttering treatment history, workplace requirements and psychological state to suggest potential approaches to the management of their stuttering.
- *Matching assessment to learning outcomes:* The learning outcomes clearly indicated to students that to pass the subject they would be required to integrate and apply theory to practice, rather than demonstrate isolated knowledge. As this was the first time a case-based exam had been used for this topic, the author also used her observations of the students' responses to the formative cases to write the new case-based exam questions. Table 20.1 provides some examples of assessment of learning outcomes using the previous traditional exam questions and the new case-based exam questions.
- *Review for fairness:* All new exam questions were reviewed by the author and a colleague to assess for clarity and bias, and to ensure that questions did not advantage some students. Older students who have more life experience or domestic students who have a better understanding of the Australian healthcare context might answer some questions at a higher level than younger or international students. For example, the question in Vignette 20.1 might have some cultural implications regarding the way parents are spoken to in relation to their children's difficulties. The question in Table 20.1 assumes that all students understand what a community health centre is in Australia. This potential bias would be appropriate if a stated learning outcome is "demonstrated knowledge of the Australian Health Care System", but in this subject this is not a stated

learning outcome. For both these questions it was decided to allow room for culturally different answers in the marking criteria.

Table 20.1. Examples of learning outcomes, traditional exam questions and case-based exam questions

Learning Outcomes	Traditional Exam Questions	Case-based Exam Questions
Demonstrate understanding and application of the consequences of stuttering Design evidence-based treatments for children and adolescents who stutter	Describe the short- and long-term consequences of stuttering for individuals who stutter. Which treatment for school-age children who stutter has the most scientific evidence and at what level is this evidence?	Steven, a 15 year old boy who stutters, is referred to you by his parents. Steven has had treatment for stuttering before which was unsuccessful. He is embarrassed about his stuttering but he is also embarrassed about coming to the clinic. Steven tells you he doesn't believe his stuttering can be fixed and he is just going to "live with it", "none of [his] friends care about it anyway". What advice would you give to Steven's parents regarding the short- and long-term consequences of stuttering? Taking an evidence-based approach, if Steven agreed to a trial of treatment, what treatment would you start with and why?
Integrate evidence-based practice with individual and/or organisational cultures or contexts to deliver effective stuttering treatments Demonstrate ethical reasoning in stuttering management	How would you adapt the Lidcombe Program, an early intervention for stuttering, for delivery in a group setting? What are the ethical issues involved in delivering treatments without strong scientific evidence?	You are working in a busy community health centre with a very long waiting list for treatment. Your manager tells you that a new service delivery model will be implemented which involves all clients under 5 years of age receiving six group treatment sessions and then 6 months later, six weekly individual sessions, to treat their communication disorder. You have three preschool stuttering children on your caseload. How will you manage these three children given the new service delivery model? What are the implications of implementing evidence-based practice in this context? Are there any ethical considerations in these circumstances?

- *Developing marking criteria:* Marking criteria should ensure that the awarding of marks in the exam is done consistently across students and markers. Often new marking criteria need adjusting during the marking process, so do not be concerned if this is not perfect on the first attempt. Marking criteria can be either criterion-based, defining specific responses required, or standards-based, defining holistic levels of performance. The choice will depend on the assessment format. In this case, the relatively short answers in an examination format lend themselves to a criterion-based marking format. Table 20.2 shows an example of marking criteria developed for two of the exam questions cited.

Table 20.2. Example of marking criteria

Question	Mark Allocation
What advice would you give to Steven's parents regarding the short- and long-term consequences of stuttering?	– Identifies 1-2 long-term consequences – Identifies 1-2 long-term consequences and presents them in "parent friendly" language – Identifies 3-4 long-term consequences and presents them in "parent friendly" language – Identifies 3-4 long-term consequences and presents them in "parent friendly" language and integrates them with Steven's current feelings about his stuttering
Taking an evidence-based approach, if Steven agreed to a trial of treatment, what treatment would you start with and why?	– Identifies an evidence-based treatment – Identifies an evidence-based treatment that can be delivered via distance or self-managed by Steven – Identifies an evidence-based treatment that can be delivered via distance or self-managed by Steven – Demonstrates integration of evidence-based practice and Steven's circumstances in the justification of treatment choice

REFLECTIONS

Several lessons were learned through the process of converting the exam component of the subject assessment from a traditional assessment of knowledge to a case-based assessment of students' ability to apply theory to practice.

– *Changing student expectations of assessment:* Despite students practising answers to case-based questions and receiving feedback, a small proportion of students seemed to fall back into "traditional exam mode". These students produced relevant theory in response to the questions but did not apply and translate the information to the individual or organisation. Subsequently, students were able to identify the lack of application but reported that case-based answers did not seem "academic enough". Qualitative feedback from a small group of students also identified that they felt the exam did not allow them to demonstrate their knowledge. The teaching team interpreted this feedback to mean that for some students, application of theory to individuals or organisations felt very much like using their common sense. Hence we concluded that in future students needed more opportunity in the exam to display their clinical reasoning rather than simply assuming that if they arrived at a correct answer their reasoning was sound. We will also provide model answers that clearly demonstrate how knowledge is applied and used to inform reasoning in response to case-based questions.

– *Allowing for several correct answers:* As the case information was quite brief students often made different assumptions to fill in gaps, influencing the ultimate answer they gave. For example in the case of Lauren (Vignette 20.1) some students assumed that Lauren had already had a full formal assessment of her speech and language skills and other students did not. Consequently in answer to the question, "What further assessment would you do?" some indicated formal speech and language testing and some indicated further in-depth assessment of her stuttering. Depending on the student's assumption, both answers are potentially correct. Hence we identified that it was important to find ways to help students identify the assumptions they had made in their clinical reasoning process, for the assessor to allow for different correct answers and again for students to have the opportunity to demonstrate their clinical reasoning.

– *Thinking like a clinician:* Student feedback regarding the use of case-based assessment has been positive. Students responded well to the authenticity of the task and recognised the alignment between the assessment and learning outcomes of the subject.

– *Teaching like a clinician:* Similarly, assessors also responded positively. Constructive alignment draws upon clinical skill sets of identifying the learning outcome (e.g. client's goals), the activities (e.g. therapy) required to reach these outcomes, and criteria by which we can identify that an outcome has been reached. Academic staff enjoyed the case-based teaching approach and reported feeling more confident in assigning grades to case-based assessment. When case-based assessment is used, students who have not achieved the learning outcomes are generally readily identifiable. Their inability to know what to do in authentic clinical situations is apparent.

WHAT HAVE WE LEARNED?

Both authors have learned much through developing and applying their understanding of the dynamic, interesting and powerful inter-relationship between learning and assessment. Furthermore, we have learned a great deal from our colleagues in their efforts to move from ensuring that students "know" to that students are able to "do". Our colleagues are implementing a range of innovative assessment strategies across our programs, including case-based assignments, case-based vivas that evaluate students' clinical reasoning, validated workplace assessments of performance, and assessment of students engaging in other authentic professional activities, such as developing critically appraised topics to answer clinical questions posed by clinicians in the field. There is also scope in the future to introduce multidisciplinary cases that encourage allied health students to work collaboratively to solve clinical problems.

Curricula also aim to provide opportunities for students to revisit clinical problems and engage with them at a more complex level. For example, cases can be integrated across subjects and years of the curriculum so that students return to early cases and deepen their understanding. The notion of "cases" is also being extended from individuals to organisations and communities, such as a class of preschool children. This approach is supporting students to move into innovative clinical placements, such as supporting childcare staff in providing an enriched communication environment for all children using the service.

The overarching lesson we have learned is that authentic assessment that focuses learning towards application of theory to clinical problems provides students with motivating learning experiences. Students experience constructive alignment of learning outcomes, activities and assessment with clarity of purpose that is congruent with their clinical experiences and future work roles.

REFERENCES

Biggs, J. (1999). What the student does: Teaching for enhanced learning. *Higher Education Research & Development, 18*(1), 57-75.

Boud, D. (2007). Rethinking assessment as if learning were important. In D. Boud & N. Falchikov (Eds.), *Rethinking assessment in higher education: Learning for the longer term* (pp. 14-27). New York: Routledge.

Boud, D., & Falchikov, N. (2006). Aligning assessment with long-term learning. *Assessment and Evaluation in Higher Education, 31*(4), 399-413.

Hager, P. (2004). Metaphors of workplace learning: More process, less product. *Fine Print, 27*(3), 7-10.

Higgs, J., & Edwards, H. (1999). Educating beginning practitioners in the health professions. In J. Higgs & H. Edwards (Eds.), *Educating beginning practitioners* (pp. 3-9). Oxford: Butterworth-Heinemann.

Kim, S., Phillips, W. R., Pinsky, L., Brock, D., Phillips, K., & Keary, J. (2006). A conceptual framework for developing teaching cases: A review and synthesis of the literature across disciplines. *Medical Education, 40*, 867-876.

McAllister, S., Lincoln, M., Ferguson, A., & McAllister, L. (2010). Dilemmas in assessing performance on practicum. In L. McAllister, M. Paterson, J. Higgs, & C. Bithell (Eds.), *Innovations in allied health fieldwork education: A critical appraisal* (pp. 247-260). Rotterdam, The Netherlands: Sense.

McCabe, P., Purcell, A., Baker, E., Madill, C., & Trembath, D. (2009). Case-based learning: One route to evidence-based practice. *Evidence-based Communication Assessment and Intervention, 3*(4), 208-219.

Michelle Lincoln PhD
Faculty of Health Sciences
The University of Sydney, Australia

Sue McAllister PhD
School of Medicine
Flinders University, Australia

SANDRA WEST, MELINDA J. LEWIS AND MARY-HELEN WARD

21. BLENDED LEARNING IN HEALTH PROFESSIONAL EDUCATION

The Intersection of Technology, Pedagogy and Content

The impact of technology in society and particularly in educational settings is extensive, challenging traditional notions of teacher-centred approaches to learning, learners and learning locations. Now embedded within the higher education sector are (a) new learning technologies including software such as learning management systems and e-portfolios, (b) collaborative learning approaches such as case- and problem-based learning, and (c) professional demands for curricula that facilitate both critical and inquiry-based learning.

This case study addresses a situation encountered by many health professionals who engage in teaching within a modern Australian university. "Sally", a newly appointed lecturer, who completed her preparation for practice degree in the early 2000s and who believes herself to be a competent user of practice-related ICT (information and communications technology) and has extensive experience in clinical teaching (experiential learning), is bemused by her students' use of technology during her first lecture. The focus here is on the determination of the intersection of technological knowledge, content knowledge and pedagogical knowledge (Shulman, 1986; Mishra & Koehler, 2006) and how these play out in the design and development of blended learning and teaching activities conducted within the formal, informal and virtual spaces available to teachers and learners.

THE SETTING

Sally is a mid-career clinician who has very recently been appointed to a discipline-based lecturer's position. Her main teaching responsibility is a large (200+ students) undergraduate unit of study requiring weekly lectures and four weekly tutorial teaching sessions, availability for student queries, and assessment design and marking. She has had only 2 weeks to prepare for the semester's lectures, so has had to use material that was prepared by her predecessor who has left the institution. Much of the content feels dated to her, but she reasons that she can start from what she has, and update it as she goes along – perhaps presenting the traditional view in class and discussing recent clinical practice in the tutorials.

*   *   *   *

S. Loftus et al. (Eds.), Educating Health Professionals:
Becoming a University Teacher, 245–254.

Sally is slightly nervous before her first lecture. But, she reasons (to calm herself), she has been a clinical educator for 3 years, and she knows her subject material inside out, theory and practice. Once she gets into her stride in front of the class she'll be fine.

But it doesn't go quite as she expected. The students don't seem to be very engaged with her. They are playing with their phones; a couple have iPads, and are paying more attention to them than they are to her. Four students sitting together have laptops; they seem to be engaged – they are taking notes rapidly as she speaks. She has spent quite a lot of time preparing her PowerPoint slides and as she clicks through them she begins to feel more confident. With about 10 minutes to go she begins to sum up, thinking she'll leave 5 minutes for questions, when a hand goes up.

"Errr, yes?"

"I was just wondering when this lecture will be up in e-learning?"

Sally is pleased she'd thought of that. It has been a struggle, working with the e-learning system at the university, but she managed to get her slides uploaded into the site along with a word document listing other useful learning resources.

"I put my slides up just before I came over to this class. You should be able to see it when you leave here."

"Why haven't you linked the readings from the library?" asks one of the students with a laptop open.

"Sorry?"

"I've just had a look in the e-learning site and you've only put a list of the readings. You should have linked them from the library."

Sally feels her throat tighten. She takes a swig from her water bottle.

"Thanks for that information. I've only been here a couple of weeks. I'll sort that out this afternoon."

That seems to satisfy the student. And really, what does it matter? She knows her material, and it is good that she could provide the readings for the students to access so easily. She clears her throat and is about to finish her summary of the main ideas when another student, one who had been tapping at his phone for most of the lecture, breaks in.

"That point you made about assessing the patient...?"

"Yes", says Sally, with a smile. This is the kind of exchange she has imagined, with students discussing the ideas she has carefully structured for them.

"That's not how we do it where I've been working. And I've just had a look online and there's at least three articles saying that the methods you outlined and explained today are outdated."

"Are they from Medline?"

"Yes."

"They are very controversial, and I intend to introduce them later in the course. I thought perhaps I'd start by giving you the traditional view on approaches to patient assessment."

People are starting to pack up and leave the room.

"Maybe we'll continue this discussion in the next class."

THE FOCUS

Although many clinicians are very familiar with the technology used in their clinical work and at home, they are often not as familiar with the specialised e-learning systems used by universities. If they graduated before 1995 they may never have engaged with the multitude of learning technologies that university staff now have at their fingertips: a learning management system like Blackboard or Moodle; a lecture capture system like Lectopia or Echo360; personal learning spaces (e-portfolios) for students such as Desire2Learn, Mahara or Pebblepad; text-matching software like TurnItIn to detect plagiarism. To these add digital repositories of articles, book chapters and images that university libraries hold (which ensure that access to material complies with a university's copyright licence). Furthermore, a bewildering array of systems, methods and concepts, and the rapidly developing conceptualisations of learning spaces, both physical and virtual (Ellis & Goodyear, 2010) need to be considered and incorporated into teaching in tertiary settings.

Unlike many clinical environments, students working within the university learning space are also now ubiquitously connected to the Internet and each other through their tablets, laptops, and smart phones. Although they are sitting in a formal lecture (physical learning space), students may be reading and replying to emails, checking their Facebook notifications and writing on their friends' walls. They may be tweeting and texting – arranging their next shift for work, organising childcare, responding to partners, children or parents – and they may or may not be taking notes on what is being presented to them. Most importantly, they may be working within the virtual learning space by using Google or the library pages to look up concepts or references that the lecturer is discussing, and sourcing further articles from these resources while they listen.

This phenomenon of the seemingly universal connectivity of younger people has seen them referred to, variously, as the digital generation, "generation e", and "digital natives". Many theories have sprung up around this connectivity, including most famously that of the digital natives – first published by journalist Marc Prensky – that has now been soundly debunked by Kennedy et al. (2009), among others, who have shown that competence in the digital world is not related solely to age. It is important to keep in mind, however, that apparent lack of attention in class does not mean that students are not engaged and learning.

When they have left the classroom, today's students can still be connected to their learning materials wherever they are physically located: on a bus or train, in a café on or off-campus, in the university library or their own living room, in a computer lab on campus. If the lecture has been recorded they will be able to listen to it again and again (and figures show that students do – at The University of Sydney for example, students download over 1,000,000 copies of recorded lectures every year). This sense that learning is not restricted to the face-to-face engagement of the lecture, tutorial or lab is generally known as "flexible" or "blended" learning. While the definitional meaning of such terms continues to evolve, it was well described by Ellis and Goodyear (2010, p. 91) as "situations in which e-learning is playing a part in a broader set of learning activities, such as those associated with lectures, laboratories, tutorials, seminars, clinics and the like."

Engaging with students in so many ways beyond the face-to-face classroom experience means, however, that teachers need even more carefully to consider the pedagogical purpose of each component of their work: the lecture, e-learning site, the tutorial, lab sessions, clinical requirements, assessments, and even their availability to students.

*   *   *   *

On returning to her office Sally is surprised to discover three emails from students in the class. One is from the student who had pointed out the new material, wanting to continue the discussion; one is asking when the first assignment is due; and one is asking for a special exam to be set because she is going to be overseas on the exam date. Sally attempts to answer them, and while she is doing this two more arrive. One is from the student who had already asked her about the assignment, asking another question about class times, and the other is from a student who had missed the lecture, had looked at the PowerPoint slides online and now wanted to come and talk to her about them – and also wanted to know why the lecture wasn't audio-recorded and why the readings weren't linked electronically from the library, where they could be accessed with only two clicks..

While Sally is staring at the screen, wondering where to start, her colleague Emma appears in the doorway.

"How did the lecture go?"

"I'm not sure… they seemed very critical … and now I've got all these emails". She finds she is breathing deeply to avoid the panicky feeling.

"Come on", says Emma kindly. "Let's get a coffee".

STRATEGY

Sally feels defensive as they settle down in the coffee shop.

"What am I doing wrong? For heaven's sake, I should know how to manage a few students. I've been a clinical educator long enough!"

"It's a bit different here," observes Emma. "In a hospital they can't use their mobiles or laptops easily, because of the firewall. I found it quite a shock when I arrived, but I read something that helped me. It's about the intersection of technology, pedagogy and content, and how to create an environment that helps to build knowledge. You've got the content knowledge, no question, and you know how to teach, but with all the technology we have available – and they expect us to use – you do have to plan your teaching a bit differently."

"In class this morning they argued with me! And then all those emails … honestly, I don't know where to start!"

"Would you like me to help you make a plan? I've been doing this for a while now, and I've survived."

"That would be really great."

Emma pulls a pen out of her bag and grabs a paper napkin from the container on the table. She draws three circles on it, and writes C in one, P in the second and T in the third.

"So there's your content knowledge" – she indicates the circle labelled C – "and there's your knowledge about teaching – about what works for learners". She indicates the circle marked P. You probably have them pretty well integrated".

She quickly redraws the two circles, overlapping.

"But there's another dimension that you'll have to take into account."

A third circle, T is added below the other two.

"That's your technology knowledge."

"I think that should be a lot smaller than the other two!" says Sally with a grin.

"Easy to fix!" replies Emma. "There's staff training and there's a helpdesk and there's a lot of 'how-to' stuff on the web, too. But I think you can see that what you need to aim at is this."

She draws the three circles overlapping.

"You really have to see these three elements as one system, and if you make changes in one it will have an effect on the other two. And, you know, there's really no part of your relationship with students that isn't in there somewhere. "

She taps the diagram with her pen.

"For instance, those emails … people wanting to know things that are in the Unit of Study Outline?" Sally nods. "Don't answer them. Announce in class, and in the e-learning site, that you won't answer any question that's covered in the Unit Outline. That's teaching them to find reliable sources of information, rather than just going to the nearest person. If you don't set some boundaries, you'll drown. That goes for office hours too. You need to set some and keep to them."

*   *   *   *

As well as clinical expertise and content knowledge, teaching in 21st century universities requires consideration of the ways that students create knowledge from the information that is so freely available to them. Although it is possible that the apparent lack of attention in Sally's class doesn't necessarily mean that students are not learning, most people, of whatever age, who are engaging with technology, are simply seeking information rather than creating deep knowledge for themselves. Teaching in healthcare contexts no longer means just selecting and presenting content from the infinite amount available; rather, it means guiding students through the available literature and the planned and unplanned learning that clinical experience provides, into a personal consideration of the key concepts that you as the teacher want them to understand, critique and apply. This is how students will come to understand concepts as more than just facts, rather as knowledge that is integrated into their future practice. As many of the information-gathering approaches commonly used by today's undergraduate students are only contributing to "surface learning" (Bluic, Ellis, Goodyear, & Hendres, 2011), teaching requires considerable pedagogical strategising to draw students toward deeper learning and understandings. This will aid the development of their personal knowledge(s) within today's complex, multi-faceted learning environments.

The TPACK Framework as Strategic Scaffold

TPACK, developed by Mishra and Koehler (2006), is a framework that many have found useful for both unpacking and integrating the types of knowledge teachers require when designing learning experiences. Its visual representation as briefly drawn by Emma and in greater detail below (Figure 21.1) provides a scaffold both for teasing out the relevant elements of technological, pedagogical and content knowledge when designing a learning experience and for reflecting upon one's teaching – be it in a particular instance or more broadly across a semester's work.

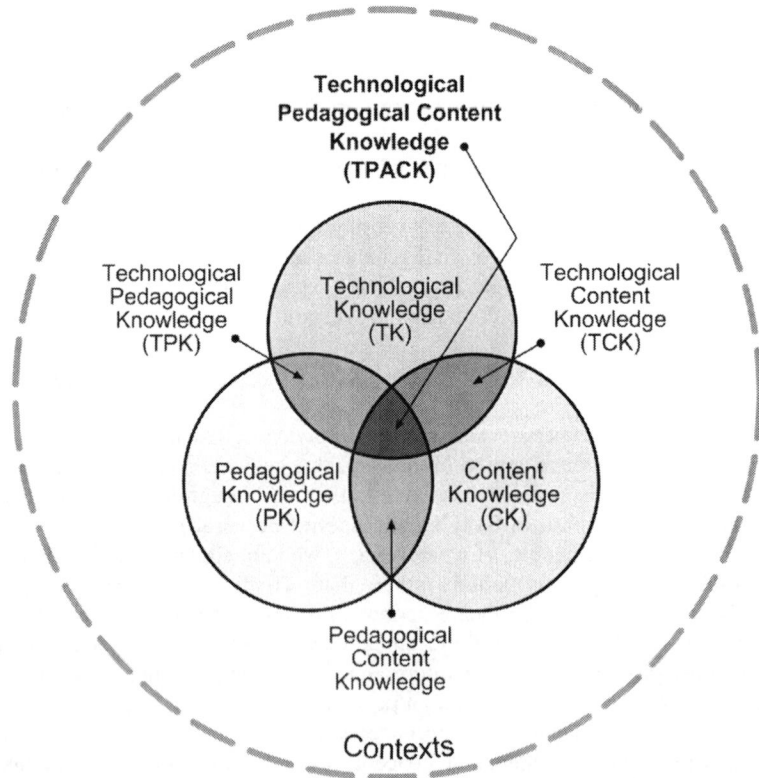

Figure 21.1. Technological, Pedagogical and Content Knowledge (TPACK) (from http://tpack.org/)

250

TPACK Elements

Technological Knowledge: This incorporates the knowledge of all of the standard technologies of the classroom (Mishra & Koehler, 2006) but it is now extending also to include knowledge of digital and virtual technologies sufficient to manage their effective use within learning situations.

Pedagogical Knowledge: Health academics frequently come to tertiary teaching with a certain way of knowing, built up over years of being inducted and educated within a discipline and practising that discipline. The epistemology (way of knowing) of practitioners within a discipline is something that, in general, serves to unite those who share it by providing a basis for a shared language and the commonalities of practice. However, the *practice* of a profession is not the same as *learning to practise* the profession; hence "the epistemology of a discipline should not be confused with a pedagogy for teaching or learning it" (Kirschner, Sweller, & Clark, 2006, p. 83). Pedagogies are essentially enacted theories of learning, such as cognitivism, behaviourism or social constructivism. Pedagogical thinking informs our decision-making about the approaches to teaching and learning; for example, planning for a lecture using the skills of explaining and information giving is inherently using instructivist pedagogy. If the learning goal were to engage groups of students in writing collaboratively in response to a topical issue/concept, you would adopt a more socially oriented constructivist pedagogy. Neither is inherently better or worse; the best choice of pedagogical approach is governed by what you want students to learn.

Content Knowledge: This is knowledge about the actual subject matter that is to be learned or taught (Mishra & Koehler, 2006) that has been gained in the context of the relevant discipline's nature of inquiry and approaches to knowledge construction i.e. its epistemology.

TPACK Intersections

The usefulness of the TPACK framework can be seen in the overlapping of the three initial circles (Figure 21.1). It is these intersections that allow the identification of existing new knowledge and also facilitate the derivation of new knowledge.

Pedagogical Content Knowledge (PCK) was first described by Shulman (1986) as "knowledge of pedagogy that is applicable to the teaching of specific content": where, for example, new clinical practices are rehearsed in a clinical lab so that students are exposed to particular learning experiences.

Technological Content Knowledge (TCK) focuses on the relationship between technology and content, which is becoming increasingly pivotal in designing learning experiences. For example, with knowledge of digital technologies students can record observational outcomes of clinical/laboratory practices, using a camera phone.

251

Technological Pedagogical Knowledge (TPK) emphasises the existence, components and capabilities of various technologies as they are used in the settings of teaching and learning. For example, one could extend the TCK example to include using the digital observational record as the basis for developing effective descriptive writing and reporting techniques, with both the recorded observation and the student's description of it then being submitted for feedback through an e-learning portal.

Technological Pedagogical Content Knowledge (TPACK) is finally created at the intersection of all the elements. This is an integrative process; Mishra and Koehler (2006, p. 1029) described it as requiring teachers to develop their "sensitivity to the dynamic, [transactional] relationship between all three" in melding their disciplinary, technological and pedagogical expertise. In our example, this is demonstrated by the feedback given to students on their written report of the digitally recorded observational material. This feedback can address the accuracy of the link (or absence of a link) between the observation and the written report, textual or diagrammatic communication about an observed phenomenon being a key skill of work in health and science. (See also *What is TPACK?*, 2011.)

CHALLENGES FACED

The aim of this chapter was to provide a framework that can be readily applied to learning and teaching situations within higher education, in particular health science curricula. The TPACK framework consists of the components of knowledge (technological, pedagogical and content) required when planning for, designing and delivering learning and teaching within a technology-rich environment. We illustrated TPACK as it applies to the climate and context of health professional education for academics entering the field of university work.

Sally's story is not atypical of the experiences and challenges new academics face today; students constitute a consumer-driven sector, with a high use of technology for information seeking, social networking and knowledge construction. Their expectations for learning and for achievable academic outcomes might not coincide with those of academic staff. Such challenges are not new or even recent, as Knight and Trowler's (1999) discussion of the mentoring and induction of new academics demonstrates. Recently, Shreeve (2011) explored "the added complications brought when one is employed within the academy because of expertise in a professional practice outside the academy" (p. 79), and Oldland (2011), in an autobiographical article, presented a novice academic's reflections on her transition from clinical manager to university lecturer. Both these articles highlight the challenges inherent in such career moves.

REFLECTIONS

At the end of semester Sally and Emma meet again for coffee.

"I feel really quite pleased with how the semester went, on balance", says Sally, "And a lot of that is thanks to you. I felt like I was drowning that day when you brought me here in the first week. But today I got two emails from students, thanking me for the unit, and hoping that I'd be teaching them again in the future.

Emma grins. "They probably thought it would help their exam mark... No, sorry, I'm joking. That's great. So what changes did you make in the end?"

"I tried to think more about how they were learning and less about what I wanted to teach. I realised I was assuming that they would need me – the physical me – more than they did, so I tried to use the technology as a kind of repository for the content, and added a lot more links and had some structured discussion boards for the key concepts that underpin the unit. The structured discussions worked really well, and didn't add to my load nearly as much as I thought they would – I just keep a kind of watching brief on them. Some of the students didn't bother with them, but those who did really seem to find it a good way to develop their ideas. I also sorted out how to manage the more demanding students. Keeping in mind that I was responsible for creating an environment for them to learn, but they were responsible for what and how much they learned really helped. I think that some of them learned not to bug me so much – I just copied the emails to the discussion list if they were looking for information I'd already provided or we'd already talked about.

"Sounds great", says Emma, "It certainly can be a challenge, moving from one very large institutional system to another. I remember myself, wondering if I'd fallen down the rabbit hole when I first started here after 10 years in the hospital system. It takes time. You've survived your first semester, and I don't expect you'll find the early weeks of next semester quite so challenging."

REFERENCES

Bluic, A-M., Ellis, R., Goodyear, P., & Hendres, D. M. (2011). The role of social identification as university student in learning: Relationships between students' social identity, approaches to learning, and academic achievement. *Educational Psychology, 31*(5), 559-574.

Ellis, R., & Goodyear, P. (2010). *Students' experiences of e-learning in higher education: The ecology of sustainable innovation.* New York: Routledge.

Kennedy, G., Dalgarno, B., Bennett, S., Gray, K., Waycott, J., Judd, T., et al. (2009). *Educating the net generation: A handbook of findings for practice and policy.* Melbourne: University of Melbourne Press.

Kirschner, P., Sweller, J., & Clark, R. (2006). Why minimal guidance during instruction does not work: An analysis of the failure of constructivist, discovery problem-based, experiential and inquiry-based teaching. *Educational Psychologist, 41*(2), 75-86.

Knight, P., & Trowler, P. (1999). It takes a village to raise a child: Mentoring and the socialization of new entrants to the academic professions. *Mentoring and Tutoring: Partnership in Learning, 7*(1), 23-34.

Mishra, P., & Koehler, M. (2006). Technological pedagogical content knowledge: A framework for teacher knowledge. *Teachers College Record, 108*(6), 1017-1054.

Oldland, E. (2011). Transition from clinical manager to university lecturer: A self-reflective case study. *Higher Education Research & Development, 30*(6), 779-790.

Shreeve, A. (2011). Being in two camps: Conflicting experiences for practice-based academics. *Studies in Continuing Education, 33*(1), 79-91.

Shulman, L. (1986). Those who understand: Knowledge growth in teaching. *Educational Researcher, 15*(2), 4-14.

What is TPACK? (2011). Retrieved from http://mkoehler.educ.msu.edu/tpack/what-is-tpack/

Sandra West RN BSc (Macq) PhD (Macq)
Faculty of Nursing & Midwifery
The University of Sydney, Australia

Melinda J. Lewis BAppSc (MRA) MHlthScEd (Syd)
Faculty of Nursing & Midwifery & Sydney e-learning
The University of Sydney, Australia

Mary-Helen Ward BA, MA(Hons), MPhil (Massey)
Sydney e-learning
The University of Sydney, Australia

PETER H. T. COSMAN

22. LEARNING PRACTICAL SKILLS

Practical, or procedural, skills in healthcare share many features with psychomotor skills in other unrelated disciplines. Since this is the case, we can refer to the published scientific literature on psychomotor skills in general in order to understand how best to teach procedural skills to students, and how best to assess them. It may then be possible to formulate the principles and objectives that govern a curriculum in procedural skills. These principles and objectives will dictate the requisite learning experiences to be included in the curriculum. Consideration may then be given to the types of training media appropriate for the objectives at each stage of the curriculum.

The pride of place given to training in technical and other clinical skills has been recognised since antiquity. In *The Canon*, Hippocrates mused:

> Want of skill is a poor thing to prize and treasure. It robs a man of contentment and tranquillity night and day and makes him prone to cowardice and recklessness, the one a mark of weakness, the other of ignorance. Science and opinion are two different things; science is the father of knowledge but opinion breeds ignorance. (Lloyd, Chadwick, & Mann, 1978, p. 69)

Hippocrates was here speaking of cognitive skills, but his remark is equally valid for psychomotor skills.

The preceptor or apprenticeship model has enjoyed a monopoly on training in healthcare since the earliest known records of medical practice. The *Edwin Smith Surgical Papyrus* (Breasted, 1927) dates back to – at the latest – the 19th century BC, and gives an account of surgical standards accepted at that time. Indirectly, it relates the traditional methods of surgical training – entrusting a young apprentice to the care and knowledge of a master of the craft – and these do not appear to diverge greatly from current methods of training. The characteristic features of this model are that it is a teacher-centred approach to education, conducted in a loosely structured manner, whenever appropriate opportunities should happen to present themselves, an aspect sometimes dubbed "education by random opportunity". Training occurs *en passant*, in the course of performing the routine duties of patient care. The mentor–student relationship is characterised by close supervision in a series of one-to-one situations, in which principles and procedures are taught on the basis of the mentor's interpretation of current standards of practice.

This model has worked well in the past, but a number of recent developments threaten its utility. Among them is the elucidation and widespread adoption of the fundamental principles of adult education, emphasising individual development, a

S. Loftus et al. (Eds.), Educating Health Professionals:
Becoming a University Teacher, 255–268.

learner-centred approach in an environment conducive to learning, and almost continuous high-quality feedback on performance.

Educational accountability as well as greater public and academic focus on the nature of medical error means that it is no longer acceptable to conduct training in a manner that compromises the safety of patients in our charge. There is a need to change from informal to formal learning of practical skills.

Minimisation of adverse outcomes requires a graduated exposure to the requisite skills. Progression from novice to expert proceeds through five levels of performance as characterised by Stuart and Hubert Dreyfus (Dreyfus & Dreyfus, 1986; Dreyfus, 2004):

Novice: Instruction begins by decomposing a task into elements that are not governed by context, which form the basis for rules or generalisations; following the rules outside the arena of instruction leads to poor performance, as a frame of reference or pragmatic context within which the rules may be applied is missing.

Advanced Beginner: Application of the rules within appropriate contexts begins to take place as the novice begins to understand how the generalisations apply in real-world examples.

Competent Performer: Broader experience is gained by increasing exposure to a wider variety of real-world situations; as this occurs, trainees learn to recognise and keep track of ever-greater numbers of potentially relevant elements, since they cannot yet predict which elements will be critical for successful performance, and so cannot selectively focus on those elements, and performance becomes so painstaking as to be emotionally overwhelming.

Proficient Performer: The resulting positive and negative emotional experiences reinforce successful sensorimotor perspectives until eventually trainees develop a sense of situational awareness or pattern-recognition; they can identify the salient aspects of the task at hand, but respond to them consciously by following explicit rules.

Expert: When enough experience has been gained with a wide variety of responses to various situations, trainees develops intimate knowledge of the outcomes of these responses, and can use this repertoire to react automatically to a wide variety of situations without application of conscious thought.

These characteristics ought to be borne in mind when assessing the skills of trainees at various stages of their training. It should also be noted that individual trainees would be at different stages of proficiency for different types of task, depending on the extent of their exposure to these tasks in the real world. For instance, a trainee may be proficient at intestinal anastomotic techniques, but be a novice in vascular anastomosis, simply because he or she has had greater exposure to colorectal surgery than to vascular surgery. Although one of the benefits of simulation-based training is to make training more homogeneous, the differences cannot be eliminated altogether. However, simulation recognises patient safety as an overarching principle and allows trainees to achieve an acceptable level of proficiency before approaching their first patient.

NOMENCLATURE AND DEFINITIONS

Although the term "skill" may have several colloquial definitions, a precise educational definition was proposed by Edwin Guthrie (1952, p. 259):

> the learned ability to bring about predetermined results with maximum certainty, often with the minimum outlay of time or energy or both.

Skills are further classified as "closed" if they predominantly rely on proprioception for successful completion, and "open" if they rely more heavily on environmental feedback (Poulton, 1957). While it is possible to train for sensory, cognitive, motor, and procedural tasks separately, it is more efficient initially to master the fundamental skills which comprise the building blocks of several tasks. This learning of task fragments is known as "part-task" training, and may be more effective than "whole-task" training in the acquisition of complex psychomotor skills. The rationale behind this notion is that learning part-tasks which are then integrated into a complete task frees the learner from becoming too focused on the minutiae of movement – the *choreography* of a task – and shifts attention towards learning control of the task as a whole (Whiting, 1972).

A single skill, such as suturing, can be applied to a number of varied, unrelated tasks, such as vascular anastomosis or closure of an abdominal incision. What differs between each of the applications of such a skill is the cognitive element; the principles of the motor aspects of the task are invariant. By corollary, tasks comprise a number of skills, coupled together in a particular order to achieve a desired outcome. In order to avoid the confusion associated with the colloquial use of the terms "ability", "skill", "task", and "procedure", we espouse the taxonomy proposed by Satava, Cuschieri, & Hamdorf (2003a) and Satava, Gallagher, & Pellegrini (2003b) (see Box 22.1).

Box 22.1. Definitions

Ability
An inherent characteristic or innate aptitude, present prior to training, which an individual brings to a given task.

Skill
An acquired (learned) proficiency of execution in a particular domain, which is the result of applying a specific combination of abilities to a given task.

Task
A piece of work to be done, usually incorporating multiple skills.

Procedure
A series of steps taken to accomplish a particular end.

After *Metrics for Objective Assessment of Surgical Skills Workshop* (Satava et al., 2003a, b).

Learning a skill within one context does not automatically allow for transfer to another. In fact, it may even interfere with learning the same skill in a different context, resulting in *negative transfer*, or *interference*. Surprisingly, however, learning the same skill initially in the second context may permit transfer to the first context! This phenomenon is known as *transfer asymmetry* (Rosenbaum, Carlson, & Gilmore, 2001). The possibility of abstraction or generalisation of a learned skill depends on a number of factors, including the variety of the trainee's previous experience with the skill (Borger & Seaborne, 1966), and the number of cognitive elements shared between the training task and the transfer task (Thorndike, 1903).

DESIGNING THE SKILLS CURRICULUM

Designing an instructional program in procedural skills requires *hierarchical decomposition* of procedures into their component skills, which begins with *training needs analysis*, itself comprising four components: mission analysis, task analysis, trainee analysis, and training analysis. The combined output of these four phases forms the basis of curriculum design. Learning   procedural   skills   in healthcare does not occur in a vacuum; to practise competently, the healthcare professional must master the relevant knowledge, skills, and attitudes (Rasmussen, 1983), elaboration of which is the purpose of *mission analysis*. These are determined by the nature of the task to be learned, its occupational context and the environment in which it is executed. A rarely performed, complex procedure with a life-or-death outcome performed by a specialist surgeon who frequently performs component elements individually in other contexts will obviously require training different from that required to train a trainee to perform a common procedure designed to increase patient comfort. The *specificity of training* principle requires that training be undertaken to the standard required for satisfactory day-to-day performance (Barnett, Ross, Schmidt, & Todd, 1973); this is a critical realisation of training needs analysis.

Task analysis outlines the knowledge required for execution of psychomotor tasks, both declarative and procedural. This distinguishes understanding how a task may be performed from actually being able to perform the task: the former does not necessarily guarantee the latter (Miller, 1990). After all …

> No one has ever managed to write the instructions for riding a bicycle or bouncing on a trampoline and then found the reader successfully engaging in these tasks based on reading alone. (Rosenbaum et al., 2001)

Task analysis takes into consideration the abilities and previous experience required of the candidate for successful completion of training.

This theme is carried further by *trainee analysis*. Current research into the nature and acquisition of expertise minimises the role played by natural, innate ability for particular tasks (Ericsson & Lehmann, 1996), or even a general aptitude for particular categories of tasks (Oxendine, 1967; Rosenbaum et al., 2001). There is good evidence, on the other hand, to indicate that in any field of endeavour – cognitive or psychomotor – an expert level of performance can be achieved by most individuals with about 10,000 hours of deliberate practice, or 10 years of *directed training* for 4 hours per day, which is the maximum duration of training sustainable over a protracted period of time (Ericsson, 1993).

In an elegant article, Fitts (1964) argued that skill learning occurs in three phases, although the entire process of learning is a continuous rather than a discrete phenomenon. The first is the *declarative stage* (or *composition stage* or *cognitive stage*), in which the basic rules of a task are articulated and learned. Next is the *associative stage* (or *proceduralisation stage*), during which the procedures of the task become more fluent. Finally, during the *autonomous stage*, the procedures become automated, being performed more rapidly and with greater immunity to disruption by external conditions. The most dramatic rapid changes in performance are seen in the first phase, and a plateau is reached by the third stage, although performance slowly continues to improve by small increments with practice over time.

Trainees in healthcare, whether at undergraduate or graduate level, are adult learners, for which reason any training program designed to cater for their needs must adhere to the four principles of adult learning (Knowles, 1990): adult learning is self-directed and autonomous, experiential, relevant and goal-directed, and heuristic. The Calman Report (Department of Health, 1993) recommended adoption of the broad principles of adult learning in order to streamline training. With respect to skills training, this means designing the curriculum so that training opportunities are presented as close as possible before tasks are required in the clinical environment, and each training encounter builds on knowledge and skills attained in previous encounters. Sufficient time must be afforded the trainee to achieve proficiency in a skill before moving to the next training exercise. Basic skills form the fundamental building blocks identified in a *task taxonomy* specific to a procedural domain. Initial teaching should be directed to mastery of these fundamental skills, with later instruction providing opportunity for *hierarchical synthesis* of more complex tasks from previously mastered components.

The task taxonomy is used in training analysis to determine the objectives to be met by trainees before training is deemed successful. It also determines the criteria by which training is evaluated, such as the Kirkpatrick and Kirkpatrick (2006) typology. Reaction criteria measure trainees' impressions of training; learning criteria measure learning outcomes by assessing the knowledge or skills gained by trainees during training; behavioural (or transfer) criteria are measures of on-the-job performance following training; and outcomes criteria indicate training program utility in terms of contribution to organisational objectives. Each successive level of evaluation is more difficult to achieve than the previous level, but it is also a more robust analysis. Some analysts also add *return on investment* as a fifth evaluation level. Data from each level of evaluation is required for complete assessment of training.

STRATEGIES IN SKILL ACQUISITION

A good curriculum must address other issues that emerge from training needs analysis. As well, curriculum designers must consider the changing emphasis in information requirements over the course of the three phases of skill acquisition (Day, Winfred, & Shebilske, 1997). Ackerman's Theory (Ackerman, 1988, 1989, 1992) states that the emphasis in each of three phases is on a different aspect of the skill. The *declarative* or cognitive phase has the highest information requirements, as the cognitive elements of learning predominate. In the *associative* phase trainees learn to correlate environmental cues with aspects of performance, while in the *autonomous* phase, the psychomotor aspects of learning are dominant. These general principles ought to underpin any learning activity.

Demonstration and Verbal Instruction

Pre-training preparation, in the form of self-instructional materials, demonstration and verbal instruction, may impart a rough mental model of the skill to be learned, but some aspects of task execution cannot be perceived by a novice armed with even the most detailed set of instructions (Borger & Seaborne, 1966; Rosenbaum et al., 2001). Previously prepared instructional materials enable trainees to prepare at their own pace, and can be used for deliberate "symbolic rehearsal" (Jarvis, 1967). This *mental practice* is defined as rehearsal of a skill in the mind, in the absence of any overt gross muscular movements (DesCoteaux & Leclere, 1995), and has been shown to improve performance on complex psychomotor tasks (Richardson, 1965a, b). Experimental evidence suggests that observing a skill being demonstrated does not lead to improved performance until after the learner has performed several iterations (Baker, 1968). On the other hand, observation mingled intermittently with practice by the observer may contribute to more rapid achievement of proficiency, but this is not maintained in transfer of training, and is not well retained after periods without practice (McCullagh & Little, 1990).

Interestingly, performance on a psychomotor task can deteriorate if the performer is concurrently engaged in a second, verbal task involving motion planning. This is thought to arise as a result of conflicting demands on a common cognitive resource. Hence, it is possible to attenuate the performance of a learner on a training task by simultaneously conveying verbal instructions for the performance or refinement of the task (Grafton et al., 1992; Baker et al., 1996).

One strategy to avoid this attenuation of learning is hierarchical decomposition, mentioned earlier (Marescaux et al., 2001). Another strategy involves combining verbal instruction with visual demonstration and additional visual cues. This technique, compared to other instructional methods, has been found to result in fewer errors during the learning phase of a psychomotor task, and in improved retention (Janelle, Champenoy, Coombes, & Mousseau, 2003).

Distributed Practice

Interposition of a period of non-practice between successive training sessions is called *distributed practice*, in contrast to concentrated or mass practice. Initially devised to avoid the negative effects of fatigue on learning (Barnett et al., 1973), it has been found to provide an additional training benefit in the form of *reminiscence*, defined as improvement in performance without practice (Borger & Seaborne, 1966). It was first noticed that testing performance immediately after a number of training trials showed results not as impressive as testing after a short delay. Further investigation showed that the effectiveness of a given number of training trials improved if the trials were separated by short periods without practice.

The benefits of distributed practice extend to cognitive tasks and tasks which generally require minimal energy expenditure, so those benefits cannot be explained merely in terms of physical fatigue. In the case of fine motor skills, for instance, short periods of continuous practice – in the order of minutes – can lead to deterioration in accuracy, although not necessarily in speed. Moreover, impaired performance is particularly pronounced in tasks involving vigilant observation – such as watching radar screens or repeatedly adjusting precision instruments – which do not require expenditure of great amounts of physical energy. Oddly enough, the benefits of distributed practice are reduced if the rest periods involve watching another perform the task (McCullagh & Little, 1990). All these features point to some kind of mental rather than physical fatigue.

A number of experiments conducted in the early 1990s further elucidated a previously unrecognised factor. Earlier studies had found that the improvement in performance which results from distributed practice does not occur immediately after the conclusion of a practice session, but some 8 to 10 hours later (Karni & Sagi, 1993; Julesz & Kovács, 1995). Subsequent investigation of this phenomenon discovered the significant role played by rapid-eye-movement sleep. Conventional and maternal wisdom emphasising the importance of a good night's rest during periods of training is thus vindicated, but an important principle is established for skills training: a distributed practice strategy is essential to optimise the rate of learning skills and for their long-term retention.

Knowledge of Results

Providing trainees with feedback on their performance serves two purposes: it plays an informational role in skill development and it plays a motivational role, which may be equally as important. Knowledge of results can be either *prescriptive* or *descriptive*. Descriptive knowledge of results can be acquired either during task execution – known as *concurrent information feedback* – or following task completion – known as *terminal information feedback*. Providing concurrent knowledge of results improves error recognition and allows modulation of task execution, whereas terminal information feedback serves as the prescription for the next iteration of the task, and is more important for skill retention (Newell, 1991). It is important that the outcome measure is perceived in substantively the same way as such information would be perceived in the real-world task (Holding, 1993).

Knowing the outcome of a task being learned serves to build a mental representation of the task, to identify errors in task execution, and to modulate internal rhythm and timing for the optimisation of task performance, thus calibrating the executed movements to the desired outcome. Each repetition of a task during practice results in more appropriate mental representation. This effect is observed on a trial-by-trial basis, but is also sustained in longer-term retention (Blackwell & Newell, 1996). The greatest benefit during acquisition of skills occurs when the feedback is immediate (Robb, 1968), although retention may be improved in the longer term by delaying feedback for one or two trials (Anderson, Magill, & Sekiya, 1994); retention is also improved if the feedback schedule is controlled by the learner (Janelle, Kim, & Singer, 1995). Decreasing the relative frequency of knowledge of results feedback does not otherwise affect performance (Ho & Shea, 1978), but summarising feedback over a large number of trials leads to a protracted skill acquisition phase and poor skill retention (Borger & Seaborne, 1966; Anderson et al., 1994).

Finally, the term "knowledge of results" is very widely used in the psychomotor skills training literature, almost to the exclusion of the term "feedback". There is an important distinction between the two terms, although they can be used interchangeably in colloquial circumstances. The distinction is that feedback is often seen as less than objective, or overly judgemental – and therefore detrimental, whereas knowledge of results emphasises awareness of the outcome of one's actions, rather than the critical evaluation of those actions by some third party. It is believed that this awareness of outcome contributes more to formulation of the mental schematic of the task at hand. Through direct experience of one's actions, an internal model is established, which cannot be created by relying on another's evaluation of one's performance (Noble, 1968).

Task Fidelity

Task fidelity is the extent to which the elements of a simulated task qualitatively resemble those of the real task. By applying the principles of *hierarchical decomposition*, it may be possible to quantify the extent of task fidelity.

Currently, the degree of task fidelity required of a simulator remains largely speculative. The value of task fidelity increases as the graphical and tactile sophistication of the simulator approaches the procedure simulated, but the utility threshold for this value has yet to be defined. It is reasonable to speculate – on the basis of Ackerman's Theory, discussed earlier – that the required level of fidelity will vary in proportion to the user's level of skill experience, or the learning phase for that task. Users with greater proficiency in the skill being taught – whether gained from real or simulated experiences – will derive less benefit than users who are less proficient at a given procedure, and this has been determined experimentally (Tracey & Lathan, 2001).

Transfer of Training

The training environment is designed to be a controlled one, with little variation from one performance of a task to the next. This is a double-edged sword: while it facilitates skill acquisition, it fails to fully expand the scope of situations to which the learned skill may eventually be applied. Training outside the operating room, for instance, would have little value if the skills learned could not be utilised in the operating room; it is rather expected that the skills acquired during training will transfer and prove useful to patients. Yet such transfer of training cannot be assumed to occur automatically, either at the generic level or at an individual level: rigorous testing must be undertaken to ensure that the learning environment and the skills a trainee acquires within it are robust.

Another simulator-related factor influencing transfer of training is the variability of the training medium. If the same task can be rehearsed repeatedly under different training conditions that simulate the various conditions under which the real-world task is performed, transfer of training is more likely to be successful (Holladay & Quinones, 2003).

A further aspect governing transfer of training may be the inherent ability of the trainee. This is not reliably predictable, and its effects are not well understood (Ackerman, 1987). It does have some bearing, however, on who will most likely benefit from a particular training exercise, and who will require remedial exercises (Tracey & Lathan, 2001).

Much broader factors also contribute to transfer of training. A notable determinant of whether or not training is implemented is workplace culture. Significantly delaying the first real-world execution of learned tasks after completion of training may result in extinction of the acquired skills prior to transfer (Arthur, Bennett, Stanush, & McNelly, 1998). There is currently a tendency for healthcare educators to emphasise teaching "one safe way" to perform the tasks being taught. If this one way does not conform to the preferences of the mentors on the clinical unit it is unlikely that the mentors will allow the trainee to continue to utilise any method other than their personally preferred one (Ford, Quinones, Sego, & Sorra, 1992). This can lead to inundation of the trainee with too many options to learn effectively at once, and so may hinder transfer. The workplace climate is also important: if pressure to complete tasks quickly is unchecked, the trainee may feel compelled to surrender transfer opportunities to other, more competent team members (Quinones, Ford, Sego, & Smith, 1995). The attitudes of trainees' work companions – including supervisors, other trainees, nursing staff, and others – and the prevailing culture of the healthcare facility have an important impact on the extent of transfer of training.

Skill Retention and Decay

Skill retention is the preservation of the effects of learning for some time after practice has ceased; *skill decay* is the loss of acquired skills after periods of non-use. The factors governing retention can be classified into one of four categories.

1. *Methodological factors* are those that can be modulated during the training period to improve retention.
2. *Task characteristics*, such as whether it is a physical or cognitive task or whether it is closed-looped or open-looped, also influence the degree of decay, but cannot be modified.
3. *Trainee characteristics* affect retention; trainees with greater ability tend toward more gradual decay than those of less ability.

4. *Retrieval conditions*, particularly the similarity between the training conditions and the testing conditions, also contribute to the extent of skill retention or decay observed.

The single most important factor influencing retention of learned material is *overlearning*. This is defined as continuing to practise a skill beyond the achievement of some competence criterion level. It is thought that the effects of overlearning result from reinforcement of the criterion state. Consider a training exercise in which the competence criterion is defined as a single errorless repetition of the training task; once this criterion is achieved, practice is halted. Prior to achieving the criterion, a trainee will usually have produced successively fewer errors in each of the repetitions prior to the last. From a retention perspective, therefore, there is no innate distinction between the errorless trial and those immediately preceding it. If, on the other hand, training continues beyond achievement of the competence criterion, additional repetitions are performed without error, so confirming the correctness of the performance. The sequence of motions that produced the competent performance is then preserved in memory. Overlearning also increases trainees' confidence in their performance and mitigates factors such as interruptability, stress and anxiety, which can hamper test performance (Arthur et al., 1998).

Decay is also affected by the *retention interval*, defined as the length of time between conclusion of training and testing for retention. Without interval practice, cognitive skills deteriorate more rapidly than psychomotor skills. Decay of both types of skill may be arrested to some extent by mental practice, although this effect is more pronounced for cognitive skills than it is for psychomotor skills. Anticipation of post-training assessment at some remote future date may motivate trainees to undertake self-directed practice to improve testing performance (Driskell, Willis, & Copper, 1992).

STRATEGIES IN SKILL ASSESSMENT

Assessment of procedural skills can occur in a variety of circumstances. Candidates for selection into training programs may be assessed to determine whether their ability is of sufficient calibre for the training ahead. At the conclusion of training, technical skills should be objectively assessed to determine whether a trainee has reached an acceptable level of professional competence. On return to clinical practice following a protracted absence, skill assessment may be a component of evaluating readiness for return to work. Periodic assessment of technical skills should also be undertaken to demonstrate currency of technique. Skill assessment in all these situations is a high-stakes venture, as a career may hang in the balance, as might the lives and welfare of many prospective patients. The assessment instruments used must, therefore, be valid and reliable.

Validity and *reliability* are empirically determined qualities of an assessment instrument, and essential. Although these two terms have fairly broad meanings in common usage, they have specific meanings in research and educational testing

(American Psychological Association, 1999). Further discussion of these constructs and their constituent elements is beyond the scope of this book, but information about how these concepts apply to skills assessment in healthcare are available (Cosman & Cartmill, 2011).

TRAINING MEDIA

A variety of training media are available for learning practical skills in healthcare. Selection of an appropriate training medium depends on the particular skills to be learned, the learning criterion, the previous experience of the trainee, the training environment, availability of resources, and local faculty expertise.

Standardised or surrogate patients are frequently used, but must be trained to minimise variability in performance. Although this is usually straightforward, the utility of surrogate patients is limited to non-invasive procedures with low risk of injury or discomfort. Use of fellow students as surrogate patients for practising invasive procedures is to be discouraged for ethical reasons. When training in such procedures is required, it may be acceptable to consider *synthetic or inanimate models*. *Computer-based instruction* may also be an acceptable alternative, although it is unlikely to provide an opportunity to practise procedural skills. *Animated mannequins* and *virtual environments* are useful for learning non-technical skills, but do not allow rehearsal of procedural skills. Highly specialised staff are needed to maintain such facilities. A combination using computer-based instruction, virtual environments, or inanimate models with the use of a surrogate patient in a *hybrid simulation* allows learning within the context of direct patient contact.

For training in more invasive procedural skills, *animal or human cadaveric tissue*, or even *live animals*, may be considered, although their use is limited by potential infectious risks and considerations of task fidelity. It may be possible to overcome these limitations by using *virtual reality simulation*, but this is costly to acquire and maintain.

The above discussion is necessarily cursory, but the evidence base and practical considerations to support selection of appropriate training media are well summarised in Cosman, Hemli, Ellis, and Hugh (2007).

TRAINING FACILITIES

Training does not typically occur in a single environment, but rather reflects the various settings in which healthcare professionals practise. Although the need for training on patients will never be fully extinguished by *ex vivo* training, major training experiences can now be satisfactorily conducted away from busy clinical settings. Not every training location will have access to all resources, but training networks can and should share resources to ensure equitable access to all trainees, using either a completely decentralised or a hub-and-spoke model. The facilities required to accommodate all forms of training include ward areas (intensive care unit, resuscitation bays, beds, stores, utilities, etc.), clinic areas, control room(s), debriefing room(s), operating room(s), surgical laboratory, animal laboratory, anatomy laboratory and seminar room(s). These facilities should be adequately staffed by technical and teaching personnel, and be resourced with appropriate models.

CONCLUSION

Initial training in the healthcare professions no longer prepares someone for a lifetime of practice. Advances in practice require re-training of qualified practitioners during the course of their career. This is often delivered in the form of continuing professional development courses, the design of which should follow the processes outlined in this chapter. The two overarching principles governing practical skills training are that patient outcomes are not compromised to accommodate training, and that trainees are afforded opportunities for training and practice until proficiency is attained. Consideration of these matters is essential in construction of a meaningful learning experience.

REFERENCES

Ackerman, P. L. (1987). Individual differences in skill learning: An integration of psychometric and information processing perspectives. *Psychological Bulletin, 102*(1), 3-27.

Ackerman, P. L. (1988). Determinants of individual differences during skill acquisition: Cognitive abilities and information processing. *Journal of Experimental Psychology: General, 117*(3), 288-318.

Ackerman, P. L. (1989). Within-task intercorrelations of skilled performance: Implications for predicting individual differences? (A comment on Henry & Hulin, 1987). *Journal of Applied Psychology, 74*(2), 360-364.

Ackerman, P. L. (1992). Predicting individual differences in complex skill acquisition: Dynamics of ability determinants. *Journal of Applied Psychology, 77*(5), 598-614.

American Psychological Association, American Educational Research Association and National Council on Measurement in Education. (1999). *Standards for educational and psychological testing.* Washington, DC: American Educational Research Association.

Anderson, D. I., Magill, R. A., & Sekiya, H. (1994). A reconsideration of the trials-delay of knowledge of results paradigm in motor skill learning. *The Research Quarterly for Exercise and Sport, 65*(3), 286-290.

Arthur, W. Jr., Bennett, W. Jr., Stanush, P. L., & McNelly, T. L. (1998). Factors that influence skill decay and retention: A quantitative review and analysis. *Human Performance, 11*(1), 57-101.

Baker, C. H. (1968). An evaluation of guidance in learning a motor skill. *Canadian Journal of Psychology, 22*(3), 217-227.

Baker, S. C., Rogers, R. D., Owen, A. M., Frith, C. D., Dolan, R. J., Frackowiak, R. S. et al. (1996). Neural systems engaged by planning: A PET study of the Tower of London task. *Neuropsychologia, 34*(6), 515-526.

Barnett, M. L., Ross, D., Schmidt, R. A., & Todd, B. (1973). Motor skills learning and the specificity of training principle. *The Research Quarterly, 44*(4), 440-447.

Blackwell, J. R., & Newell, K. M. (1996). The informational role of knowledge of results in motor learning. *Acta Psychologica (Amsterdam), 92*(2), 119-129.

Borger, R., & Seaborne, A. E. M. (1966). *The psychology of learning.* Harmondsworth, England: Penguin.

Breasted, J. H. (1927). *The Edwin Smith surgical papyrus.* Chicago, IL: University of Chicago Press.

Cosman, P. H., Hemli, J. M., Ellis, A. M., & Hugh, T. J. (2007). Learning the surgical craft: A review of skills training options. *ANZ Journal of Surgery, 77*, 838-845.

Cosman, P. H., & Cartmill, J. (2011). *Simulation in surgical education*. Saarbrücken, Germany: Lambert Academic Publishing.

Day, E. A., Winfred, A. Jr., & Shebilske, W. L. (1997). Ability determinants of complex skill acquisition: Effects of training protocol. *Acta Psychologica, 97*(2), 145-165.

Department of Health. (1993). Hospital doctors: Training for the future. In *The report of the Chief Medical Officer's Working Group to advise on specialist medical training in the United Kingdom* (The Calman Report). London: HMSO

DesCoteaux, J. G., & Leclere, H. (1995). Learning surgical technical skills. *Canadian Journal of Surgery, 38*(1), 33-38.

Dreyfus, H. L., & Dreyfus, S. E. (1986). *Mind over machine: The power of human intuition and expertise in the era of the computer*. New York, NY: Free Press.

Dreyfus, S. E. (2004). The five-stage model of adult skill acquisition. *Bulletin of Science, Technology and Society, 24*(3), 177-181.

Driskell, J. E., Willis, R. P., & Copper, C. (1992). Effect of overlearning on retention. *Journal of Applied Psychology, 77*(5), 615-622.

Ericsson, K. A. (1993). The role of deliberate practice in the acquisition of expert performance. *Psychological Review, 100(*3), 363-406.

Ericsson, K. A., & Lehmann, A. C. (1996). Expert and exceptional performance: Evidence of maximal adaptation to task constraints. *Annual Review of Psychology, 47*(1), 273-305.

Fitts, P. M. (1964). Perceptual-motor skill learning. In A. W. Melton (Ed.), *Categories of human learning* (pp. 243-285). New York, NY: Academic Press.

Ford, J. K., Quinones, M. A., Sego, D. J., & Sorra, J. S. (1992). Factors affecting the opportunity to perform trained tasks on the job. *Personnel Psychology, 45*(3), 511-528.

Grafton, S. T., Mazziotta, J. C., Presty, S., Friston, K. J., Frackowiak, R. S., & Phelps, M. E. (1992). Functional anatomy of human procedural learning determined with regional cerebral blood flow and PET. *Journal of Neuroscience, 12*(7), 2542-2548.

Guthrie, E. R. (1952). *The psychology of learning* (Rev. ed.). New York, NY: Harper.

Ho, L., & Shea, J. B. (1978). Effects of relative frequency of knowledge of results on retention of a motor skill. *Perceptual and Motor Skills, 46*(3 Pt 1), 859-866.

Holding, D. H. (1993). Sharing verbal and visuospatial resources in working memory. *Journal of General Psychology, 120*(3), 245-256.

Holladay, C. L., & Quinones, M. A. (2003). Practice variability and transfer of training: The role of self-efficacy generality. *Journal of Applied Psychology, 88*(6), 1094-1103.

Janelle, C. M., Champenoy, J., Coombes, S., & Mousseau, M. (2003). Mechanisms of attentional cueing during observational learning to facilitate motor skill acquisition. *Journal of Sports Sciences, 21*(10), 825-838.

Janelle, C. M., Kim, J., & Singer, R. N. (1995). Subject-controlled performance feedback and learning of a closed motor skill. *Perceptual and Motor Skills, 81*(2), 627-634.

Jarvis, L. (1967). Effects of self-instructive materials in learning selected motor skills. *The Research Quarterly, 38*(4), 623-629.

Julesz, B., & Kovács, I. (1995). *Maturational windows and adult cortical plasticity*. Reading, MA: Addison-Wesley.

Karni, A., & Sagi, D. (1993). The time course of learning a visual skill. *Nature, 365*(6443), 250-252.

Kirkpatrick, D. L., & Kirkpatrick, J. D. (2006). *Evaluating training programs: The four levels* (3rd ed.) San Francisco, CA: Berrett-Koehler.

Knowles, M. S. (1990). *The adult learner: A neglected species* (4th ed.). Houston, TX: Gulf.

Lloyd, G. E. R., Chadwick, J., Mann, W. N. (1978). *Hippocratic writings*. Harmondsworth, NY: Penguin.

Marescaux, J., Leroy, J., Gagner, M., Rubino, F., Mutter, D., Vix, M. et al. (2001). Transatlantic robot-assisted telesurgery. *Nature, 413*(6854), 379-380.

McCullagh, P., & Little, W. S. (1990). Demonstrations and knowledge of results in motor skill acquisition. *Perceptual and Motor Skills, 71*(3 Pt 1), 735-742.

Miller, G. E. (1990). The assessment of clinical skills/competence/performance. *Academic Medicine,* *65*(9 SuppL), S63-S67.

Newell, K. M. (1991). Motor skill acquisition. *Annual Review of Psychology, 42,* 213-237.

Noble, C. E. (1968). The learning of psychomotor skills. *Annual Review of Psychology. 19,* 203-250.

Oxendine, J. B. (1967). Generality and specificity in the learning of fine and gross motor skills. *The Research Quarterly, 38*(1), 86-94.

Poulton, E. C. (1957). On prediction in skilled movements. *Psychological Bulletin, 54,* 467-478.

Quinones, M. A., Ford, J. K., Sego, D. J., & Smith, E. M. (1995). The effects of individual and transfer environment characteristics on the opportunity to perform trained tasks. *Training Research Journal, 1*(1), 29-48.

Rasmussen, J. (1983). Skills, rules, and knowledge; Signals, signs, and symbols, and other distinctions in human performance models. *IEEE transactions on systems, man, and cybernetics, SMC, 13,* 257-266.

Richardson, A. (1965a). Mental practice: A review and discussion. Part I. *The Research Quarterly, 38*(1), 95-107.

Richardson, A. (1965b). Mental practice: A review and discussion. Part II. *The Research Quarterly, 38*(2), 263-273.

Robb, M. (1968). Feedback and skill learning. *The Research Quarterly, 39*(1), 175-184.

Rosenbaum, D. A., Carlson, R. A., & Gilmore, R. O. (2001). Acquisition of intellectual and perceptual-motor skills. *Annual Review of Psychology, 52*(1), 453-470.

Satava, R. M., Cuschieri, A., & Hamdorf, J. (2003a). Metrics for objective assessment. *Surgical Endoscopy, 17*(2), 220-226.

Satava, R. M., Gallagher, A. G., & Pellegrini, C. A. (2003b). Surgical competence and surgical proficiency: Definitions, taxonomy, and metrics. *Journal of the American College of Surgeons, 196*(6), 933-937.

Thorndike, E. L. (1903). *Educational psychology.* New York, NY: Science Press.

Tracey, M. R., & Lathan, C. E. (2001). The interaction of spatial ability and motor learning in the transfer of training from a simulator to a real task. *Studies in Health Technology and Informatics, 81,* 521-527.

Whiting, H. T. A. (1972). Overview of the skill learning process. *The Research Quarterly, 43*(3), 266-294.

Peter Hani Tawfik Cosman BA, MBBS, PhD, FRACS
School of Medicine
University of Western Sydney, Australia

MEGAN SMITH, STEPHEN LOFTUS AND TRACY LEVETT-JONES

23. TEACHING CLINICAL REASONING

Clinical reasoning skills are essential to the everyday practice of health professionals. Clinical reasoning distinguishes independent, thinking and decision-making professionals from individuals who implement technical activities under instruction from others. Teaching health professional students to engage in clinical reasoning requires explicit attention and strategy by teachers and strategies designed to model this skill. In this chapter we explore our collective research and practical experience to present an understanding of clinical reasoning that beginning teachers can draw upon in their practice. We begin by highlighting what we believe are the key contemporary understandings of clinical reasoning and then explore and comment on a case example from Megan's experience of researching and teaching clinical reasoning to physiotherapy students. We then reflect upon the key messages for those with an interest in teaching clinical reasoning.

UNDERSTANDING CLINICAL REASONING

"Clinical reasoning (or practice decision making) is a context-dependent way of thinking and decision making in professional practice to guide practice actions" (Higgs & Jones, 2008, p. 4). The term *clinical reasoning* is often used synonymously and interchangeably with the notions of professional judgement, problem solving, clinical decision making and critical thinking. Over the last decade there has been an increased interest in understanding the nature, significance and teaching of clinical reasoning (Norman, 2005; Loftus & Smith, 2008). Key elements of clinical reasoning identified are that individuals require a well-developed, multi-dimensional knowledge base, flexible cognitive abilities, and metacognitive abilities in order to adapt reasoning according to the task and situational demands (Ajjawi & Smith, 2010). The cognitive processes used in reasoning have been identified as involving analytical as well as non-analytical processes. Analytical processes involve deliberate thinking, whereas non-analytical processes involve more intuitive processes that draw on recognition of similar prior cases (Eva, Hatala, LeBlanc, & Brooks, 2007). Although analytical processes were typically thought to be used by novice practitioners and non-analytical processes as the domain of expert, or highly experienced and high performing practitioners, it is now accepted that novices and experts use both processes depending on the nature of the task (Norman, Young, & Brooks, 2007).

Ryan and Higgs (2008) noted that educational strategies to teach and facilitate learning clinical reasoning rely on understanding "the nature and context" of reasoning as it occurs in practice, and applying this to teaching strategies.

S. Loftus et al. (Eds.), Educating Health Professionals:
Becoming a University Teacher, 269–276.

Consequently, approaches to teaching clinical reasoning have reflected the complexity of understanding we now have of clinical reasoning; a range of strategies are considered rather than an accepted "best" approach. In classrooms this involves students working through examples from practice such as cases and clinical problems, integrating experience and knowledge from clinical placements through reflection, and using simulation and role playing as enactments of clinical reasoning. In this chapter we reflect upon current approaches and present our experience of researching clinical reasoning and applying our deepening understanding of this phenomenon to our teaching practice.

THE SETTING

The case example of teaching clinical reasoning we present was set in Charles Sturt University, Australia. This university offers educational programs in a broad range of health disciplines, including a bachelor of physiotherapy preparing students for entry-level practice as physiotherapists. Physiotherapy graduates are expected to practise independently upon completion of their studies and to have developed independent skills in clinical reasoning (Australian Physiotherapy Council, 2006).

On campus, students study theoretical and practical subjects relevant to the practice of physiotherapy. They then undertake clinical placements in which they apply and extend their capabilities in clinical reasoning by working with clients in practice settings. The discipline of physiotherapy involves practice in a range of specialist areas and this is reflected in the curriculum, with teaching directed at each of these specialist areas. Clinical reasoning is not taught as a discrete topic in physiotherapy; rather, the process of clinical reasoning is integrated with teaching of the knowledge and clinical skills required for practice. The example outlined here relates to Megan's experience in teaching physiotherapy students in the specialist area of cardiorespiratory and acute care physiotherapy.

THE FOCUS

The focus of this case is to describe Megan's experience of researching clinical reasoning as part of her doctoral studies and to describe how this research impacted on her teaching of clinical reasoning to physiotherapy students. Megan describes the educational approaches that were generated from her deepening insights about clinical reasoning and then reflects upon the challenges that emerged. Stephen and Tracy then offer their reflections from the perspective of their personally constructed understandings of clinical reasoning.

THE STRATEGY

Megan's Research

In my doctoral research I sought to address the contextual influences on clinical decision making. During clinical experience as a physiotherapist I had observed

270

that decisions and actions by physiotherapists varied according to the context in which the decision was made. The findings from my research contributed increased knowledge of clinical reasoning by revealing the dimensions of context and its impact on decision making (Smith, Higgs, & Ellis, 2007), the process of decision making (Smith, Higgs, & Ellis, 2008) and the effect of enhanced experience of practitioners on decision making (Smith, Higgs, & Ellis, 2010).

Megan's Teaching Approaches

Although my research into clinical reasoning did not lead to a novel and specific pedagogical approach it generated ideas that could be integrated into my teaching. The evolution of teaching clinical reasoning for me can be mapped against three phases. The first phase related to the approach I used prior to researching clinical reasoning. The second phase was during and immediately following my research and involved my emerging understanding of clinical reasoning as a phenomenon that could be incorporated into my teaching. The final phase was a reflective phase in which I reviewed the lessons I had learned about teaching clinical reasoning.

When I began teaching I drew upon my understanding of how I had used clinical reasoning during my practice as a physiotherapist. In terms of understanding clinical reasoning, I had limited access to the hidden or tacit use of clinical reasoning that I had developed. My approach to teaching thus emphasised that students should acquire knowledge of clinical information, interpret clinical facts, perform clinical skills and choose appropriate treatments. However, I had a poor understanding of how to optimally convey the manner in which these were blended in actual practice as a reasoning process. I assumed that students would be able to "do" the reasoning by having learned about the various elements of the process.

During and immediately following my research, my teaching changed as I began to use teaching approaches aimed at specifically developing students' abilities to use clinical reasoning. A key insight I gained was that clinical reasoning is a complex construct which is dependent on the nature of the task, the context in which it occurs and the characteristics of the person making the decision. Key aspects of reasoning in physiotherapy are also the presence of uncertainty and a time-dependent evolving understanding of the clinical situation. Identifying these features revealed that teaching and learning clinical reasoning both require the manipulation of multiple concepts and ideas and are as complex as the construct itself. In this chapter, while I have selected three examples from my teaching to describe, there were many nuanced ways in which my teaching developed during that time and since.

Example 1: Giving Students Frameworks for Clinical Reasoning

Students learning to use clinical reasoning have limited insight into the shape and purpose of the cognitive processes that are used in their discipline and in the course of clinical practice. Through my research I was able to identify the various types of decisions that physiotherapists make and the reasoning pathways they use in clinical practice. This approach assumes that students need to learn to think like experts (Vermunt & Verloop, 1999; Radomski & Russell, 2010). My ability to communicate patterns of reasoning to students gave them a structure and purpose to use as the basis for their own decision making. Cardiorespiratory physiotherapists make decisions that balance the risks and benefits of potential treatments (e.g. sitting a patient out of bed following surgery where there are risks of the patient becoming hypotensive and falling). I discovered that physiotherapists use a process of determining whether physiotherapy is indicated and then considering the positive and negative effects. They balance these considerations with their own feelings of confidence in the situation before deciding on a course of action. Using case studies I created scenarios that required students to work through this process, and was able to guide them through the decision making process required for action. My research also found that decision making for cardiorespiratory physiotherapists was not a case of a single decision between fixed alternatives but a process of ongoing decision action cycles. This insight helped me to develop teaching tasks that provided students with evolving information, replicating clinical reasoning as it would be required in practice.

Example 2: Clinical Reasoning Occurs in a Context

My research revealed that clinical reasoning is dependent on the context in which it occurs. Learning clinical reasoning requires students to understand that it does not always result in a single right answer; rather it requires students to have the ability to recognise and balance the contextual factors that impact on their decision making and actions. Students also need to learn the contextual influences on the sources of knowledge they develop during practice and how to be critical of their developing knowledge base.

I had always used case studies extensively in my teaching because I believed that students needed to learn to think about realistic clinical problems. This approach was reinforced as I learned more about clinical reasoning. My research emphasised the importance of thinking carefully about the contextual factors that affect the decisions being made. For example, when asking students to plan exercise programs for patients, rather than leaving them to assume unlimited resources, I defined, controlled and varied these aspects of the context to help them understand the impacts on their decision making.

Example 3: Making Simple and Complex Decisions

In my research, practitioners indicated that some decisions were more difficult than others. It was the range of factors about the decision that influenced its complexity. This was an important insight as it allowed me more effectively to design learning tasks that progressively added complexity. Previously I had been less conscious about the tasks I gave students, tending to focus on the client condition and the provision of authentic cases rather than being able to vary the characteristics of the case to control and progress its complexity for students, enabling them to develop their clinical reasoning skills. Some of the factors that added complexity which I learned to vary were the number and relevance of clinical variables, the urgency of the situation, the emotional and ethical issues, and the congruence and conflict in the information.

CHALLENGES FACED

Reflecting back on my experience of researching and teaching clinical reasoning I have concluded that clinical reasoning does need to be explicitly taught to students. What becomes intuitive to expert practitioners is not intuitive to beginning practitioners. Both teaching and learning clinical reasoning are challenging.

Through research, educators are better able to develop teaching strategies that give students access to how practitioners think in the reality of practice. Further research is needed, however, into how students learn to reason, how learning to reason varies among individuals, and the optimal strategies for assisting students to learn clinical reasoning. There is no single most effective way to teach clinical reasoning (Rochmawati & Wiechula, 2010). This is not surprising given the complexity of clinical reasoning as a process.

> The more one studies the clinical expert, the more one marvels at the complex and multidimensional components of knowledge and skill that she or he brings to bear on the problem, and the amazing adaptability she must possess to achieve the goal of effective care. (Norman, 2005, p. 426)

A further challenge in academic settings lies in how to teach clinical reasoning in a way that is transferable to clinical practice (Le Maistre & Pare, 2004). Although a better understanding of clinical reasoning allows teachers to identify foundational elements, the complexity of reasoning means that immersion in clinical practice reveals the true nature of clinical reasoning to students. We can be confident that our efforts in the classroom are rewarded only when students apply their clinical reasoning skills in clinical practice.

REFLECTIONS

Reflections from Stephen

Clinical reasoning, like education, is best seen as an umbrella term for a range of different and complex activities. As pointed out, it is not always useful to see clinical reasoning in isolation. The same applies to education. Education is always *about* something and *for* some purpose. Likewise, clinical reasoning is always for a purpose and always in a context, such as diagnosing *this* patient in *these* circumstances in the *here* and *now*. However, as with education, it can be useful to think of clinical reasoning as a collection of different practices and to consider what they might have in common. For example, medical students eventually realise the relevance and usefulness of problem-based learning as a way of thinking through clinical cases, but generally only after they have been immersed in some real-world practice and had the chance to reflect upon the connections between what happens in the classroom and what happens in the clinic. As one medical student reflected:

> I think it's a really good idea [problem-based learning]. It's how you think clinically ... it's how you should think clinically. (Loftus, 2009, p. 152)

As with many complex activities, it can be useful to consider clinical reasoning at different levels of abstraction. For example, biology can be studied at different levels of abstraction, from the level of molecular biology through to the level of the study of ecosystems of whole continents. In the same way, we can study clinical reasoning from the perspectives of different disciplines. A cognitive science approach studies clinical reasoning as information processing, and this can be useful. Other approaches, based on the social sciences, see clinical reasoning as a complex and personal interaction that focuses on the relationship between patient and clinician. For example, a hermeneutic approach (Svenaeus, 2000; Montgomery, 2006) focuses on whole/part relationships and asks questions such as: how are the bits of information gathered in the assessment (the parts) related to the final diagnosis (the whole)? A narrative inquiry approach (Loftus & Greenhalgh, 2010) asks: what stories are patients living out? In chronic pain cases, for example, patients might be living out the story of the invalid on a downward spiral because they can find no solution for their pain which seems overwhelming and never seems to get better. Treatments, such as cognitive behavioural therapy, can then be seen as a means of persuading such patients to start living out a new life story, one in which the pain is managed and consigned to the background so that a relatively normal life can continue (Loftus, 2011).

These are just some examples of the disciplines that can be used to reflect on clinical reasoning. When it comes to teaching clinical reasoning, it is important to encourage students to reflect on the cases they have seen and been involved in. We can use a multidisciplinary approach and use ideas from different disciplines to encourage such reflection. For example, if we wish to adopt a cognitive science approach to clinical reasoning, we can ask students to consider what information was gathered and how it was processed. If we adopt a narrative medicine approach, we can ask students to think through the stories that were being told or acted out and how these stories shaped the ways participants thought through the issues. If we adopt a hermeneutic approach, we can ask how the parts of the case were related to the whole and how the relationship between participants in the clinical encounter developed, what interpretations and meanings emerged, and how they emerged. The list goes on. To understand a complex activity like clinical reasoning, and to teach it, we need a range of disciplines to provide us with the conceptual tools to open up its complexity so that our students can begin to appreciate what it involves.

Reflections from Tracy

Competent professional practice requires not only knowledge and skills but also sophisticated thinking abilities. Safe and effective health professionals use disciplined and systematic thought processes to guide their practice and inform their decision making. Although teaching clinical reasoning can be complex and challenging it is nevertheless an imperative. There is evidence that clinical reasoning ability is a key factor in the provision of quality care and the prevention of adverse patient outcomes. Health professionals who do not possess clinical reasoning skills can fail to detect patient deterioration, resulting in "failure-to-rescue" (Aiken, Clarke, Cheung, Sloane, & Silber, 2003). In fact, cognitive errors have been identified as a factor in over 57% of adverse events in healthcare (Wilson et al., 1995); this includes failure to collect, process and act on clinical data.

To become competent health professionals, students must be taught the process and steps of clinical reasoning as well as the connections between cues, decisions and patient outcomes. Learning to reason effectively does not happen serendipitously. It requires practice, determination, and students' active engagement in deliberate learning activities; it also requires reflection, particularly on activities designed to improve performance (Levett-Jones, 2013). The facilitation of clinical reasoning requires educators to model, teach and assess student's developing skills, in both academic and clinical settings, on many occasions. To develop clinical reasoning skills, students should be exposed to intellectually challenging situations in clinical, simulated and classroom settings that will cause them to re-examine many taken-for-granted assumptions and reflect on their emerging clinical reasoning skills and professional understandings.

REFERENCES

Aiken, L. H., Clarke, S. P., Cheung, R. B., Sloane, D. M., & Silber, J. H. (2003). Educational levels of hospital nurses and surgical patient mortality. *JAMA, 290*(12), 1617-1620.

Ajjawi, R., & Smith, M. (2010). Clinical reasoning capability: Current understanding and implications for physiotherapy educators. *Focus on Health Professional Education: A Multi-disciplinary Journal, 12*(1), 60-73.

Australian Physiotherapy Council. (2006). *Australian standards for physiotherapy*. Canberra: Australian Physiotherapy Council.

Eva, K. W., Hatala, R. M., LeBlanc, V. R., & Brooks, L. R. (2007). Teaching from the clinical reasoning literature: Combined reasoning strategies help novice diagnosticians overcome misleading information. *Medical Education, 41*(12), 1152-1158.

Higgs, J., & Jones, M. (2008). Clinical decision making and multiple problem spaces. In J. Higgs, M. Jones, S. Loftus & N. Christenson (Eds.), *Clinical reasoning in the health professions* (3rd ed., pp. 3-17). Edinburgh: Butterworth-Heinemann.

Levett-Jones, T. (Ed.). (2013). *Clinical reasoning: Learning to think like a nurse*. Sydney: Pearson.

Le Maistre, C., & Pare, A. (2004). Learning in two communities: The challenge for universities and workplaces. *Journal of Workplace Learning, 16*(1-2), 44-52.

Loftus, S. (2009). *Language in clinical reasoning: Towards a new understanding*. Saarbrücken: VDM Verlag.

Loftus, S. (2011). Pain and its metaphors: A dialogical approach. *Journal of Medical Humanities, 32*(3), 213-230.

Loftus, S., & Greenhalgh, T. (2010). Towards a narrative mode of practice. In J. Higgs, D. Fish, I. Goulter, S. Loftus, J.-A. Reid & F. Trede (Eds.), *Education for future practice* (pp. 85-94). Rotterdam. The Netherlands: Sense.

Loftus, S., & Smith, M. (2008). A history of clinical reasoning research. In J. Higgs, M. A. Jones, S. Loftus & N. Christensen (Eds.), *Clinical reasoning in the health professions* (3rd ed., pp. 205-212). Amsterdam: Butterworth-Heinemann.

Montgomery, K. (2006). *How doctors think: Clinical judgment and the practice of medicine.* Oxford: Oxford University Press.

Norman, G. (2005). Research in clinical reasoning: Past history and current trends. *Medical Education, 39*(4), 418-427.

Norman, G., Young, M., & Brooks, L. (2007). Non-analytical models of clinical reasoning: The role of experience. *Medical Education, 41*(12), 1140-1145. doi:10.1111/j.1365-2923.2007.02914.x

Radomski, N., & Russell, J. (2010). Integrated case learning: Teaching clinical reasoning. *Advances in Health Sciences Education, 15*(2), 251-264. doi:10.1007/s10459-009-9195-x

Rochmawati, E., & Wiechula, R. (2010). Education strategies to foster health professional students' clinical reasoning skills. *Nursing & Health Sciences, 12*(2), 244-250. doi:10.1111/j.1442-2018.2009.00512.x

Ryan, S., & Higgs, J. (2008). Teaching and learning clinical reasoning. In J. Higgs, M. Jones, S. Loftus & N. Christenson (Eds.), *Clinical reasoning in the health professions* (3rd ed., pp. 379-387). Edinburgh: Butterworth-Heinemann.

Smith, M., Higgs, J., & Ellis, E. (2007). Physiotherapy decision making in acute cardiorespiratory care is influenced by factors related to the physiotherapist and the nature and context of the decision: A qualitative study. *Australian Journal of Physiotherapy, 53*(4), 261-267.

Smith, M., Higgs, J., & Ellis, E. (2008). Characteristics and processes of physiotherapy clinical decision making: A study of acute care cardiorespiratory physiotherapy. *Physiotherapy Research International, 13(*4), 209-222.

Smith, M., Higgs, J., & Ellis, E. (2010). Effect of experience on clinical decision making by cardiorespiratory physiotherapists in acute care settings. *Physiotherapy Theory and Practice, 26*(2), 89-99.

Svenaeus, F. (2000). *The hermeneutics of medicine and the phenomenology of health: Steps towards a philosophy of medical practice.* Dordrecht: Kluwer Academic.

Vermunt, J. D., & Verloop, N. (1999). Congruence and friction between learning and teaching. *Learning and Instruction, 9*(3), 257-280. doi:10.1016/s0959-4752(98)00028-0

Wilson, R., Runciman, W., Gibberd, R., Harrison, B., Newby, L., & Hamilton, J. (1995). The quality in Australian health care study. *Medical Journal of Australia, 163*, 458-471.

Megan Smith PhD
Faculty of Science
Charles Sturt University, Australia

Stephen Loftus PhD
The Education For Practice Institute
Charles Sturt University, Australia

Tracy Levett-Jones PhD
School of Nursing and Midwifery
The University of Newcastle, Australia

ANDREW KILGOUR, TANIA GERZINA, MIKE KEPPELL
AND JANET GERZINA

24. UNDERSTANDING THE PLACE OF
ASSESSMENT STANDARDS

A Case Study in Medical Diagnostic Radiography

A major problem confronting the education of students in many health professions is assessing what they do on clinical placements in (often) non-university clinical facilities. Like campus-based assessment, such assessments need to be conducted in a manner that is objective and fair, and is seen to be objective and fair. These assessments are usually undertaken by non-university staff working at the clinical placement. One clinical site might also have students from different universities, and each university may have different expectations and guidelines about assessment. Even when a university provides assessment guidelines and criteria, there is a need to interpret them in the context of service requirements of the clinical facility. When students are directly involved in providing patient care, the clinical facility will have standards and demands that directly and complexly impact on assessment of students. Many staff conducting assessments feel they have to navigate a "minefield" with conflicting demands and different reporting requirements that often seem disconnected from each other (Kilgour, 2011). This issue is now seen as a major challenge facing the education of health professionals, as more education is completed in clinical placements (as in work-integrated learning) and such placements are competitively sought.

This chapter presents a case study of an attempt to deal with this issue of assessment in clinical placements. A solution was to establish an Australian national standard in assessment for all educators involved in the particular discipline of medical diagnostic radiography. Rather than reinventing the wheel, the Australian national standard already established for speech pathology (Ferguson, McAllister, McAllister, & Lincoln, 2006) was used as a guideline. This chapter, therefore, summarises of the experience of developing national assessment standards in the discipline of medical diagnostic radiography. We believe the lessons learned can be applied to many other health professions.

S. Loftus et al. (Eds.), Educating Health Professionals:
Becoming a University Teacher, 277–286.

THE SETTING

Medical Radiography Science

The professional skill of medical radiographers is to provide diagnostic images that support precise medical decisions made by a medical team. Formal courses in radiography in Australia began in the late 1920s. The education featured early placement of trainee radiographers (students) in radiology departments of hospitals under the supervision of hospital-based staff. Students also attended evening classroom-based learning sessions in college. Learning was practically-focused, with early emphasis on the development of clinical skills supported by education in medical and physical sciences in the classroom learning environment.

Education and training of radiographers, as with many health professions worldwide, has undergone substantial change in Australia over the years. The contemporary approach to medical care based on the bio-psychosocial model of health, first theorised by Engel in 1977, has been a significant driver of the evolution and elaboration of many health professions. The transition for health professions in terms of enculturation, specific implications for hospital service and of course for educational and curriculum reform was equally significant. Radiography was one such health profession which underwent transition into a university-based program.

The Medical Diagnostic Radiography Degree

Medical diagnostic radiography education in Australia has much in common with similar education programs throughout the Western world. This education is now typically offered as a 4-year university degree program in tertiary institutions across Australia. As with many health professions, accreditation for medical radiography programs is nationally imposed. In this case, accreditation comes from the Australian Institute of Radiography Professional Accreditation and Education Board. Like many health professionals, medical radiographers are registered with the Australian Health Professions Regulation Agency. Education is university campus-based, and clinical placements are provided in a variety of hospital and clinical settings.

The Degree at The University of Sydney

The undergraduate degree of Bachelor of Applied Science (Medical Radiation Science) Diagnostic Radiography, has been offered since 1988 as a degree program through the discipline of medical radiation science in the Faculty of Health Sciences at the university. This is typical of the degree programs in Australia and serves as a useful case study to illustrate the key points we wish to make. For students who are already practising in radiography, the discipline offers a range of specialist masters programs in the category of graduate entry toward degrees such as the Master of Health Sciences (MRS). The program provides theoretical skill acquisition and clinical placements to assist students in achieving prescribed professional competencies.

The University of Sydney students attend clinical placements in two geographical locations: a city urban area and a rural area. Placements are located in a mix of small and large private practices and small and large public and private hospitals. Undergraduate students (those who enter the program from high school) complete 25 weeks of clinical placement over 3 years. Postgraduate students (those with previous tertiary education experience) complete 22 weeks of clinical placement over 2 years. Supervision of students in clinical placements is by trained radiology department educators employed at the site and/or by radiographers. Assessments used include written assessments and assignments, observation of practice and practical assessments, achievement manuals (log books) and specialty reports that target knowledge, skills and professional behaviour.

THE FOCUS

Successful learning in the clinical placement is largely dependent upon the ability of clinical supervisors to provide authentic mentorship, experiential advice and a willingness to guide and empathise with students in the privilege of patient care. Supervisor ability to reliably assess a number of students in clinical placements is a challenge found in many health profession programs, including radiography. Besides competing placement duties, added complexity comes with the need for supervisors to apply different assessment formats with different standards for students from different universities.

This challenge is a core issue for the pedagogy of work-integrated learning. In the case of medical radiography, specific problems have been identified (Kilgour, 2011):

- significant variations about assessment objectives
- internal variations in regard to accountability for assessment
- clinical supervisors being uncomfortable with failing poorly performing students
- different interpretations among placement-based supervisors as to what constitutes competence
- confusion as to use of assessment tools among supervisors who accept students from more than one university, due to differences in assessment paperwork from the different universities
- lack of reliability of the grades ascribed by supervisors compared with those of university educators.

Local solutions to these problems have included applying complex algorithms to equate assessment inputs and improving educator briefing on assessment tools. As student numbers rise and supervisor numbers fall, these local solutions have not been sustainable and assessment practice can decline as a result.

THE STRATEGY

The approach taken was to consider standards-based assessment and the alignment of assessment practices with nationally recognised standards within a professional field. This approach was used by the profession of speech pathology, for example. COMPASS® Online (Competency Assessment in Speech Pathology) is a national speech pathology assessment tool used across many universities in Australia (Ferguson et al., 2006). Endorsed by the Speech Pathology Association of Australia, that assessment is a validated tool for determining levels of competency of speech pathology students, and is web based. The website is:
http://www.speechpathologyaustralia.org.au/resources/compassr

An aim, then, was to develop an assessment strategy for medical diagnostic radiography that would be nationally integrated and widely accepted in the educational community. A process using elements of naturalistic educational action research and ethnographic methodology was thought best to achieve this aim. The primary goal of action research is not simply to generate new knowledge or understanding but to have an immediate effect on reforming and improving what is being done in the practice setting (Kemmis & McTaggart, 1992). This enquiry paradigm was chosen as it lends itself to educational environments and has, for example, often been associated with professional teacher development (e.g. Winter, 1996). It is conducted both in and about the workplace (Collins & Duguid, 1989). Essentially, the research features cycles of planning, acting, observing and reflecting, in the current case, about teaching and learning in medical radiography. In this case study, action research techniques were organised into the framework shown in Table 24.1.

The literature analysis highlighted areas of assessment in higher education of specific application to clinical education. These included standards-based assessment (e.g. O'Donovan, Rust, Price, & Carroll, 2005; Sadler, 2005; Woolf, 2004; Yorke, 2011), where standards of quality are applied to grading and achievement. This highlighted the need to improve the reliability and validity of clinical assessment in diagnostic radiography academic programs by developing an evidence-based assessment strategy designed with input from the profession. Other themes in the literature were types of knowledge and understanding, alignment to curriculum, teacher's role, competence, assessment type (formative vs. summative and analytic vs. holistic), and professional judgement.

Table 24.1. Strategy framework to develop a national clinical assessment standard framework in medical radiography

---

Systematic literature and current practice review. Key words: assessment, competency, clinical assessment, radiography, diagnostic radiography. Databases: e.g. Medline, ERIC©, from 2001 to 2011. Major themes organised using NVivo8™ qualitative data analysis software.

Search conference. This is the analysis and discussion of narrative data seeking to derive themes from impressions and experiences. The narrative data came from interviews and focus groups with radiography students, clinical placement supervisors (national and international), current practitioners, practising radiographers and managers, education providers.

Reflexive critique. This is a process in which researchers become aware of their perceptual biases (Winter, 1996). Being aware of their own biases helps researchers to analyse the qualitative data concerning educational practice in a detached and objective manner.

Analysis of current competency benchmarks. These are the professional competencies required by the Australian Institute of Radiography, which are used as a benchmark for the standard required for entry into and accreditation within the profession.

Iterative analysis … of qualitative data to plan alignment of educational practice to meet assessment requirements of professional competencies and to work towards a national clinical assessment standards framework.

Reporting of synthesis of search and review information

Development. Background for a National Clinical Assessment Standard Framework in Medical Radiography (NCASMR) based on the assessment framework.

Trial/pilot qualitative study … of assessment framework within the academic and training community.

Iterative analysis. Refinement of framework and development of national assessment.

Implementation and evaluation … of effectiveness of the NCASMR framework to structure a national assessment.

The search conference provided discussion on mapping of the assessment of student competency against standards developed and published by the Australian Institute of Radiography (AIR) and the National Registration Authority. Another matter raised was the need for a consistent nationwide process. A national set of educational standards of assessment of competence in medical radiography is seen as the key to meeting the assessment challenge and ensuring uniformity across

281

Australia as to the standard expected of a graduating radiographer. This point is illustrated in the following quotes from clinical supervisors in medical radiography.

> What reference point do we use for that standard? You go to Paris and you have the standard for a metre. Where do we go to determine what is the standard?

And further,

> Do we set the standard, or is it the clinics out there, that say, well we don't need radiographers out there with a diploma or a degree, we just need somebody that knows how to push a button, so X is right about setting standards, but he's right again about who sets the standard that we've got to measure? Is it us? And the AIR? Or is it the employers?

Lifelong learning was also discussed:

> I think then you've got to look at what is the scope of practice, which is a different question altogether, which is once they've qualified, what then are the skills there that need to be maintained, to still have them defined as a radiographer?

A degree of frustration was also noted among students and academics alike at the apparent inconsistencies in grades achieved in clinical units of study:

> I think the problem with a lot of students at clinical [placement] is that they either lack the opportunities they need, to actually get the areas that they're after, or they actually, for some reason or another, have issues with the supervisor, not that only bad students have issues, but sometimes people just don't click, and you've basically nowhere to go.

Reporting and presentation of the synthesised data was undertaken in several forums: the Australasian Association of Educators in Medical Radiation Science, the Australia and New Zealand Association for Health Professional Education, the Australian Institute of Radiography's Annual Scientific Meeting of the Medical Imaging and Radiation Therapy, and in The University of Sydney Work-Integrated Learning Research Unit meetings. These conference meetings provided important engagement with the radiography community (in both benchmarking and iterative analysis of case study data), especially with members of the Professional Accreditation and Education Board of the AIR. The AIR provides *Competency Based Standards for the Accredited Practitioner* to successfully apply for practice through the national Australian Health Practitioner Regulation Agency, found at http://www.air.asn.au/. Educational assessment standards for students in the profession, though, are a focus of ongoing consideration by AIR, and their development was the core aim of the case study described in this chapter.

Several challenges were faced in the project. To a large extent, they centred on the problems of clinical supervisors in providing valid and reliable assessment of students in clinical settings, noted by Kilgour (2011). To reach the objective of valid assessment through a national standardised strategy of assessment, the supervisors themselves had to be engaged and willing partners in the development of those standards.

Clinical supervisors' apparent discomfort with failing poorly performing students was one such challenge. Anecdotal evidence from reviewing clinical assessment forms for student radiographers suggested that the grades awarded on clinical placement were artificially high. Burchell, Higgs, and Murray (1999) suggested that this is a common phenomenon for two reasons: the combination of assessor and mentor roles among people working in small groups with a common culture leads to a reluctance to criticise or fail colleagues with whom they work; the nature of the occupational culture in a caring profession can lead to resistance to the idea of judging people negatively. If we are to take this seemingly common inflation of grades into account, we must find a way to address these largely cultural issues. This is not as simple as scaling the grades of all students enrolled in the unit of study, because although the grade inflation phenomenon is common it is not universal. Students who are graded without artificial inflation would therefore be unfairly penalised should such scaling of marks be implemented.

Supervisors themselves were confused in their definitions of "competent". Miller (1990) distinguished several hierarchical layers of competence as a framework for assessment. Biggs and Collis (1982, p. 88) defined competence as "firstly a quantitative accrual of the components of a task, and then the qualitative restructuring of these components". This is what seems to happen in practice. Most supervising radiographers have seen beginning students who see radiographic theory as a series of disjointed facts, and have then watched as these same students piece the facts together when given a chance to apply the theory in real-world practice. In order to truly assess competence, measurement of how well students are able to "restructure the components" is required, but this needs to be applied consistently.

An insight (by AK), gained by observing many clinical placements, was that clinical supervisors interpreted assessment criteria differently, and had different expectations of students' clinical performance. This suggested that assessment of competence should have structure, reflect progression and development through the course, and explore natural issues of professional conduct. Hager, Gonczi, and Athanasou (1994) referred to the concept of an integrated assessment of competence, defining it as conceptualised in terms of knowledge, abilities, skills and attitudes displayed in the context of a carefully chosen set of realistic professional tasks. Applying this to the assessment of a student radiographer's clinical performance, we can see that all four of these vital factors need to be present for the student to be considered competent. Not only should these features be present, however; they should be as highly developed as possible.

As a consequence of our teaching, we want our students to exhibit highly developed skills, such as cognitive skills. Sadler (1989) suggested that engagement in the practice of the skills of integration of knowledge, complex problem solving, critical opinion forming, lateral thinking and innovative action together fosters the development of sophisticated cognitive abilities in a learner. Adopting assessment approaches that expressly target these higher cognitive skills is an important educational goal. The SOLO Taxonomy (Structure of the Observed Learning Outcome), as described by Biggs and Collis (1982) helps us understand how a learner's performance grows in complexity when mastering tasks. The clinical assessment framework should not only measure the level a student has reached in SOLO, but should also provide a means for assisting and encouraging the student to progress to the "extended abstract" level. That is the level at which a student can truly be considered competent. Sometimes the assessor defers to the judgement of a senior, as in this quote:

> It was usually the clinical coordinator, or clinical director, or whatever you called it, that would sign them off at the end of the thing. So they would sign them off, saying, "in my opinion", and they took advice from chiefs, from other colleagues, "in my opinion, this person is competent to practise", you know, and that carried a lot of weight... This was the opinion of a well-qualified person that in his opinion, this person was competent to practise.

The intuitive or experiential approach taken by assessors may, however, be inconsistent with pedagogical assessment practice that is more structured (O'Donovan et al., 2004; Sadler, 1989), and effort should be made to integrate the value of intuitive and pedagogical assessment feedback for students. Some supervisors do attempt this, again quoting a clinical supervisor:

> A combination of regular feedback, but then a[n intuitive] judgment I'd say, maybe because that's the system I was used to, but a[n intuitive] judgment at the end, after all this analytic feedback which they get, which helps them improve...

Another significant challenge for clinical supervisors has been developing a teacher identity, the place of the "self" in emotional connectivity and related issues of agency as an educator or clinical supervisor. Beauchamp and Thomas (2009, p.186) concluded:

> In order to anticipate the reshaping of professional identity that will come, we must continue to consider the situation of teachers in the early years of practice, where the influence of their surrounding context – the nature of the educational institution, teacher colleagues, school administrators, their own students and the wider community – is strongly felt.

The project is ongoing and continues to challenge all involved to think more deeply about all these issues such as teaching and learning in clinical environments, as well as teacher identity.

REFLECTIONS

This project has become an ongoing endeavour but has already yielded important insights.

Learners are considered competent when they demonstrate that they understand and can act upon the essential similarities and differences between clinical situations that are superficially the same but have subtle differences.

The literature has demonstrated that professional development and support enhance clinical supervisor confidence and consistency. Such support also encourages supervisors to share with each other and form networks of learning and teaching communities. At the same time, this support can provide a means by which important information about the curriculum can be disseminated. It is also clear that clinical supervisors have unique development needs and interests and that these individual needs must be catered for as far as possible.

Integrated assessment, described by Hager et al. (1994, p. 8) as "where competence is conceptualised in terms of knowledge, abilities, skills and attitudes displayed in the context of a carefully chosen set of realistic professional tasks" allows the assessor to apply assessment in the context of a realistic professional setting. As well as judging how well students can master the key aspects of their profession it is also now clear that good assessment is an important learning process in itself.

The notion of national and common standards for assessment of performance in clinical placements is a compelling ideal for any health profession. To achieve this ideal we have learned that it is important to have widespread consultation and discussion in order to articulate and resolve the many differences of opinion that inevitably occur. We have also learned that improving the standards will be an ongoing exercise for the foreseeable future. However, this is a worthwhile effort as supervisors, students and ultimately patients will all benefit.

REFERENCES

Beauchamp, C., & Thomas, L. (2009). Understanding teacher identity: An overview of issues in the literature and implications for teacher education. *Cambridge Journal of Education, 39*(2), 175-189.

Biggs, J. B., & Collis, K. F. (1982). *Evaluating the quality of learning: The SOLO taxonomy.* New York: Academic Press.

Burchell, H., Higgs, T., & Murray, S. (1999). Assessment of competence in Radiography education. *Assessment and Evaluation in Higher Education, 24*(3), 315-326.

Collins, J. S., & Duguid, P. (1989). Situated cognition in the culture of learning. *Educational Researcher, 32*, 32-42.

Engel, G. L. (1977). The need for a new medical model: A challenge for biomedicine. *Science, 196*, 129-136.

Ferguson, A., McAllister, L., McAllister, S., & Lincoln, M. (2006). *Benchmarking clinical learning in speech pathology to support assessment, discipline standards, teaching innovation and student learning.* Australian Learning and Teaching Council/Priority Projects Program.

Hager, P., Gonczi, A., & Athanasou, J. (1994). General issues about assessment of competence. *Assessment and Evaluation in Higher Education, 19*(1), 3-16.

Kemmis S., & McTaggart, R. (Eds.). (1992). *The action research planner* (3rd ed.). Geelong, VIC: Deakin University Press.

Kilgour, A. J. (2011). Assessment of competency in radiography students – A new approach. *The Radiographer, 58*(3), 32-37. Retrieved from
http://search.informit.com.au/documentSummary;dn=897620052350752;res=IELHEA

Miller, G. E. (1990). The assessment of clinical skills/competence/performance. *Academic Medicine, 65*(9 Suppl), S63-S67.

O'Donovan, B., Rust, C., Price, M., & Carroll, J. (2005). "Staying the distance": The unfolding story of discovery and development through long-term collaborative research into assessment. *HERDSA News 27*(1), 12-15.

Sadler, D. R. (1989). Formative assessment and the design of instructional systems. *Instructional Science, 18,* 119-144. Retrieved from http://www.michiganassessmentconsortium.org/sites/default/files/MAC-Resources-FormativeAssessmentDesignSystems.pdf

Sadler, D. R. (2005). Interpretations of criteria-based assessment and grading in higher education. *Assessment and Evaluation in Higher Education, 30*(2), 175-194.

Winter, R. (1996). Some principles and procedures for the conduct of action research. In O. Zuber-Skerritt (Ed.), *New directions in action research* (pp. 16-17). London: Farmer.

Woolf, H. (2004). Assessment criteria: Reflections on current practice. *Assessment and Evaluation in Higher Education, 29*(4), 479-493.

Yorke, M. (2011). Summative assessment: Dealing with the measurement fallacy. *Studies in Higher Education 36*(3), 251-273.

Andrew Kilgour PhD candidate
School of Dentistry & Health Sciences
Charles Sturt University, Australia

Tania Gerzina PhD
Faculty of Dentistry
The University of Sydney, Australia

Mike Keppell PhD
Australian Digital Futures Institute
University of Southern Queensland, Australia

Janet Gerzina RT
Specialist Magnetic Radiation Imaging
Royal Prince Alfred Medical Centre, Australia

PATRICIA MCCABE AND BELINDA KENNY

25. INDIGENOUS ISSUES – A PRACTICAL EXAMPLE

The Byalawa Project

The need for health professions to work safely and effectively with patients and clients who come from diverse social and cultural backgrounds is an international issue of concern. Tertiary educators understand that cross-cultural competence requires specific attention in health sciences professional preparation programs (Purden, 2005). Furthermore, teaching students to work with Indigenous peoples is an essential component of such programs. In Australia, the *Closing the Gap Initiative* focuses on reducing disparities between Indigenous and non-Indigenous Australians' life expectancy and morbidity (http://www.fahcsia.gov.au/our-responsibilities/indigenous-australians/programs-services/closing-the-gap). This government initiative has implications for curricula across the health professions. For example, the Deans of Australian and New Zealand Medical Programs Council has committed to inclusive training of pre-practice medical students, which includes cultural safety in all aspects of medical education (http://www.medicaldeans.org.au/projects-activities/indigenous-health/cdams-indigenous-health-curriculum-framework).

In response to the need for curriculum development in Indigenous health, educators must seek resources that facilitate students' cross-cultural communication skills. The Byalawa project (http://www.byalawa.com) is a web-based resource for health professionals and health professional students to develop culturally safe interviewing practices. The multimedia resources are research-based and include six video case studies, learning outcomes and themes, sample lesson plans, learning and teaching resources and links to other relevant materials.

THE SETTING

The Faculty of Health Sciences at The University of Sydney provides undergraduate and postgraduate professional preparation degrees in 10 allied health disciplines including speech pathology, occupational therapy, exercise physiology and diagnostic radiography. The Faculty has a long tradition of providing specialised tertiary education to Aboriginal health workers and support to students of Aboriginal or Torres Strait Islander heritage through the Yoorang Goorang Indigenous Education unit.

In 2008, as part of a curriculum renewal process, educators from the Faculty of Health Sciences critically reflected upon our approaches to learning and teaching in Indigenous health across the curriculum. Our aim was to incorporate Indigenous health issues in interdisciplinary learning and teaching activities across all

S. Loftus et al. (Eds.), Educating Health Professionals:
Becoming a University Teacher, 287–296.

programs, not just those which focused upon Indigenous issues. Following this reflection, we recognised that we were not adequately preparing our students to work with Indigenous populations during their professional preparation. Our next step was to search for existing learning and teaching resources to build cross-cultural learning activities. We discovered limited resources and an absence of clear guidelines in the literature to support the development of content for such resources. The absence of quality, evidence-based learning and teaching resources posed a major challenge to preparing students for working with Indigenous people. We also surmised that educators from beyond our Faculty and university might be experiencing similar challenges. This led to the concept of the Byalawa project.

THE FOCUS

The focus of the Byalawa project was twofold. We aimed firstly to investigate best practice in interviewing Indigenous patients, and secondly to create and test resources that could be used to teach these concepts. To address these aims, we decided to develop online video resources that could be adapted for use in a range of tertiary professional preparation programs. Essentially, in creating the resources, we planned to increase educators' access to learning and teaching materials that might facilitate effective communication between graduating health professionals and their Indigenous clients and patients.

In summary, two major tasks underpinned the development of Byalawa resources:

- Investigation of appropriate content for the resources through qualitative research.
- Creation and testing of the resources for use by educators and students.

In completing these tasks we adopted a research-enhanced approach to learning and teaching (Brew, 2003), creating evidence-based materials with demonstrated learning outcomes.

THE STRATEGY

The project emerged from discussions between the first author and academic colleagues during formal meetings. Ideas were then shaped by informal discussions with colleagues who expressed commitment to Indigenous healthcare and frustration with the apparent resource limitations. A project team evolved from these discussions. The team included the educators who had participated in the reflective process which sparked the project. Other colleagues were specifically recruited because their research and/or teaching expertise matched the needs of the project. We wanted to include as many professions as we could, and we sought team members who could contribute either through their contacts and experience with Indigenous Australians or through their passion for learning and teaching research. We also sought Indigenous and non-Indigenous health professionals so that our team could represent a range of perspectives. We wanted to avoid an insular approach whereby the resources developed were relevant only to a specific institution or profession. Finally, in Australia, most Indigenous people live in cities and large towns (ABS, 2010), but the limited materials we had unearthed focused on working with rural and remote communities; therefore we wanted our materials to have an urban focus.

A project team was assembled from all health faculties at The University of Sydney (Health Sciences, Medicine, Dentistry, Nursing and Pharmacy) and from James Cook University (Townsville, Australia). Our team was successful in obtaining funding from the Australian Learning and Teaching Council to (1) research the needs of Indigenous patients and clients in initial interviews with health professionals, (2) create learning and teaching resources to address these needs, and (3) trial the resources with pre-qualification students in a range of health professions. We chose interviewing because it is a skill that many health professionals use on a daily basis. After careful deliberation, the undertaking was named the Byalawa project. *Byalawa* in the Dharug language means "to talk" and was chosen to reflect our emphasis upon communication.

The Byalawa project was an action research project comprising four phases, with each phase consisting of observing, planning, acting and reflecting (Kember & Kelly, 1993). Action research approaches are well suited to projects where there is a desired change in practice or learning environment. Although our team members had previous experience with quantitative and qualitative research paradigms, this was the first action research project completed by anyone in our team.

Action research provides for cycles of action and reflection. Each subsequent stage of a project is dependent upon what has been learned in previous stages. Hence continuous improvement is inbuilt and evaluation is cyclically built into the action research methodology. In the Byalawa project, each cycle of action and reflection corresponded with the four stages of the project:

1. *Planning and consultation*: This stage focused on developing relationships with Indigenous communities and identifying strengths and support needs within the team. Our large team was organised into subgroups that contributed to the research, community engagement and resource development components of the project.
2. *Design and production Part A – Working with Indigenous people*: The first component of the design and production stage focused on gathering qualitative data about the process of conducting health-related interviews with Indigenous Australians. Data were collected through individual interviews with Indigenous health researchers, community consultation, and a number of focus groups with stakeholders. During this stage, key members of our team visited Indigenous communities to discuss the aims of the research and to share ideas about how to develop appropriate resources.
3. *Design and production Part B – Working with health professionals and university teachers.* During the second component of the design and production stage, we examined pedagogy, curricula and recommendations from research in

higher education to inform our recommendations for implementing new curricula. We also consulted widely with potential consumers to determine whether our resources met specific learning needs and could be adapted in response to students' (and educators') knowledge, experience and professional roles.

4. *Implementation and evaluation.* In this stage, we filmed, edited and trialled the newly developed materials. We sought feedback from university educators and students who used the draft materials during classes and group learning activities. During this stage we focused on producing high-quality resources that were designed to maintain student interest and stimulate discussion and reflection on Indigenous health issues. In contrast to learning resources that provide a "recipe" for working with Indigenous people, we sought to develop resources that facilitated reflection and discussion of strategies for effective communication.

Our action research approach was guided by five overarching principles which the team agreed upon from the outset of the project. These five principles underpinned each stage of the project:

- to be culturally appropriate through consultation with Indigenous people and communities. We recognised that we were both learners and educators in this research process.
- to involve a wide range of stakeholders, including Indigenous people, health professionals, university lecturers and students. We understood that this was a multifaceted project and collaboration was an important feature in resource development.
- to be academically rigorous, adaptable for different curricular pedagogies, for novice to advanced students, in interdisciplinary or single-discipline contexts. We acknowledged that health sciences educators teach within time and curriculum constraints and need user-friendly resources. At the same time, resources must have scope for creative and stimulating learning experiences.
- to present a range of urban and regional stories that represented real and frequently occurring interactions between Indigenous people and health professionals. We wanted to build the resources based upon lived experiences, not on assumptions about healthcare interactions.
- to use real health professionals in the learning materials to give authenticity. We had observed in our own teaching that students are adept at recognising "actors" portraying health professionals and that this affected their responses to audio-visual resources.

Clearly, these five principles reflected the project team's perceptions of quality educational resources. To deliver the final website and videos we adopted a number of specific strategies which were consistent with these principles. Our strategies included:

a) *Engagement of Indigenous communities* to inform the background, settings and the nature of interactions.

b) *Recruitment of experts* including a project manager, Indigenous staff members, and an expert production company. Experts co-ordinated the project's operations and contributed specific skills to the project.

c) *Regular meeting times* to facilitate communication across institutional settings and between stakeholder groups. The regular meetings provided opportunities for problem solving and for celebrating achievements. Teleconferencing enabled team members to participate in a range of diverse settings.

d) *Working parties* for specific components of the project, providing opportunities to capitalise upon strengths of team members and to distribute project workload.

e) *Presentation of progress* at education forums along the way, which provided us with formative feedback from academics/educators. Presentations facilitated dissemination of information about the project's aims and expected outcomes to potential resource consumers.

f) *Flexibility*: Consistent with action research, goals for the project were refined in response to community and stakeholder input and challenges encountered along the way.

g) *Being open to learning from our Indigenous participants and actors*. We needed to identify and put aside our preconceived ideas and listen to our participants' stories.

h) *Marketing and publicity activities*. Importantly, we wanted educators to become familiar with our project and educational resources. Marketing and publicity activities provided opportunities for sharing enthusiasm for resources that addressed Indigenous health issues and for offering colleagues a new approach to this important area of curriculum development.

Our guiding principles and strategies were integrated with each stage of the project. For example, during our planning stage, we consulted a number of educational design professionals and examined existing resources, including the *Health and Disability: Partnerships in Action* learning and teaching package (http://www.cddh.monash.org/health-and-disability.html). We accepted advice from our production company about strategies that had previously been successful in recording healthcare interactions. Consultation helped us to develop curriculum materials such as learning objectives and themes, and sample lesson plans.

As a project team we then participated in a curriculum development workshop in which we brainstormed our aspirations for the curriculum resources, established interim objectives and allocated roles in curriculum development to various team members. To support design and production, we conducted two workshops, one each at the 2010 and 2011 ANZAHPE (Australian and New Zealand Association for Health Professional Educators) conferences. During the workshops we explored the approaches health academics would be likely to adopt when using the proposed materials. Workshops also provided a forum for professional colleagues to review and provide guidance on the first draft of the video materials (McCabe et al., 2010; Sheepway et al., 2011). Diverse educational needs were identified during the workshops. Educators requested resources that could be adapted to meet case-based and problem-based learning environments and materials that were appropriate for lecture, tutorial, independent and online learning experiences.

To support implementation and evaluation, we trialled project materials with five cohorts of students in two universities. We asked university teachers to provide us with feedback on the materials and a detailed description (using a proforma) of how the materials were used and with whom. In response to this feedback we developed a range of cues/prompts/questions that educators might choose to adopt when they were implementing the resources with their students.

These strategies resulted in the Byalawa website, which contains six video vignettes, sample lesson plans, learning outcomes, links and other resources, and a quick-start guide for using the site.

CHALLENGES FACED

Developing a research-based learning and teaching resource in the area of Indigenous health was far more challenging than we anticipated when we commenced the project. Challenges centred on the qualitative processes associated with establishing what we should teach, the need for authentic engagement with a wide range of stakeholders, and maintaining team member commitment over a 3-year period from initial idea to launch of the resource.

(1) Qualitative Research

In developing these resources as a research-led learning and teaching project we imposed two research layers upon ourselves. This led to two separate and complex ethics processes. In the first ethics submission process, we needed to engage the relevant Indigenous community and gain their consent, obtain approval from our respective universities, and submit our proposal to the peak Aboriginal health research agency. During the second ethics process, we engaged with multiple student cohorts and teachers on four campuses in five degree programs at two universities. These administrative requirements impacted upon project timelines as the team needed to address diverse issues and requirements at each participating site. Inevitably, it became more challenging to achieve parallel progress across sites and smooth stepwise progression with the two research layers.

(2) Authentic Engagement with a Range of Stakeholders

Indigenous communities and individuals
At the commencement of the project, our team included Indigenous health and education professionals who introduced us to a range of Indigenous communities in the hope that the communities might partner us in the project. Each community we spoke with was interested but reported being overwhelmed by the amount of research being conducted with them and on them. We searched for opportunities for direct community involvement, including employing Indigenous research workers. In the end, our most effective relationships were founded upon existing

networks between one of our team members and an Indigenous community. Where the relationship between team member and community was more distant we were unable to form a sufficiently firm arrangement for the project to proceed. Because relationships were so important, any change in personnel in the project team or in the Indigenous community sent us "back to square one" in developing effective and productive relationships.

From our experiences, it became clear that long-term professional relationships and engaging Indigenous communities during the planning stages of the project were keys to their future involvement. From the community-based qualitative research we learned about the importance of professional relationships in effective health interviewing. Our research experiences were aligned with comments from our focus group participants that emphasised the need for trust to develop between Indigenous patients and health professionals.

We have used this knowledge as one of the themes in the Byalawa project http://www.byalawa.com/learning-materials#relationships. For example, our participants told us that health practitioners need to:

- more fully introduce themselves: who they are, where they come from, what their experience is, and also share a little of themselves, their family, interests, etc. Even a comment about the footy will break the ice.
- explain WHY they want even basic information BEFORE they ask the question.
- understand why Indigenous patients may be reluctant to share information if they do not know how it will be used.

Developing and maintaining a relationship with the Indigenous actors used in our video materials was an important factor in the final success of the project. In order to engage them with the materials we ran two separate days of workshop and storytelling. From their stories and the focus groups we developed the scripts that were then enacted for our videos.

Politics of inter-university collaborations
Cross-institutional collaboration was an important and rewarding aspect of our project. Nonetheless, the institutions had different philosophies and practices regarding curriculum that covered Indigenous health issues. We needed to manage expectations by explaining that we were contributing innovative resources but it was unrealistic for us to provide a "one size fits all" curriculum package.

Difficulty establishing/recruiting mentors, champions, communities of practice
We acknowledged the importance of mentorship and guidance in conducting research with Indigenous communities. But we experienced barriers to recruiting such mentors. We consistently received encouragement and feedback that supported the relevance and importance of developing our learning and teaching materials. Practical, problem-solving advice that covered the "how to?" and "what other options?" needs posed by our project was sometimes unavailable.

(3) Team Commitment

When we began this project the core project team recruited other members we thought would be interested in the project topic and would contribute knowledge and skills to the project. This led to a large and diverse team. Our diversity of locations, disciplines, skills, employers and agendas was both the strength of our team and one of its major challenges.

Over the 3 years that it took to complete the project we had varying engagement from team members as their other roles and responsibilities changed. The lesson from this is that team relationships are better managed via a small core group and achievement of individual goals is best achieved through a size-limited project team, each member having specific accountable outcomes. Finally, relationships of team members with the wider university community were invaluable in finding champions for the project and in marketing the resultant website to the wider community.

REFLECTIONS

Feedback from a range of stakeholders has been overwhelmingly positive. What has been surprising is the diversity of people and programs using the resources. In particular, we have had many requests from Indigenous community agencies who want to use the video in their professional development or staff training activities. However, when we have presented the materials at learning and teaching forums comments have been made about the urban settings not being representative of all Indigenous health experiences. These criticisms have caused us to change how we explain our purpose on the site and subsequently some of the wording of the support materials.

As part of the educational research process we surveyed students after exposure to the materials. It was pleasing that students valued the use of real health professionals in the video, although the fact that these clinicians made "mistakes" was an irritant to more junior students. A number of students commented that they would have expected the clinicians to do a better job. Such comments have been used to refine the explanatory materials and to make the website more user-friendly. Many students said the video would not replace real clinical experience but they felt a little better prepared after completing the associated classes.

Reflections. As health professionals and academics, we strive to be reflective practitioners (Schön, 1987). Tricia McCabe, the team leader, reflected:

> Initially I was dismayed that no resources existed which would meet the need. It was puzzling why no-one else had seen it, especially when improving Indigenous health is a national priority. Now it has been successfully completed, I can see why it might be the case. It was plain hard work maintaining everyone's energy across so many ups and downs while at the same time maintaining my own focus and purpose. However, when we made progress it was an exhilarating project. Writing this chapter has been an

opportunity to recognise we have done a good job. The remaining challenges are to write up the research so that our materials are truly an example of research-enhanced learning and teaching. It will be challenging to re-engage the team now that they have moved on to other issues.

Belinda Kenny, who was a member of the project committee, reflected:

Although we were from diverse professional backgrounds, it was immediately clear that everyone on the project team shared a commitment to developing resources to facilitate health professions' students learning about Indigenous health. We all had a vision for the final resources and this vision needed to be negotiated and adapted in response to the challenges of the project and the need to develop a resource that could be used cross-disciplinary and cross-institutionally. The opportunity to brainstorm options for learning and teaching Indigenous health issues in a creative and constructive way with professional colleagues was one aspect of the project that I found very enjoyable. Experiencing the challenges of engaging Indigenous communities in research projects was an eye-opener and revealed that good research outcomes are grounded in long-term planning, effective communication and flexibility.

CONCLUSIONS

Our learning and teaching/action research experiences are summarised in seven tips for future researchers or academics who identify the need to develop new community-focused curricula or resources.

1. Build in a considerable foundation time. You will need early buy-in from communities – invest time and energy early in the project to establish and consolidate these relationships.
2. When there is no evidence on which to base learning and teaching practice, translation of a research-enhanced learning and teaching philosophy into action is more complex than it appears.
3. Know your own strengths and pay for expertise, such as digital video editing.
4. The Indigenous communities with whom we worked all asked what immediate opportunities there were for community members in terms of employment, training or mentoring. Next time we would build this into the project design.
5. When working with specific communities you may find yourself "competing" with projects that will deliver immediate, short-term benefits to community members. Plan for this.
6. The research burden on communities was an issue of which we were unaware and that needs to be considered.
7. Have a smaller project team which is enhanced by an advisory committee.

We learned that (1) filming and editing professional quality video is time-consuming and best achieved with the help of a professional production company, (2) our health students knew a lot about remote and regional Indigenous

Australians but not about urban Indigenous peoples; this is concerning, as most Indigenous Australians live in cities, (3) the materials were generally well accepted by the students who viewed them in a range of learning and teaching activities and provided excellent stimulus to discussion and reflection both in class and online.

ACKNOWLEDGEMENTS

We acknowledge the ongoing custodianship of the Dharug people of the Eora nation over the land on which the Cumberland Campus of the The University of Sydney stands. Byalawa means "to talk" in Dharug and we thank Richard Green for his suggestion of this word to be our title.

The Byalawa project was funded by the Australian Learning and Teaching Council (ALTC). The opinions expressed in this chapter are the authors' own and do not represent those of the ALTC or the Australian government.

Thanks to the members of the Byalawa project team and our Indigenous participants for their contributions.

The project can be found at http://www.byalawa.com

REFERENCES

Australian Bureau of Statistics (ABS). (2010). *Demographic, social and economic characteristics overview: Aboriginal and Torres Strait Islander people and where they live.* Retrieved from http://www.abs.gov.au/AUSSTATS/abs@.nsf/lookup/4704.0Chapter210Oct+2010

Brew, A. (2003). Teaching and research: New relationships and their implications for inquiry-based teaching and learning in higher education. *Higher Education Research & Development, 22*(1), 3-18. doi:10.1080/0729436032000056571

Kember, D., & Kelly, M. E. (1993). *Improving teaching through action research.* HERDSA green guide 14. NSW: Higher Education Research and Development Association of Australasia.

McCabe, P., Sheepway, L., Morrison, S., Miller, A., Brown, L., Gerzina, T. et al. (2010). *Development of learning strategies and resources to teach health care students cross-cultural interviewing skills.* PeArL session presented at the ANZAME Conference, Townsville, Australia.

Purden, M. (2005). Cultural considerations in interprofessional education and practice. *Journal of Interprofessional Care, Supplement 1*, 224-234. doi:10.1080/13561820500083238

Schön, D. A. (1987). *Educating the reflective practitioner: Toward a new design for teaching and learning in the professions.* San Francisco, CA: Jossey-Bass.

Sheepway, L., McCabe, P., Farrington, S., Kenny, B., Pont, L., Mackenzie, L. et al. (2011). *Introducing the Byalawa Project resources: Teaching health professional students how to communicate effectively with Indigenous people.* Workshop presented at the ANZAHPE Conference, Alice Springs, Australia.

Patricia McCabe BAppSc(SpPath), PhD
Speech Pathology
The University of Sydney, Australia

Belinda Kenny BAppSc(SpPath), PhD
Speech Pathology
The University of Sydney, Australia

CLAIRE MACRAE, SUSIE SCHOFIELD AND ROLA AJJAWI

26. PROFESSIONAL DEVELOPMENT FOR MEDICAL EDUCATORS

THE SETTING

The Students

Dundee University Medical School, on the east coast of Scotland, delivers a 5-year undergraduate medical program with about 160 students per year. Approximately 15% of the students are from Dundee and the surrounding area, 50% from the rest of Scotland, and 25% from England, Wales and Northern Ireland, with the remaining 10% being international students.

In common with most UK medical schools, the course attracts mainly school leavers aged 17-18 years, with only a small number of mature age students; 60% of the students are female. At this stage, most students would not have clearly defined career goals, and part of the role of the School is to offer experience in a range of clinical specialities in order to support career choices. Dundee is committed to a widening access policy, and offers opportunities for students from a diverse range of social and economic backgrounds.

The Program

The program is delivered in three phases: Phase 1 (a short, introductory period in semester 1) provides an introduction to basic principles underpinning clinical medicine; Phase 2 (years 1-3) delivers integrated teaching based around body systems; and Phase 3 (years 4-5) consists primarily of teaching in the clinical setting, following the apprenticeship model of training.

In common with other UK medical schools, the school designs its own curriculum and assessments in line with General Medical Council (GMC) guidance, and is subject to regular quality assurance visits by the GMC (the UK regulator for the medical profession). Throughout the course, a range of educational approaches and delivery methods is employed, including lectures, small group teaching, traditional "bedside" teaching encounters, elements of problem-based learning (PBL), team-based learning (TBL) and e-learning. Assessment strategies including objective structured clinical examinations (OSCEs), portfolios, online exams and workplace-based assessment are utilised to assess knowledge, skills and professional behaviour throughout the course.

S. Loftus et al. (Eds.), Educating Health Professionals:
Becoming a University Teacher, 297–310.

The Organisation

The Medical School is part of the College of Medicine, Dentistry and Nursing, which offers opportunities for interprofessional teaching and learning as well as potential for joint staff development initiatives. The School also has a close relationship with its partner health board, National Health Service (NHS) Tayside, and is based within Ninewells Hospital, Tayside's main teaching hospital. The vast majority of the clinical teaching is delivered on-site at Ninewells, or in other Tayside hospitals and general practices, although students in later years have the opportunity to undertake placements in other Scottish health boards. NHS Tayside also provides postgraduate medical training in a wide range of clinical specialities. Dundee has a much higher rate of unemployment than other Scottish cities, and it is estimated that around 29% of the population live in areas flagged as the most deprived in Scotland based on a range of factors such as income, crime rates, access to training, etc. In the 2009 Census, 24% of the population was aged over 60. Linked to this, instances of cardiovascular and respiratory problems are higher than in the general Scottish population, and students and teachers need to be aware of both the additional risks to health carried by deprivation and the barriers to effective health promotion within these groups (Dundee City Council, 2012).

The Staff

Of the School's academic staff, around 100 are directly involved in undergraduate teaching; these individuals have various levels of research, administrative and managerial duties. Academic staff members are primarily clinicians who maintain their clinical practice through delivery of a fixed number of NHS sessions. Academics deliver around 70% of the teaching in Phases 1 and 2, and around 20% in Phase 3 as students are increasingly exposed to clinical practice. The remainder of the teaching is delivered by a wide range of NHS teachers, including doctors, nurses and other healthcare professionals.

NHS Tayside employs around 450 consultants and 850 trainee doctors, any of whom may be involved in teaching undergraduate students at some point. Although new academic staff are required to hold a postgraduate teaching qualification (or to have completed this within 3 years of taking up the post), most clinical staff have no formal teacher training and many have limited experience of teaching undergraduates.

The Funding

The course is funded through a mix of student fees and government subsidies. The subsidies are in two parts: funds paid to the Medical School via the Scottish Higher Education Funding Council and funds paid to the NHS via NHS Education for Scotland (NES) known as ACT funding (additional costs of teaching). Both these are allocated on a per capita basis. NHS ACT funds are allocated and reviewed against strict criteria and must be used to support delivery of undergraduate medical education within the NHS. This includes provision of support and development opportunities for NHS teaching staff.

The Context

Between 2002 and 2006 an NHS Workforce review (NHS National Workforce Projects, 2006) concluded that an aging educator workforce combined with poorly articulated career pathways for new educators was creating a situation where clinical academic posts were hard to fill. Furthermore, if this trend continued it could lead to a shortage of clinician-educators in the future. The review group made a number of specific recommendations, including the need to more clearly define entry and exit points for an academic career and the need for generic teaching and research skills to be taught throughout medical training.

Recent guidance from the GMC (2009a) has emphasised the importance of selecting, supporting and training ALL staff involved in teaching and assessment. In *Good Medical Practice*, the GMC (2006) states, "if you are involved in teaching you must develop the skills, attitudes and practices of a competent teacher". Whereas clinical academics are selected by the University on a competitive basis and are required to undertake a formal qualification in teaching as well as receive regular performance appraisal, NHS clinical teachers are on-the-job doctors who have generally had no training for their educational role.

The trend for producing a better selected, better skilled clinical teaching workforce is set to continue. The GMC is currently consulting on a "trainer approvals framework" which will set basic standards for all medical educators. Individuals listed as trainers would be expected to provide evidence of ongoing professional development for their teaching role at appraisal. Alongside this project, NES is developing a *National Framework for Faculty Development*, identifying a core set of competences and minimum training requirements for clinical teachers across Scotland.

The Stakeholders

Staff development initiatives must be planned to address the needs of a range of stakeholders. NHS teaching staff need a basic set of teaching skills; academic and potential academic staff require development opportunities which will allow for future career progression; both the Medical School and NHS Tayside need to be confident that they will meet current and future regulatory requirements; the funding providers are concerned with cost-effectiveness and return on investment; and not least, patients and the public want to know that the doctors who will be treating them in future have been trained to deliver high-quality care in a professional manner. Increasingly, UK students are seen as consumers, as government subsidies are reduced or withdrawn; many of them will self-fund their education. This is reflected in their comments on quality assurance surveys indicating that they have high expectations in terms of both quantity and quality of the teaching they receive in return for fees paid.

The Team

Delivering our staff development initiatives is a team of experienced educationalists based in Dundee's Centre for Medical Education. As well, ACT has funded an NHS Director of Medical Education (DME) and a staff development officer to co-ordinate provision of training within NHS Tayside, and a number of senior academic staff also have an interest in faculty development. The role of each is discussed further below.

THE FOCUS

Timeframe

This case study focuses on staff development opportunities introduced over the period 2008 to the present.

Main Challenges

The context presented a number of challenges to be addressed, including: clinicians having little or no formal educational training; teaching being a low priority compared to patient care, administration and research; and teaching being done by employees of two completely separate organisations (Schofield et al., 2010). To address these challenges we needed to provide:

- appropriate training and support for a diverse group of educators with a wide range of prior knowledge, skills and experience
- training that is robust enough to meet current and future regulatory requirements
- opportunities for NHS teachers wishing to make the transition to academia
- opportunities grounded in real practice, based on existing literature and designed to meet the needs and preferences of participants.

THE STRATEGY

In their guide to faculty development, McLean and colleagues (2008) advocated conducting a systematic needs assessment before planning any interventions. This process includes: (1) identifying the desired state of affairs; (2) examining the current position, including existing provision and available resources; (3) considering the forces driving the intervention, as they will influence participant attitudes; and(4) researching the needs of the target audience.

As described above, the Medical School desired all faculty members to be appropriately trained and supported, taking account of their current roles and future development plans. *Tomorrow's Doctors* (GMC, 2009a) states, "Everyone involved in educating medical students will be appropriately selected, trained, supported and appraised". *Appropriate* is a key term here, as we need to account for the current roles and future development plans of individuals.

Mapping of Existing Initiatives

Before planning any new initiatives, it was important to identify existing educational opportunities.

Table 26.1. Initiatives in place pre-2008

Provider	Initiative	Format
Centre for Medical Education	Accredited medical education training (PGCert, PGDip, MMEd)	Modular distance learning or face-to-face awards bearing degrees
Centre for Medical Education	Discovery course in medical education	Week-long face-to-face course introduction to medical education
Medical School	Centrally provided workshops	½ day face-to-face workshops (primarily on assessment)
Medical School	Departmentally delivered workshops	1 hour – ½ day training sessions booked from a menu of options
University central professional development unit	Centrally provided workshops	½ day workshops covering a range of generic topics (e.g. presentation skills)

The courses on offer by CME were popular and well subscribed nationally and internationally but had a low uptake locally. Training opportunities provided on the main university campus were also poorly attended by medical faculty; anecdotally, reasons included geographical difficulties of attending off-site training, related both to travel time and the need to be on site in case of clinical emergencies; perceptions that generic training did not adequately address specific needs of medical teachers; and poor communication between the main University and the Medical School.

The primary source of staff development was through a series of workshops offered annually to clinical departments and facilitated by senior academic staff with an interest in faculty development. Interest in and uptake of these opportunities had gradually tailed off, as had availability of suitable facilitators with the time and expertise to deliver the sessions.

Driving Forces

McLean et al. (2008) described forces driving the introduction of staff development initiatives as either *internal* (of benefit to the individual/institution, e.g. orienting new faculty members; supporting individuals to improve; encouraging career progression; or *external* (conforming with public expectations; accountability requirements). Although external drivers may be the strongest, having potential penalties attached for non-compliance, it is important to ensure that individuals see the benefit to themselves of taking part, otherwise uptake will be low. In our case, there was significant external pressure from both the regulator and the funding providers to introduce a more robust model of staff development, so it was particularly important not to lose the perspective of the individual and what he/she would gain from the process.

Needs Assessment

Needs assessment surveys were conducted to identify perceived training needs for the clinical teachers' educational roles, attitudes to training, preferences for delivery of training and barriers to training within the workforce. This was published as part of a national survey (Schofield et al., 2009, 2010) and Tayside data were extracted for local use (Schofield et al., 2010). The survey identified a number of educational areas where consultants felt that training would be valuable, and also indicated that their preference for delivery was via short workshops or a blended approach incorporating a mix of face-to-face delivery and self-directed study. By far the greatest barrier to participation was time, and less than a third of consultants felt that undertaking an educational degree would help them perform their educational role. This could go some way to explaining the low uptake of accredited training locally.

Following this we examined the needs of doctors in training. This was primarily accomplished by scrutiny of the various specialist training curricula with respect to teaching competences the trainee was required to have demonstrated on completion of training. Although there was significant variation between specialities, the exercise identified six generic topics with which all trainees were expected to engage regardless of speciality, including small group teaching, presentation skills, assessment, appraisal, feedback, and mentoring and student support.

We then looked at the needs of specialist groups of teachers, including OSCE examiners, student support tutors and admissions interviewers, where specialist skills might be required. Alongside this, the career development needs of potential academics were given consideration.

Putting Together the Program

Having identified the needs of our diverse staff groups, we planned interventions to meet the continuum of needs. Steinert et al. (2006) conducted a systematic review of faculty development initiatives and identified a number of features of effective interventions. These included learning through experience, receiving feedback on teaching performance, valuing peer relationships, applying educational principles when designing the intervention, and using a range of educational methods within the intervention. These guidelines informed the development of our program.

Our initial efforts were focused on ensuring that adequate formal training was available to each group of teachers, and the provision is summarised in Table 26.2. We also implemented a number of strategies to make a career in academic medicine more appealing and accessible. Medical training in the UK generally follows the same pattern: 5-6 years undergraduate training, 2 years Foundation training (where trainees follow a rotation of general medical / surgical posts under close supervision) and then 3-7 years specialist training in their chosen field, after which they take up a career-grade post, most commonly as a consultant or general practitioner (GP). Nationally, a number of entry and exit points have been identified to allow practitioners to move in and out of academia with minimal disruption to the progression of their clinical careers. We developed initiatives at each of these stages in line with national guidance, and they are also summarised in Table 26.2. GPs were not included as they are subject to different regulations and manage their own training budgets.

Educational Qualifications

The opportunity to complete formal postgraduate qualifications in Medical education remains (certificate/diploma and master's). The program is specifically designed with busy clinicians in mind, with a mix of practical and theoretical modules. The program is mapped onto the Academy of Medical Educators' (2012) framework, with the certificate catering for teachers as practitioners, the diploma for teachers as educational leaders and the master's for teachers as educational researchers.

Table 26.2. Faculty development opportunities on offer in 2012 to particular groups based on identified need

Staff group	Specific considerations	Training offered to clinical teachers	Academic career development opportunities
Foundation doctors	Limited experience and opportunity to teach formally but involved in bedside teaching. Heavy clinical workload and steep learning curve leave little time for non-clinical training.	Foundation Year (FY – newly graduated) doctors welcome to attend core teaching skills workshops.	Six places offered as part of academic Foundation program – in addition to the regular curriculum academic trainees develop skills in teaching, research, leadership and management. One post-holder supported by ACT to undertake accredited modules from the PG Certificate Medical Education course.

Table 26.2. (continued)

Staff group	Specific considerations	Training offered to clinical teachers	Academic career development opportunities
Specialist trainees	Trainee doctors expected to demonstrate competence in teaching by end of program. Often delegated teaching responsibilities by busy seniors. More protected time for study leave.	"Core skills" workshops offered covering key areas identified across training curricula – e.g. teaching small groups, principles of assessment.	3 x 2-year teaching fellowships offered (ACT-funded) including funding to undertake an educational qualification. Part-funding for an educational degree available to other trainees demonstrating commitment to / aptitude for teaching.
Consultants	Teaching expected as part of role and often included in the job plan. Often expected to take on leadership or curriculum planning roles with little experience or training.	"Specialist" workshops offered to support those in specific roles such as examiners, student support tutors, etc. Standalone workshops based on topics identified in consultant survey.	Full funding available for those with a heavy teaching workload to undertake an educational qualification (ACT-funded).
Other healthcare professionals	Increasing number of other professionals delivering training within the undergraduate medical curriculum.	Departmental training sessions offered, tailored to specific needs of the group.	Those in leadership roles supported through ACT to undertake a relevant educational qualification (e.g. certificate of advanced practice: education for nurses).
Academic teaching staff	Expected to hold an educational qualification or to complete one within 3 years of taking up post.	Encouraged to participate in workshops for consultants.	Those with the aptitude encouraged to become involved in design and delivery of faculty development workshops.

ACT funding is available to support clinicians undertaking the course – annually this covers 10 fully-funded places or more part-funded places. To qualify for full funding, clinicians would generally be expected to hold a career-grade post and to demonstrate ongoing commitment to teaching in NHS Tayside.

To make the academic work of the Centre more appealing to clinical staff, periodic opportunities are also provided for them to attend "taster" sessions, such as enrolling in an individual module of the face-to-face program without undertaking the associated assessment, or attending a week-long Discovery Course which provides a comprehensive introduction to medical education and the opportunity to network with other educators. Participants who attend our 1-week courses have the option of completing an assessment which then gives them Accreditation of Prior Learning on a module of the Certificate. These alternative pathways for entry into the Postgraduate Certificate provide flexibility for busy clinicians who are not sure that a full Master's is the right path for them. The trend towards professionalisation of medical education (Irby et al., 2010) can be seen in the increasing popularity of the degree programs.

Academic FY Program

In Dundee we created six academic Foundation posts and developed a teaching skills program designed to meet the specific needs of these newly graduated doctors. Foundation doctors are clinically very busy with patient care and routine ward work. They have limited contact with students in formal teaching opportunities but tend to deliver the majority of the bedside/informal learning.

With this borne in mind, the developed program included minimal theory, focusing on practical elements which the trainees would have the opportunity to use almost immediately. In the first year, four discrete training sessions of 2 hours each cover a range of topics, including teaching a clinical skill or practical procedure; managing a small group; assessing performance in the clinical context; identifying struggling students; and giving feedback on performance. The second year will run for the first time in 2012-13 and sessions will become more practical, with trainees given opportunities to deliver teaching to medical students and have their performance assessed. As part of this program, one trainee has the opportunity to "specialise" in teaching and is funded to complete an accredited training course.

Specialist Training

During specialist training, trainees are developing specific skills and expertise in their chosen clinical specialty. This phase of training lasts 3-7 years depending on specialty. During this time, trainees have the opportunity to undertake "out of program" experience, which would generally be spent in a recognised 2 or 3year program, e.g. as a research fellow. Using ACT funding we have created three teaching fellowships where trainees engage in various teaching activities and educational research while completing the Postgraduate Certificate in Medical Education. During this time they are still clinically active, and on completion they are able to re-enter their training program at the point they left it. So far six trainees have completed the program, with a further three currently enrolled. All who completed the fellowship are still very involved in teaching, and one has moved into an educational leadership role.

The trainees who remain in clinical training also become more involved in teaching. All UK specialist training curricula now include a teaching component, and most trainees will be required to have their teaching performance assessed. We have developed a series of half-day "core teaching skills" workshops which are open to all, but primarily aimed at giving trainees a basic grounding in teaching theory and practice. The workshops have been developed to include practical activities and to cater for a range of learning needs and preferences, including more advanced topics that extend learners beyond the introductory workshops.

Consultants

All consultants in the UK are expected to undertake an educational role. Many consultants have significant practical experience but very limited formal training for their teaching role. A survey of Scotland's NHS consultants (n=2246 respondents) in 2006 identified that although 98% of respondents had a teaching role, 94% had no educational qualification (Schofield et al., 2009). Moreover, 48% had not attended any educational workshops and a further 42% had attended 1-2 educational workshops.

We used the information from the needs assessment questionnaire to offer a number of workshops on topics of interest as well as a series of "specialist" workshops for those who hold specific roles, such as OSCE examiners or portfolio reviewers. These workshops are marketed specifically to consultants, often on a named-invitation basis as a way of indicating that their contribution is valued by the Medical School.

As described above, we have also made funding available as an incentive for consultants with a special interest to undertake a qualification in medical education. Uptake of funding is still low and we are working on ways of promoting this initiative. It is likely that unless holding an educational qualification is tied to NHS pay awards and promotions schemes this figure will remain low.

Communities of Practice

Given our diverse group of teachers, we were also keen to encourage interaction between groups and to build a sense of community where teachers felt appreciated and supported in their roles. Steinert (2010) advised that staff development programs can play a pivotal role in developing communities of practice through helping to nurture both new and experienced educators. In order to promote the more academic aspects of the role and to provide a forum for educators to meet each other and make connections, we have also introduced a series of educational research seminars. They develop a collegiate spirit and a shared language, hopefully improving recruitment and retention and fostering enthusiasm for teaching. A range of local, national and international speakers present their educational research projects and there is opportunity for discussion and reflection. While the focus is on research, a number of the topics are identified as having particularly strong practical applications and these are supported by ACT funding and promoted to clinical teachers.

We have also run a 1-day in-house education conference for the past 2 years in which we aim to give clinical teachers a more academic perspective on their role. This event provides opportunities for those who are involved in research or educational projects locally to disseminate their work more widely and to network with colleagues who share an interest in education, as well as providing workshops in educational topics.

CHALLENGES FACED

Uptake

As with any new initiative, we have faced a number of challenges. Uptake of opportunities provided has generally been good, but we still struggle to interest consultants in accredited training. We will continue to promote the training to this group – as national developments move on, it is likely that a teaching qualification will be seen as more valuable in the future.

Time

Time to attend training does not seem to be as much of a problem at individual level as our survey would suggest. At institutional level, however, there is recognition that any degree of mandatory training that might be required in future will require commitment to release staff to attend. The NHS Director of Medical Education has established a teaching and training management group which negotiates with the NHS Tayside Board to ensure that teaching and training are given consideration when prioritising clinician time and setting clinical targets.

Resourcing

We have been very lucky in Dundee as ACT funding has allowed us to implement many initiatives that would not have been possible otherwise. However, finite resourcing does limit what we are able to offer. Most of our staff development workshops are delivered by the staff development officer or existing academic staff, as external trainers are beyond our budget. Events are generally run on-site so as not to incur room hire charges; this ensures high attendance but also means that participants may leave midway to answer bleeps or attend to clinical duties.

External Pressures

Initiatives from the GMC and NES have raised awareness of faculty development issues, ensuring that institutional leaders give them serious consideration. However, considering the time scales involved, it is often unrealistic to implement the changes needed in a sustainable, planned fashion. Moreover, careful change management is required as those involved are often suspicious of schemes they see as being "imposed" on them.

Personal Versus Professional Development

Individuals want to know how they will benefit personally from the training as opposed to how they will meet someone else's tick-box checklist. We have attempted to focus our training courses on very practical skills that teachers will be able to apply to immediate effect in the workplace. We provide attendance certificates for short courses to enable recognition at appraisal, and the staff development officer is available to advise those who wish to develop an individual training plan.

Institutional Culture

The final challenge is the change required in institutional culture. At the start of our project, even academic staff felt that research and management activity was more highly valued than teaching. Thanks to very supportive higher management in the Medical School, this has been mostly reversed, but for NHS staff there is still significant conflict between clinical and educational duties. Reversing this will be a slow process but the teaching and training management group led by the DME are working to this effect. Dialogue with clinical directors is now taking place, and ACT is auditing the type of teaching and amount of time NHS staff are involved in delivering.

REFLECTIONS

Feedback

Kirkpatrick's model of evaluating educational outcomes describes four levels of outcome (McLean et al., 2008): participant reaction, participant learning, change in participant behaviour and impact of changed behaviour on students. We collect participant feedback from all sessions, and use it to modify future events. Yet this is only really indicative of participant satisfaction, or at best self-reported changes in attitude or behaviour.

We are also able to look at results – e.g. student assessment outcomes, retention data, etc. This is of limited value, however, as it is very difficult to ascribe causality to this type of data which has multifactorial origins. One measurable outcome which may be more directly linked to the initiatives described here is the number of those supported in career development positions who then go on to become academics. We have not been conducting the program long enough for longitudinal follow-up but this will happen in the future.

In the future we hope to work on measuring learning and behavioural change through, for example, a peer review of teaching scheme and longitudinal follow-up of participants using observations, video diaries and/or teaching portfolios.

Benefits

We have seen a gradual shift in attitudes towards teaching and willingness to attend training among NHS staff. Our NHS managers are much more aware of the importance of teaching and the need to protect time for those involved in teaching and training. As an institution, we can be confident that we are meeting the requirements of the regulator, as the collaborative approach described here has been commended by the GMC review process (GMC, 2009b).

Learning Points

The major learning point has perhaps been the critical role of change management when introducing new, potentially unpopular initiatives. We found it vital to keep people informed of impending changes through an effective communication strategy and to illustrate the benefits to them of engaging with the changes. According to Steinert (2010), critical to the development of a community of medical educators are a common purpose, open communication and opportunities for dialogue, guidance and institutional support.

Next Steps

Returning to the challenges we identified, we have gone a considerable distance towards meeting the first three points on our list. We still have some way to go to provide real experiences, grounded in practice and with measurable changes in behaviour as a result. By introducing additional interventions such as peer review, regular observation and feedback of teaching episodes or teaching portfolios, we may be able to address this. Given the number of staff involved, this is not a realistic prospect for everyone any time soon. However, we should be able to pilot some of these initiatives over the next few years and gradually build up a bank of individuals with the skills and expertise to support them on a wider scale.

REFERENCES

Academy of Medical Educators. (2012). *Professional standards.* Retrieved from
    http://www.medicaleducators.org/aome/index.cfm/profession/profstandards/
Dundee City Council, Information & Research Team. (2010). *About Dundee 2010.* Retrieved from
    http://www.dundeecity.gov.uk/dundeecity/uploaded_publications/publication_2005.pdf
General Medical Council. (2006). *Good medical practice.* Retrieved from
    http://www.gmc-uk.org/guidance/good_medical_practice.asp
General Medical Council. (2009a). *Tomorrow's doctors.* Retrieved from
    http://www.gmc-uk.org/education/undergraduate/tomorrows_doctors_2009.asp
General Medical Council (2009b). *Quality assurance of basic medical education: Report on Dundee Medical School, University of Dundee.* Retrieved from
    http://www.gmc-uk.org/static/documents/content/2008_09_Dundee_report_and_response.pdf
Irby, D. M., Cooke, M., & O'Brien, B. C. (2010). Calls for reform of medical education by the Carnegie Foundation for the advancement of teaching: 1910 and 2010. *Academic Medicine, 85*(2), 220-227.

McLean M., Cilliers F., & Van Wyk J. M. (2008). Faculty development: Yesterday, today and tomorrow. *Medical Teacher, 30*(6), 555-584. doi:10.1080/01421590802109834

NHS National Workforce Projects. (2006). National Health Service, Workforce Review Team, Workforce hot topic briefing paper: The Education Workforce. April.

Schofield, S. J., Bradley, S., Macrae, C., Nathwani, D., & Dent, J. (2010). How we encourage faculty development. *Medical Teacher, 32*, 883-886.

Schofield, S. J., Nathwani, D., Anderson, F., Monie, R., Watson, M., & Davis, M. H. (2009). Consultants in Scotland: Survey of educational qualifications, experience and needs of Scottish consultants. *Scottish Medical Journal, 54*(3), 25-29.

Steinert, Y. (2010). Developing medical educators: A journey, not a destination. In T. Swanwick (Ed.), *Understanding Medical Education* (pp. 403-418). Oxford, UK: Association for the Study of Medical Education and Wiley-Blackwell.

Steinert, Y., Mann, K., Centeno, A., Dolmans, D., Spencer, J., Gelula, M., et al. (2006). A systematic review of faculty development initiatives designed to improve teaching effectiveness in medical education: BEME Guide No. 8. *Medical Teacher, 28*(6), 497-526.

Claire Macrae BMSc (Hons), PGCE
Medical Education Institute
University of Dundee, Scotland

Susie Schofield BSc (Hons), PGCE, MSc, PhD
Medical Education Institute
University of Dundee, Scotland

Rola Ajjawi BAppSc (Physiotherapy) Hons, PhD
Medical Education Institute
University of Dundee, Scotland

SECTION 5: FUTURE DIRECTIONS

ELAINE DUFFY AND MEGAN SMITH

27. MAJOR CURRENT THEMES IN HEALTH PROFESSIONAL EDUCATION

Reflecting on the current state of the art of health professional education evokes a mixture of conflicting thoughts and feelings, uncertainty and challenges on one hand and excitement and opportunity on the other. These sentiments have been expressed throughout this book by colleagues from a range of disciplines and contexts. The authors have shared with you their personal experiences, research and personal reflections on what it is to be a teacher/researcher in the academy. In this chapter we shed light on the major themes in health professional education, with the inherent interplay between the dynamic changes and reforms in healthcare and the trends in health professional education. We have observed three major themes: the progressive redefining of universities as business entities, the urgent necessity to realise effective education for interprofessional and primary care health, and the implications for university education of interactions between characteristics of contemporary students and changes in education technologies.

Contemporary Universities as Places of Health Professional Education

Universities are now characterised by increasing diversity, policies promoting wider access to higher education, decreasing funding and greater oversight through quality assurance (Meyer, 2012). The contemporary university needs to operate as a business to survive. In the context of gradually reduced government funding, universities are forced to seek alternative funding from non-government sources, yet still remain viable in a highly competitive marketplace. Universities have become, often supersized, competitive corporations with the executive level of management increasingly concerned with metrics, e.g. student enrolments, student retention and completions, and the numbers of dollars a university can attract.

The Australian government's initiative in 2012 to uncap student numbers, especially for the health professions, has made much more obvious to health professional educators the business motives that underlie university decisions. Such business-driven decisions can be at odds to the traditions and values of educators more motivated to contribute to the development of a high-quality health workforce. The business of health professional education has meant that proportionally larger numbers of students are offered places and universities vie for the largest numbers of students possible, sometimes reducing the entry level scores to levels much lower than previously experienced by educators.

Although we have drawn particular attention to the business motives of universities as a driver of increased student numbers, there are parallel drivers to

S. Loftus et al. (Eds.), Educating Health Professionals:
Becoming a University Teacher, 313–322.

increase student training numbers to meet future health workforce needs (e.g. through Health Workforce Australia). Regardless of these drivers, we are seeing students who were not previously gaining entry to higher education level, sitting in classrooms. This has resulted in new cohorts of students with diverse and different learning needs and for whom traditional methods of education may not be as effective. With increased numbers of enrolments, there is a parallel immense pressure on faculties and schools to retain students. There is growing concern among university educators and administrators that the changing context of education is adversely impacting on the student experience, particularly in the first year of university life and increasingly throughout the student's life cycle in the academy. A broad and comprehensive range of perspectives of the student experience is detailed in Chapter 13.

The only constant in the health and education environments is change. A myriad of factors currently influence healthcare systems nationally and globally. Changing community needs and expectations, coupled with the increasing complexity of care and chronic illness will continue to impact on healthcare delivery and health professional practice and education. The landscape of healthcare is changing continuously, impacting the ways in which healthcare is delivered and how healthcare professionals should be educated to meet these demands.

Changing Landscapes: Collaborative Practice and Interprofessional Education

In an environment of increasing complexity in healthcare there is an imperative that health professionals collaborate to meet the total needs of the client/patient. No one health professional can meet the wide ranging needs of all patients. Consumers and families are demanding they are involved in decision making about their care and they expect to receive the highest quality of care when they need it.

A reform recommended by the World Health Organization (WHO) in 1978, *Health for All by the Year 2000*, through Primary Health Care (PHC) has been revived. The PHC initiative was adopted by almost every country in the world. The primary healthcare philosophy promoted universal access, affordability, appropriate, community-based preventive and curative services with extensive community involvement, within a social justice and equity framework. The World Health Organization (WHO) set global goals and targets to achieve marked improvements, however enthusiasm for the initiative diminished largely because of changes in ideology towards market-driven health reforms. The primary healthcare concept has been re-visioned for the 21st century. Thirty years on, the WHO report (2008), *Primary Health Care Now More Than Ever,* calls for four reforms: universal coverage to end exclusion, improved service delivery - by reorganising health services around people's needs and expectations to make services more socially relevant, public health policy through integration of public health with primary healthcare, and leadership, through inclusive, participatory, negotiated leadership at all levels of health.

Many countries are struggling with how best to address the issues outlined above. In response, countries such as New Zealand, the United Kingdom, Canada and Australia have made a commitment to invest in reform processes directed at strengthening the primary healthcare sector (Commonwealth of Australia, 2009). In Australia, these reform processes have predominantly centred on encouraging a population health focus, increased accountability for performance, greater use of interprofessional teams and improved access to services for the whole population. In both acute and primary care settings, patients report higher levels of satisfaction, better acceptance of care and improved health outcomes from treatment and care by collaborative teams (Xyrichis & Ream, 2008; Mickan, 2005).

Collaborative practice works most effectively when it is organised around the needs of the population and takes into account local healthcare systems. According to McNair, Stone, Sims, and Curtis (2005) collaborative practice occurs when members of two or more professions work together in a team with commitment, mutual respect and a common purpose to improve quality care. This concept was elaborated upon by the World Health Organization (WHO, 2010) adding that collaborative practice in healthcare occurs when multiple health workers provide comprehensive services by working together synergistically with patients, their families, carers and communities to deliver the highest quality of care across settings. While preparing a team-oriented workforce is central to collaborative practice, alone it will not guarantee optimal health services. Critical changes in the workforce are necessary to enable collaborative practice to become a reality in healthcare; this presents challenges to those organisations that are trapped in outdated cultural milieus.

In the WHO (2010) report: *Framework for Action on Interprofessional Education and Collaborative Practice,* three practice level mechanisms are recommended to enable effective collaborative practice: institutional supports, work culture and the environment. A critical component of institutional support for staff is that management supports collaborative teamwork and truly believes in sharing the responsibility for healthcare service delivery among team members. A work culture that enables collaborative practice is effective when there are opportunities in the workplace for shared decision-making and regular communication through team meetings. This leads staff to make joint decisions and commitments on common goals and patient management plans, balance their individual and shared tasks, and negotiate shared resources. In the environment, space design and facilities can significantly augment or hinder collaborative practice in an interprofessional setting. Most importantly, physical space should not reflect a hierarchical structure.

There is evidence to indicate that interprofessional education (IPE) enables effective collaborative practice which in turn optimises health services, strengthens health systems and improves health outcomes (Xyrichis & Ream, 2008; Mickan, 2005). These authors found evidence in their study that there was a positive impact for patients, staff and organisations. For staff there was job satisfaction, recognition of individual contribution, motivation, and improved mental health. Patients found that teamwork improved quality of care, value-added patient outcomes and satisfaction with services. From an organisational perspective the authors claim

315

that teamwork led to a satisfied and committed workforce, improved cost control and improved workforce retention and reduced staff turnover.

A number of reviews and inquiries in healthcare, such as the *Garling Special Commission of Inquiry into Acute Care in New South Wales Public Hospitals* (Garling, 2008), highlight the negative impacts of breakdowns in communication and decision making between the different professions and the serious gaps in understanding the role of other health professions. The Garling report points to the need for health to shift from a focus on service characterised by independent professional silos to a business that centralises excellence in patient care through collaborative practice:

> Health needs to move from a craft based industry of many individual professionals practising independently to a managed business where the main goal is excellent patient care provided by multidisciplinary teams and assessed by patient outcomes and patient experience. (Garling, 2008, p. 14)

At the practice level, Garling made recommendations to reform work practices and create a modern hospital workforce where each member of the clinical workforce should be prepared to work within a multidisciplinary environment as a "member of, or as a contributor to an interdisciplinary team responsible for the delivery of patient centred care" (p. 19). A framework to conceptualise these processes and concepts was developed by the WHO (2010) and appears in Figure 27.1.

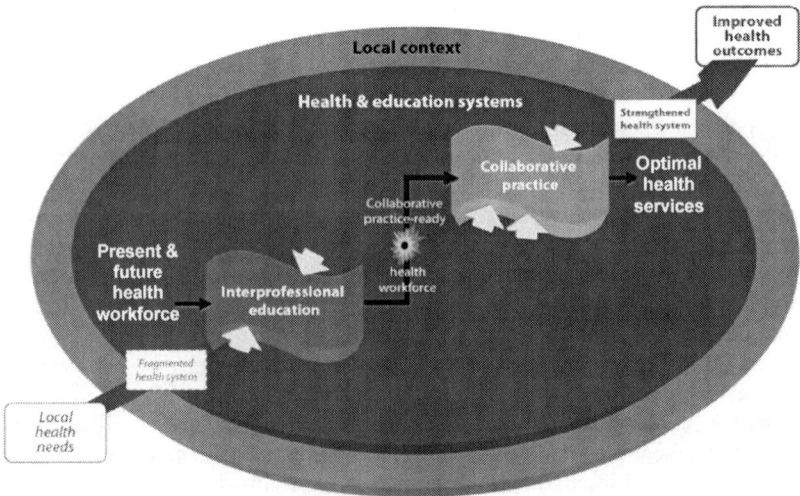

Fig. 27.1 Framework for action on interprofessional education &
collaborative practice. Reprinted with permission from:
World Health Organization (WHO). (2010, p. 18)

Interprofessional education (IPE) is becoming a more prominent feature of health professional education at both undergraduate and postgraduate levels however there is much debate about when IPE should be introduced in the educational process. The strongest argument is that it should commence at the undergraduate level prior to students becoming socialised into their individual disciplines. The opposing view is that students should be socialised into their primary discipline area prior to being exposed to other disciplines. The latter argument could be interpreted to mean that particular disciplines wish to establish a clear delineation of roles prior to exposure to other professions. Despite the prominence of policies, frameworks and position statements regarding collaborative practice and IPE, debates continue about the conceptualisation, design and implementation of interprofessional practice and IPE.

In a report to Health Workforce Australia, the Interprofesssional Curriculum Renewal Consortium (2013) undertook an Australia-wide audit and analysis of pre-registration IPE in health occurring in the Australian higher education sector during 2011 and 2012. This report is the first attempt in Australia, and globally, to present a national profile of IPE activity in higher education. The report concludes that the development of IPE within Australian universities and jurisdictions has been piecemeal and uncoordinated. Activities were found to be localised, opportunistic, adaptive and inventive yet they exist at the margins of the curriculum, are inadequately resourced and consequently unsustainable. IPE is fragmented both within and across universities and the higher education sector and there are no mechanisms to share information and learning, nor to develop research and build knowledge and capacity.

The *National Audit Report* makes seven recommendations that identify specific areas of national capacity building including the development of a common language and national IPE learning outcomes and the development of professional standards and their adoption in health professional accreditation schemes. The language of "learning outcomes" rather than "competencies" is interesting to note though the report does refer to *core* competencies that would be appropriate across all health professions. The report also highlights the importance of continuing professional development, faculty capacity building, research development and knowledge management, and the development of a nationally co-ordinated approach to IPE (ICRC, 2013, p. 14).

The Interprofessional Education Collaborative Expert Panel (IECEP) (2011), comprising international professionals across all fields of health were also inspired by a vision of interprofessional collaborative practice as central to the safe, high-quality, accessible, patient-centred care. The IECEP identified four competency domains for interprofessional collaborative practice: values/ethics for interprofess-ional practice, roles/responsibilities, interprofessional communication, and teams/teamwork (2011).

The IECEP advised that to achieve their vision for the future requires the continuous development of interprofessional competencies by health professional students as part of the learning process, so that they enter the workforce ready to practise effective teamwork and team-based care. The intent is to build on each profession's expected disciplinary competencies in defining competencies for interprofessional collaborative practice.

The Canadian Interprofessional Health Collaborative (2010) recommended that a unifying concept was required for development of core competencies for interprofessional collaborative practice. The concept of *interprofessionality* was articulated by D'Amour and Oandasan (2005) as part of the foundation work for initiatives by Health Canada to cultivate interprofessional education and interprofessional collaborative practice. They define *interprofessionality* (p. 9) as:

> The process by which professionals reflect on and develop ways of practicing that provides an integrated and cohesive answer to the needs of the client/family/population ... [I]t involves continuous interaction and knowledge sharing between professionals, organized to solve or explore a variety of education and care issues all while seeking to optimize the patient's participation ... Interprofessionality requires a paradigm shift, since interprofessional practice has unique characteristics in terms of values, codes of conduct, and ways of working. These characteristics must be elucidated.

The CIHC propose six competency domains for interprofessional collaborative practice in Canada and the Canadian government has invested significant funding to assist with implementing interprofessional education and practice initiatives. The six domains are: interprofessional communication, patient/client/family /community-centred care, role clarification, team functioning, collaborative leadership and interprofessional conflict resolution. The WHO (2010) adopted a learning outcomes frame to education which does account for the values and ethics of collaborative practice and recommends six interprofessional learning domains: teamwork, roles and responsibilities, communication, learning and critical reflection, relationship with, and recognising the needs of, the patient, and ethical practice (p. 26).

The greatest challenge in this field in Australia (if IPE were considered a priority) is the adoption of IPE requirements in the accreditation standards of all Australian health professions. The health professions have only recently moved to national registration and competency requirements are discipline-specific and stringent. Currently accreditation requirements are a barrier to the acceptance of IPE. Successful interprofessional education relies on curricula that link learning activities, expected outcomes and an assessment of what has been learned. Attention to the preparation of teachers for their roles in developing, delivering and evaluating interprofessional education is also important (Hammick, Freeth, Koppel, Reeves, & Barr, 2007). For many educators, teaching students from different disciplines how to learn about, from and with each other is a new and challenging experience and it is beneficial if teaching staff have been exposed to collaborative teamwork in practice.

In the ICRC (2013) report, of 70 IPE activities, the majority (40) did not involve patients or carers. Since survey participants were able to provide more than one response it is unclear as to how the roles of respondents overlapped. A cross-sectional review was undertaken by Abu-Rish et al. (2012) of IPE activities based

318

on 83 studies published between 2005 and 2010. Of note from this review was the finding that in 20% of the studies, students, patients and families played a role in developing IPE educational experiences. This is a growing trend internationally and Canadian colleagues Farrell, Towle and Godolphin (2006) point to five inter-related movements driving the change from passive to active patient involvement in health professional education through simulation and through real-life experiences that apply across the professions. The first is the recognition by academic institutions of the importance of partnerships with communities and community engagement. The second is patient-centred care that responds to patient preferences and involves patients in decision-making about their care. Third, healthcare reform and the involvement of patients and carers as partners in healthcare is identified as an important component of patient safety.

> If we are to really hear patients, we must learn to listen in circumstances where their authentic and autonomous voices are not attenuated by our professional privilege or drowned by the clamour of our care. (Farrell, Towle & Godolphin, 2006, p. 9)

The fourth driving force in curriculum reform and policy change (for example in the UK and Canada), is the need for health professional students to have a better understanding of the patient's experience of illness, the social determinants of health and disease and the needs of the community. Finally, the consumer movement and the dissatisfaction with traditional paternalistic relationships in healthcare is another dimension of interprofessional education that requires further research.

Health Professional Students: Generational

A vital element and central to the health professional education debate is the student. Academics have a responsibility to be aware of changing demographics in the student population, student diversity, a broad range of learning styles and students' varying expectations of university life.

Characteristics of current university students have been identified as markedly different to students in previous generations. However the most significant change that we see is that health student populations are immensely diverse, not only in generational terms, but also in gender, nationality, social status, expectations and modes of study. It is of prime importance to understand the student population abilities and needs coming into universities; universities must adapt some of their outdated strategies of "one size fits all" to facilitate a flexible, student-centred approach to learning and teaching in the academy. Taking an in-depth look at the generational differences among our student population is informative, though we need to be acutely aware of the tendency of such information becoming stereotypical and generalisable and therefore requires caution.

In the health professional disciplines we find classes consisting of high school leavers and mature age students, increased numbers of students doing part-time studies, students studying by distance learning, Aboriginal and Torres Strait

Islander students and students whose parents are migrants. There are more students entering university who are "first in family" to enter the higher education domain. This is due in part to the emphasis on access to education, equity, social inclusion and increased participation of students from low socioeconomic backgrounds as recommended in the Bradley Review (Commonwealth of Australia, 2008).

Generational descriptions are based upon significant events in the formative years of a generation, which influence the individuals' social values and attitudes and are relative to the social changes that occurred. Generations are described as: "Silent Generation" (born 1925-1945), "Baby Boomers" (born 1945-59), "Generation X" (born 1960s-1970s) and "Generation Y" (born 1977-1984). The traditional, silent or mature generation, experienced the Great Depression and World War II during their childhood. They grew up in a period of major changes such as the Women's Liberation movement, the civil rights movement and the Vietnam War. The Generation X's were raised in an era of recession, "latch key" kids, hands-off parenting and the AIDS crisis. This group is also technologically confident.

"Gen Y" is labelled, "techno-savvy" due to the explosion of easily accessible technology, Internet, mobile phones, iPods, computer games and the like. Instant text messaging is central to their lives and they expect instant responses and feedback. This group is described as: the "Nexters", the "Millenials", the "Digital Generation" and the "Me Generation" (Oblinger, 2003). What do these generational differences mean for health professional education? There are wide ranging implications for both teachers and students.

Equally we need to reflect on the generational differences of current academic staff, many of whom hail from the "baby boomer" generation as do many of our senior health practitioners. As an example, a number of studies have explored the generation Y student population in different health professional contexts. Through a cross temporal meta-analysis of undergraduate student's responses to IQ questionnaires, personality traits, attitudes, reading, preferences and expectations, Twenge (2009) concluded that "Generation Me" scored higher on assertiveness, self-liking, narcissistic traits and unrealistic expectations and goals. The researcher also concluded that Gen Y students showed some measures of stress, anxiety and poor mental health and scored lower on self-reliance. From a teaching viewpoint this suggests that students in this generation require structure and precise unambiguous instructions. Do academic staff consider generational differences and student diversity when developing courses and facilitating learning activities? This question could require a whole chapter to answer it; suffice to say that a sound understanding of the learners entering the classroom is fundamental to facilitating learning for students.

SUMMARY

There are many diverse challenges for the development and delivery of interprofessional education (IPE) through all aspects of curriculum development and its subsequent sustainability. These include: lack of curriculum space as specialty areas within the professions compete to include their speciality into shrinking curriculum. Of critical importance is the challenge to well entrenched cultural practices within education and health, which includes professional boundaries/silos, professional status and hierarchy. The lack of familiarity amongst educators about IPE pedagogy has been highlighted by a number of researchers (Jacob, Barnett, Missen, Cross, & Walker, 2012; Thistlethwaite & Moran, 2010). One of the key criticisms in higher education is the lack of a clear theoretical base though critical reviews of the literature suggest that the educational theories can be linked to adult learning theory, reflective practice theory, social psychology theory and biopsychosocial theories (Pockett, 2010).

This chapter has highlighted the dynamic nature of health professional education and practice in today's climate. The most exciting movement currently is the vision of healthcare organised with the patient at the heart of it and an interprofessional team providing excellent care and health outcomes, through true collaborative practice. The importance of appropriately preparing the next generation of health professionals for the changes in healthcare delivery cannot be underestimated. To traverse the divide between today and the possibilities of tomorrow requires visionary, transformational leadership in both the practice and educational arenas.

REFERENCES

Abu-Rish, E., Kim, S., Choe, L., Varpio, L., Malik, E., White, A. A., Craddick, K., Blondon, K., Robins, L., Nagasawa, P., Thigpen, A., Chen, L-L., Rich, J., & Zierler, B. (2012). Current trends in interprofessional education of health sciences students: A literature review. *Journal of Interprofessional Care*, pp. 1-8. doi:10.3109/13561820.2012.715604. Retrieved from http://ipe.utah.edu/content/current-trends-ipe

Canadian Interprofessional Health Collaborative. (2010). *A national interprofessional competency framework*. Retrieved from http://www.cihc.ca/files/CIHC_IPCompetencies_Feb1210.pdf

Commonwealth of Australia. (2008). *Review of Australian higher education: A discussion paper*. Canberra, Australia. Retrieved from http://www.dest.gov.au/HEreview

Commonwealth of Australia. (2009). *Primary health care reform in Australia: Report to support Australia's first national primary health care strategy*. Canberra, Australia.

D'Amour, D., & Oandasan, I. (2005). Interprofessionality as the field of interprofessional practice and interprofessional education: An emerging concept. *Journal of Interprofessional Care*, Supplement 1, 8-20.

Farrell, C., Towle, A., & Godolphin, W. (2006). *Where's the patient's voice in health professional education?* A report from the first international conference, Division of Health Care Communication, College of Health Disciplines, University of British Columbia, Canada, 3 Nov 2005. Retrieved from http://www.chd.ubc.ca/dhcc/ourwork/patients_as_educators/conferences

Garling, P. (2008) Final report of the special commission of inquiry: Acute care in NSW public hospitals. Retrieved from http://www.dpc.nsw.gov.au/__data/assets/pdf_file/0003/34194/Overview-Special_Commission_Of_Inquiry_Into_Acute_Care_Services_In_New_South_Wales_Public_Hospitals.pdf

Hammick, M., Freeth, D., Koppel, I., Reeves, S., & Barr, H. (2007). A best evidence systematic review of interprofessional education: BEME Guide No. 9. *Medical Teacher*, 29(8), 735-751. doi:10.1080/01421590701682576

Health Workforce Australia. (2012). *Health workforce 2025: Doctors, nurses and midwives – Volume 1*. Retrieved from http://www.hwa.gov.au/work-programs/information-analysis-and-planning/health-workforce-planning/hw2025-doctors-nurses-and-

Interprofessional Curriculum Renewal Consortium, Australia. (2013). *Interprofessional education: A national audit*. Report to Health Workforce Australia, Canberra, Australia.

Interprofessional Education Collaborative Expert Panel. (2011). *Core competencies for interprofessional collaborative practice: Report of an expert panel*. Washington, D.C: Interprofessional Education Collaborative. Retrieved from https://www.aamc.org/download/186750/data/core_competencies.pdf

Jacob, E., Barnett, T., Missen, K., Cross, M., & Walker, L. (2012). Australian clinician's views on interprofessional education for students in the rural clinical setting. *Journal of Research in Interprofessional Practice and Education, 2*(2), 219-229. Retrieved from http://www.jripe.org/index.php/journal/article/view/68

McNair, R., Stone, N., Sims, J., & Curtis, C. (2005). Australian evidence for interprofessional education contributing to effective teamwork preparation and interest in rural practice. *Journal of Interprofessional Care, 19*(6), 579-594.

Meyer, L. (2012). Negotiating academic values, professorial responsibilities and expectations for accountability in today's university. *Higher Education Quarterly, 66*(2), 207-217.

Mickan, S. M. (2005). Evaluating the effectiveness of health care teams. *Australian Health Review, 29*(2), 211-217.

Oblinger, D. (2003). Boomers, gen-xers and millennials: Understanding the "new students". *EduCause Review, 38*(4), 37-47.

Pockett, R. (2010). Interprofessional education for practice: Some implications for Australian social work. *Australian Social Work, 63*(2), 207-222.

Thistlethwaite, J., & Moran, M. (2010). Learning outcomes for interprofessional education (IPE): Literature review and synthesis. *Journal of Interprofessional Care, 24*(5), 503-513.

Twenge, J. M. (2009). Generational changes and their impact in the classroom: Teaching generation me. *Medical Education, 43*, 398-405.

World Health Organization, & Lerberghe, W. van. (2008). *Primary health care: Now more than ever*. World Health Organization, Geneva, Switzerland. Retrieved from http://www.who.int/whr/2008/08_overview_en.pdf

World Health Organization. (1978). *Health for all by the year 2000*. Geneva, Switzerland.

World Health Organization. (2010). *Framework for action on interprofessional education and collaborative practice*. Geneva, Switzerland: World Health Organization. Retrieved from http://www.who.int/hrh/resources/framework_action/en/index.html

Xyrichis, A., & Ream, E. (2008). Teamwork: A concept analysis. *Journal of Advanced Nursing, 61*(2), 232-241.

Elaine Duffy RN, RM, DipAppSc(CHN),BAppSc(AdvNsg),MN, PhD, FRCNA
School of Nursing and Midwifery
Griffith University

Megan Smith PhD
Faculty of Science
Charles Sturt University, Australia

STEPHEN LOFTUS AND JOY HIGGS

28. HEALTH PROFESSIONAL EDUCATION IN THE FUTURE

We live in interesting times in higher education; times that are especially interesting for those of us involved in preparing new generations of health professionals. This is because there are great changes in motion. The last few decades have seen major upheavals in the ways in which we understand and practise higher education. Changes are likely to continue for the foreseeable future for a number of reasons. There are also clear trends emerging that indicate something of what we might expect in the years to come.

Bokor, preparing a report for international consultancy firm Ernst & Young (2012) made some thought provoking forecasts in a report titled: *University of the future: A thousand year old industry on the cusp of profound change.* They describe the dominant university model as a broad-based teaching and research institution, supported by a large asset base and a large, predominantly in-house back office (p. 14). The authors predict that a transformation of university business models is expected in the future despite a long history of a slow rate of change in the sector. Ernst & Young aimed to identify the major forces impacting the higher education industry globally and locally and to explore the opportunities, challenges, and implications for Australian universities.

In this chapter we begin by discussing the reasons for continuing change and explore what we believe are the most important emerging trends and their implications. Firstly, why is there, despite all the upheavals of recent years, still an impetus for yet more change?

A GROWING SENSE OF UNEASE

Health professional education continues to be controversial. In the latter half of the twentieth century there were widespread changes, ranging from the introduction of new curricula such as problem-based learning, to the decision of many health professions to move their initial education to the universities and to the proliferation of graduate entry programs. All of these changes have been controversial for numerous reasons and many of these issues have been explored in depth in earlier chapters of this book. Many of the initial controversies have quietened down to some extent. Problem-based learning, for example, is now widely accepted as part of the mainstream of professional education. There are, however, still a number of issues that are troubling many educators of health professionals that have yet to be resolved. The resolution of these issues is likely to dominate the field of health professional education for several years to come.

S. Loftus et al. (Eds.), Educating Health Professionals:
Becoming a University Teacher, 323–333.
© 2013 Sense Publishers. All rights reserved.

A number of these issues can be seen as a sense of unease about how we understand and practise health professional education. One explanation for this sense of unease is that the current ways of discussing and understanding the whole enterprise of higher education are limited. The vocabularies we use often fail to capture what needs to be conceptualised in the depth we want or with the subtlety we want. In other words there is dissatisfaction with the discourses we use to articulate what health professional education is and how it is to be conducted.

An important discourse that has dominated the field and a growing source of dissatisfaction is the technical rational approach to education. This approach assumes that education is a precise science that is best studied in terms of cause and effect. The implication is that the findings of such an approach can then be applied in a relatively simple manner. From this perspective an educational intervention is seen as a cause that will have a distinctive and measurable effect, easily quantified by pre- and post-test measures of some sort. The most obvious example of the technical rational approach in action is the dominance of competency-based training, where what health professionals do, and how they learn to do it, is effectively reduced to straightforward technical procedures that can be observed and measured in a neutral and completely objective manner. The idea that professional practice or education can be reduced in this way is a big assumption and a growing number of voices are pointing out the considerable weaknesses of this approach (e.g. Fish, 2012).

A competency-based approach can standardise technical performance and how it is judged and this is clearly a good thing. However, the objection is that being a health professional is not the same as being a technician (Fish & Coles, 2005). The competency-based approach assumes that professional practice is little more than the application of a great many technical procedures. There are important aspects of professional practice that do not lend themselves to being conceptualised as technical procedures. A technical rational approach tends to ignore these aspects and they become effectively invisible. These aspects include critical thinking, ethicality, reflexivity, and the ability to deal with complexity, uncertainty and ambiguity. It can be argued that these aspects are qualities that reflect underlying professional values and are best understood and discussed in such terms (de Cossart & Fish, 2005; Fish & de Cossart, 2007). The technical rational approach has a vocabulary that is poorly equipped to deal with these qualities in any meaningful way and so they have tended to fade into the background of health professional education when, arguably, it is these very qualities that should be at the forefront and providing the foundation of our educational activity. When there are attempts to articulate these qualities they are often labelled as competencies (e.g. Association of American Medical Colleges, 2013). Such labelling distorts their nature and makes it difficult to engage with these qualities in ways that can be seen to reflect the true nature of professional practice.

Closely related to this is a growing tendency for the discourse of managerialism to dominate, not only education, but also the professional practice of the health professions. It has been pointed out that one of the dangers of the managerialist approach is that important educational activities, such as assessment, become seen as management "tools" to be used merely to control what health professionals do (Fish, 2012). The profound educational possibilities of assessment to help students truly engage with their professions then become hidden and lost. For example, assessment that encourages students to reflect deeply on what they are doing with a patient enables students to learn many different lessons from the one clinical encounter. These other lessons range from understanding and coping with the values underpinning professional practice to interpreting the importance of context for this *particular* patient at this *particular* time in this *particular* place and in these *particular* circumstances. These current deficiencies in health professional education have prompted a number of responses. It is these responses that we see as providing key trends for the education of all health professionals for some time to come. What characterises many of these responses is that they adopt ideas and vocabularies from a range of disciplines. In other words, these responses adopt a range of different discourses that allow us to articulate new directions in health professional education. Many of these responses can be summarised under the headings of professional identity and integration.

PROFESSIONAL IDENTITY

There are a growing number of voices calling for higher education, in general, and professional education in particular, to be seen as a process of personal formation (e.g. Cooke, Irby, & O'Brien, 2010; Sullivan & Rosin, 2008; Walker, Golde, Jones, Conklin Bueschel, & Hutchings, 2008). The idea of formation was deliberately adopted from the discourse of theology where higher education has long been seen as a process that must form a particular sort of person; the sort of person who can undertake a religious ministry (Foster, Dahill, Golemon, & Wang Tolentino, 2005). This idea has been adopted by other disciplines to refer to the formation of professional identity. From this viewpoint, a professional practitioner is someone, who not only knows about issues such as ethics and the values of their profession, but is someone who embodies these in their person and in their practice, knowing full well that they do so and why they have chosen to do so.

There is a clear trend emerging towards providing educational experiences that encourage and foster the development of professional identity. Clinical placements can provide opportunities for students to start identifying with the practitioners who supervise them; practitioners who provide the role models. This has always happened but now there is more of a trend to ensure that the participants in clinical placements are aware that this is happening. One important aspect of identity formation is the sharing of practice stories ("war stories") by which practitioners pass on to colleagues the knowledge and wisdom they gain from engagement with practice itself. A discourse that allows us to articulate what is happening in these situations is that of communities of practice (Loftus, 2010; Wenger, 1998). In the UK, the work of Della Fish and colleagues provides examples of practical measures that educators can adopt to foster the formation of health practitioners who are true professionals.

Fish and de Cossart (2007) provide resources in the form of heuristics that they claim can develop what they call the "invisibles" of professional practice. These invisibles are precisely the qualities of professionalism that the technical rational approach has such difficulty in articulating. The invisibles include a sensitivity to: professional values themselves, context, the different forms of knowledge that might be needed to manage a case, the clinical reasoning and professional judgments that health professionals need in complex cases, the therapeutic relationship established with a particular patient and the ability to reflect deeply about a case to extend one's understanding of all the social and clinical aspects of practice. The last item on the list, reflection, is one to which they pay particular attention.

Fish and de Cossart (2007) recommend regular reflective writing with the intention of encouraging learners to see a clinical situation from different perspectives and to articulate possible value conflicts, for example. The invisibles are beginning to gain acceptance from a growing number of practitioners and institutions (D. Fish, personal communication, 2012). While the invisibles are primarily intended for junior doctors, it is clear that the principles apply to any health professional student who must engage with patients in any serious manner. It is claimed that approaches such as this foster a much greater awareness of the importance of professionalism and ethical behaviour as a foundation of professional practice beyond a mere knowledge that they are required (Fish, 2012). Part of the process of identity formation requires role modelling and mentoring.

There appears to be a growing awareness that if our future graduates are to embody the professionalism we want of them then we, as educators, are going to have to provide the role models that embody that professionalism. Our students will need to see us, their teachers, acting professionally and, more importantly, *being* professional in our practice. We are a key part of their professional socialisation (see Chapter 8). We will need to actively mentor students to be sensitive to the values of our professions and our professionalism in action. This will require sufficient numbers of staff who can engage with students and have the time and opportunity to provide the in-depth mentoring needed. In an age of the so-called massification of higher education where universities are being expected to "turn out" larger numbers of new graduates with the same resources and numbers of staff as we have in the past then this poses a serious problem. This is probably one reason why managerialism and the competency-based approach are so popular. They provide a false promise of generating new professionals at a low cost. This is a current and future trend that will engage and challenge health professional educators for some years to come. Role modelling and mentoring are also important for encouraging new graduates to start developing practice wisdom.

Practice wisdom (see Gates & Higgs, 2013) builds on the idea that there are several different kinds of knowledge needed for professional practice and that wisdom extends beyond knowledge and knowing.

Practice wisdom is the possession of practice experience and knowledge together with the ability to use them critically, intuitively and practically. Including characteristics of clarity, discernment and caring deeply from an objective stance, practice wisdom is a component of professional artistry. (Titchen & Higgs, 2001, p. 275)

The need to develop practice wisdom is another emerging trend that will exercise the minds of educators in years to come. Higher education has traditionally been concerned only with propositional knowledge, the formal knowledge found in textbooks and typified by the evidence-based practice movement that privileges information generated from randomised controlled trials above all else. There is a growing awareness that other ways of knowing are also important for professional practice. These other ways include knowledge that is generated from practice itself, sometimes called practice-based evidence (Livingston & McNutt, 2011; Nevo & Slonim-Nevo, 2011).

One discourse that attempts to articulate such practice knowledge is neo-Aristotelianism, based on the work of Aristotle (trans. 2012). Neo-Aristotelianism recognises traditional propositional knowledge (*episteme*) but also technical knowledge of how to do things (*techne*) and in addition, the knowledge that comes directly from engaging in practice (*phronesis*). While phronesis cannot be taught directly our education needs to provide opportunities for students to meet the challenges of practice and thus develop phronesis for themselves. When combined with reflective practice, as described above, phronesis can help professionals develop a sense of praxis. Praxis has been defined as morally informed and morally committed action (Kemmis & Smith, 2008). However, in order for students to develop a professional identity in this way they need to engage in relevant practice in sufficient depth, with sufficient frequency, and with sufficient mentoring and reflection. As Davey observed:

> What makes a practice a practice rather than a method is precisely the fact that it is based upon acquired and accumulated experience. The acquisition of discernment, judgment, and insight is based not so much upon what comes to us in a given experience but upon what comes to us by involvement and participation in a whole number of experiences. ... Experience of this order affords a wisdom. (Davey, 2006, p. 245)

Practice wisdom then becomes a part of who and what we are as people and as professionals. This insight comes from yet another discourse. In this case the philosophical hermeneutics of Gadamer (1989). Philosophical hermeneutics is just one example of the many discourses that are now offering new ways of understanding health professional education and practice (e.g. Gadamer, 1996; Svenaeus, 2000). An overarching trend emerging for the future is the need to integrate a range of different discourses in ways that combine the strengths of each.

INTEGRATION

Some forms of integration already exist in health professional education. These include problem-based learning and interprofessional education and practice. In

327

problem-based learning the basic health sciences are integrated with clinical sciences so that students can see just how they are related and relevant to each other and in interprofessional education, students can learn how other health professions conceptualise and approach clinical cases. An important point of such integration is not to merge the different approaches into one overall clinical health science or profession but to appreciate how the different approaches can support each other so that the whole becomes greater than the sum of its parts. Through the integration of problem-based learning each science can become more relevant to clinical practice and through the integration of interprofessional education each profession can become more effective in its clinical practice. One discourse that offers a vocabulary to conceptualise what happens in this form of integration is the dialogism based on the work of the Russian scholar, Mikhail Bakhtin (1982). A growing number of scholars are using Bakhtin's ideas to develop a sophisticated understanding of how moral and ethical perspectives are intimately related to the technicalities of what happens in clinical practice (e.g. Frank, 2004). There is a trend for integration in other aspects of health professional education.

The scientific approach that has dominated health professional education is now being integrated more and more with other disciplines. These other disciplines include the social sciences and the humanities which offer distinctive perspectives from which to improve education and practice. According to Sullivan and Rosin (2008) the natural sciences help us to establish relative certainty making the world, "more amenable to rational understanding and effective action" (p. 94-95). The social sciences can, "open up for examination the diversity of human possibilities and experience" (p. 94) while the humanities can, "provide means of understanding and interpreting the complexities of purpose and meaning" (p. 94). The integration of the different disciplines opens up the possibility of developing professionals who can combine scientific analytical thought and the critical thinking of the humanities into what can be called practical reason. One indication of this trend towards integration is the growing interest in narrative medicine.

The advocates of narrative medicine (Charon, 2006; Loftus & Greenhalgh, 2010) claim that it is an example of how scientific thinking can be integrated with humanities thinking. Clinical cases can be seen as following generic narrative formats that can help us organise vast amounts of scientific knowledge. A narrative mode of thinking may not provide scientific certainty but it does provide a means of exploring and making sense of situations and contexts of action where scientific thinking and discourse falter. A narrative approach, such as employed by medical anthropologists (e.g. Moerman, 2002) can open up the sources of human meaning and value that may permit us to see why some patients are resistant to what seems so scientifically obvious. These insights can then open up the possibility of engaging with these patients in ways that might permit us to provide care that they find acceptable within their worldview. Approaches, such as this, that use integrated ways of thinking are ethical in that the humanity of others is fully recognised and a scientific approach is not imposed on people, simply because it is known to be scientifically effective.

Integrated ways of thinking allow ethical approaches to be incorporated naturally into professional practice and its education rather than as something to be included after the scientific information has been processed and decisions have been made. This demand for ethical practice seems to be another clear trend. Other disciplines outside of science can help us bring this about. For example, from a purely scientific perspective, health is little more than the absence of disease and a clinician's job is to repair the biological machine that is the body. Insights from other disciplines allow us to see health as a subjective sense of "homelike being-in-the-world" (Svenaeus, 2000, p. 100) which is how patients experience health. As Svenaeus points out

> Doctors in the clinic do not meet with agents who evaluate their pain and take a rational stand upon what they want to have done with their biological processes, but with worried, help-seeking persons, who need care and understanding in order to be brought back to a homelike being-in-the-world again. (Svenaeus, 2000, pp. 173-174)

It is insights like this that help us to see that clinical reasoning needs to be ethical from the beginning and that scientific analysis needs to be blended with the hermeneutic/interpretive thinking of the humanities. As Montgomery (2006) realised, doctors are often under the illusion that they are thinking scientifically when in reality they are thinking interpretively. They must think interpretively because they have to deal with a great deal of complexity and uncertainty.

It was an attempt to deal with uncertainty and complexity that drove the evidence-based practice movement. One emerging trend is a growing dissatisfaction with this movement and this is likely to affect health professional education. The original pioneers of the EBP movement called for the best scientific evidence to be integrated with the personal experience and expertise of the practitioner (Sackett, Richardson, Rosenberg, & Haynes, 1996). This call for integration was largely ignored while a great deal of attention has been devoted to ways of securing the best evidence and providing this to practitioners. The reason that the integration with personal expertise has been mostly ignored probably goes back to our earlier argument that without a vocabulary and an adequate discourse it simply has not been possible to engage adequately with the issue. The integration of humanities and social sciences with medical sciences, however, gives medical practice the conceptual resources to engage with the issue of personal experience and how it can be brought into dialogue with the best scientific evidence (Loftus, 2012). Along with the explosive growth in the amount and availability of scientific information for educators and students has been a concomitant increase in the use of technology, both in the practice of the health professions and their education.

The integration of technology into health professional education is a continuing trend. Simulations are just one example of a technology that continues to grow in sophistication. Simulations, whether simple or hi-tech, have great advantages as they provide students with opportunities to practise a great many skills and procedures without harming patients (Hutchings & Loftus, 2013). However, simulations do not involve real patients and there is a need to be aware that while simulations can be a great help to education they can never replace contact with real people.

This leads us to another trend of developing technology that affects both the education and practice of health professionals. This trend is the increasing availability of information, both background information, often in the form of the best evidence mentioned earlier, and detailed information about individual patients.

Electronic medical records of patients are growing in sophistication and ease of access. There are dangers that may catch out the inexperienced; particularly students and junior practitioners. Educators need to be aware of these dangers and address them because these dangers are likely to grow as the technology develops. The main problem is that test results and electronic records can come to substitute for real patients.

Verghese (2008) for example, refers to the danger of the "iPatient" (p. 2748) becoming more "real" to students and novices than the patients who are occupying the beds. Verghese claims that he had to make a concerted effort to get his junior staff to spend sufficient time on the wards interacting with real patients rather than relying on information such as test results provided online. The growing reliance on more and more sophisticated diagnostic tests and computer-based information seems to be part of a long-standing trend that some scholars (e.g. Dunnington, 2000) claim has been continuing for decades. Dunnington even coined the term "clinical skills deficiency syndrome" to describe this trend (p. 71). The risk posed to many health professionals is of losing important observational skills that can only be developed by prolonged and intensive interaction with patients under close supervision by teachers who can help students and junior practitioners develop these skills. The question arises of exactly who these teachers are going to be.

It can be argued that all health practitioners will need to become teachers in their profession in some form or other. The clinical teaching that needs to occur seems to be growing far beyond the capacity (in relation to time availability and recency of practice experience) of the available academics, even in well-staffed departments.

It has long been accepted that all health professionals must become lifelong learners in order to keep up-to-date. There now seems to be a growing expectation that they will also become lifelong teachers, starting not long after graduation. This is partly because of the growing acceptance of practice-based education where students are expected to spend ample time on clinical placements away from university settings.

A current trend is that clinical placements are increasing in number, duration and diversity of location. More and more of our students will be taught and supervised by non-academic staff. All these practitioners will need support if they are to do this well. They will need to understand what education in their profession entails. They must know *how* to teach as well as *what* to teach and they must understand the importance of the role models and the mentoring they will be providing to newcomers who are striving to establish their own sense of professional identity.

For all this to happen education needs to become a much more important core value of each health profession than it is at present. Education needs to be more central to the culture and ethos of all health professions. Our students will need to accept that they will become teachers of one sort or another soon after graduation and, therefore, having some understanding of professional education and how to conduct it is likely to become a capability expected of all graduates and junior practitioners. This trend is already present in medicine where junior doctors, only recently qualified, have long been expected to teach medical students. We can expect to see this trend spread to all health professions. A challenge arising from this is to provide standardised educational experiences for all students.

Standardisation is an emerging trend throughout higher education and has been dealt with in earlier chapters of this book. All we will add here is that some of the measures mentioned earlier, such as problem-based learning, lend themselves to addressing standards in education because of their focus on a core of knowledge and the key skills of clinical reasoning. They can also provide a standardised emphasis on the underlying professional values needed in each case. There is, however, a realisation that while standards are important we do not want to pursue standardisation to the point of expecting "one-size-fits-all" graduates. There remains the necessity to provide education that is individualised to the learning needs of different students (Cooke et al., 2010). This will be an ongoing challenge for the educators of health professionals for some time to come.

CONCLUSION

Being an educator of health professionals requires an awareness and engagement with many issues. With some issues there are clear trends into the future that seem to be taking particular directions, such as the move to integrated approaches of education, typified by practice-based education such as problem-based learning and the move to clinical placements that are longer, more frequent and more diverse.

Other trends are more problematic in that we cannot be certain how they will develop. For example, will the advance of technology continue a trend towards diminishing real time contact and interaction with patients and a decline in clinical skills? The answers to questions such as these depend on a number of factors, only some of which are under the control of educators.

Factors that educators cannot control include the funding of higher education that might affect the provision of one-to-one mentoring and the customisation of education to suit the learning needs of individual students. However, being aware of these factors means that educators can, at the least, campaign for better funding with a well-reasoned case.

There are other trends that educators can directly engage with in ways that powerfully affect the educational experience of students. These include being aware of underlying professional values and making a conscious effort to role-model these values in their own practice as well as encouraging students to adopt such values as part of their own emerging professional identity. The education of health professionals has always been a complex business. It involves professional socialisation not just technical competencies development (see Chapter 8). We now have access to a range of discourses and vocabularies that are enabling us to articulate that complexity in exciting new ways. Being a health professional who becomes a university teacher is to undertake a serious but fascinating task. We live in interesting times!

REFERENCES

Aristotle. (2012). *Aristotle's Nicomachean Ethics* (R. C. Bartlett & S. D. Collins, Trans.). Chicago: The University of Chicago Press.

Association of American Medical Colleges. (2013). *Teaching for quality: Integrating quality improvement and patient safety across the continuum of medical education.* Washington DC: AAMC.

Bakhtin, M. (1982). *The dialogic imagination: Four essays* (K. Brostrom, Trans.). Austin, TX: University of Texas Press.

Bokor, J. (for Ernst & Young). (2012). *University of the future: A thousand year old industry on the cusp of profound change.* Australian Policy Online. Retrieved from http://apo.org.au/research/university-future-thousand-year-old-industry-cusp-profound-change

Charon, R. (2006). *Narrative medicine: Honoring the stories of illness.* Oxford: Oxford University Press.

Cooke, M., Irby, D. M., & O'Brien, B. C. (2010). *Educating physicians: A call for reform of medical school and residency.* San Francisco: Jossey-Bass.

Davey, N. (2006). *Unquiet understanding: Gadamer's philosophical hermeneutics.* Albany, NY: State University of New York Press.

De Cossart, L., & Fish, D. (2005). *Cultivating a thinking surgeon: New perspectives on clinical teaching, learning and assessment.* Shrewsbury: T/m Publishing.

Dunnington, G. L. (2000). Adapting teaching to the learning environment. In L. H. Distlehorst, G. L. Dunnington & J. R. Folse (Eds.), *Teaching and learning in medical and surgical education: Lessons learned for the 21st century* (pp. 69-83). New York: Psychology Press.

Fish, D. (2012). *Refocusing postgraduate medical education: From the technical to the moral mode of practice.* Cranham: Aneumi Publications.

Fish, D., & Coles, C. (2005). *Medical education: Developing a curriculum for practice.* Maidenhead: Open University Press.

Fish, D., & de Cossart, L. (2007). *Developing the wise doctor: A resource for trainers and trainees in MMC.* London: Royal Society of Medicine Press.

Foster, C. R., Dahill, L., Golemon, L., & Wang Tolentino, B. (2005). *Educating clergy: Teaching practices and pastoral imagination.* San Francisco: Jossey-Bass.

Frank, A. W. (2004). *The renewal of generosity: Illness, medicine and how to live.* Chicago: University of Chicago Press.

Gadamer, H.-G. (1989). *Truth and method* (J. Weinsheimer & D. G. Marshall, Trans. 2nd revised ed.). New York: Continuum.

Gadamer, H.-G. (1996). *The enigma of health* (J. Gaiger & N. Walker, Trans.). Stanford: Stanford University Press.

Gates, A., & Higgs, J. (2013). Realising wise practitioners: Through lifelong practice-based education. In J. Higgs, D. Sheehan, J. Baldry Currens, W. Letts, & G. Jensen (Eds.), *Realising exemplary practice-based education* (pp. 43-56). Rotterdam, the Netherlands: Sense.

Hutchings, M., & Loftus, S. (2013). Practice-based education outside the workplace: Simulations, role plays and problem-based learning. In J. Higgs, R. Barnett, S. Billett, M. Hutchings & F. Trede (Eds.), *Practice-based education: Perspectives and strategies* (pp. 161-174). Rotterdam: Sense.

Kemmis, S., & Smith, T. J. (2008). Personal praxis: Learning through experience. In S. Kemmis & T. J. Smith (Eds.), *Enabling praxis: Challenges for education* (pp. 17-35). Rotterdam: Sense.

Livingston, E. H., & McNutt, R. A. (2011). The hazards of evidence-based medicine: Assessing variation in care. *Journal of the American Medical Association, 306*(7), 762-763.

Loftus, S. (2010). Exploring communities of practice: Landscapes, boundaries and identities. In J. Higgs, D. Fish, I. Goulter, S. Loftus, J.-A. Reid & F. Trede (Eds.), *Education for future practice* (pp. 41-50). Rotterdam: Sense.

Loftus, S. (2012). Rethinking clinical reasoning: Time for a dialogical turn. *Medical Education, 46*(12), 1174-1178. doi: 10.1111/j.1365-2923.2012.04353.x.

Loftus, S., & Greenhalgh, T. (2010). Towards a narrative mode of practice. In J. Higgs, D. Fish, I. Goulter, S. Loftus, J.-A. Reid & F. Trede (Eds.), *Education for future practice* (pp. 85-94). Rotterdam, The Netherlands: Sense.

Moerman, D. (2002). *Meaning, medicine and the placebo effect.* Cambridge: Cambridge University Press.

Montgomery, K. (2006). *How doctors think: Clinical judgment and the practice of medicine.* Oxford: Oxford University Press.

Nevo, I., & Slonim-Nevo, V. (2011). The myth of evidence-based practice: Towards evidence informed practice. *British Journal of Social Work, 41*(6), 1176-1197.

Sackett, D. L., Richardson, S. W., Rosenberg, W., & Haynes, R. B. (Eds.). (1996). *Evidence-based medicine: How to practice and teach EBM.* New York: Churchill Livingstone.

Sullivan, W. M., & Rosin, M. S. (2008). *A new agenda for higher education: Shaping a life of the mind for practice.* San Francisco: Jossey-Bass.

Svenaeus, F. (2000). *The hermeneutics of medicine and the phenomenology of health: Steps towards a philosophy of medical practice.* Dordrecht: Kluwer Academic.

Titchen, A., & Higgs, J. (2001). Towards professional artistry and creativity in practice. In J. Higgs & A. Titchen (Eds.), *Professional practice in health, education and the creative arts* (pp. 273-290). Oxford: Blackwell Science.

Verghese, A. (2008). Culture shock: Patient as icon, icon as patient. *New England Journal of Medicine, 359*(26), 2748-2750.

Walker, G. E., Golde, C. M., Jones, L., Conklin Bueschel, A., & Hutchings, P. (2008). *The formation of scholars: Rethinking doctoral education for the twenty-first century.* San Francisco: Jossey-Bass.

Wenger, E. (1998). *Communities of practice: Learning meaning and identity.* Cambridge: Cambridge University Press.

Stephen Loftus PhD
The Education For Practice Institute
Charles Sturt University, Australia

Joy Higgs AM PhD
The Education For Practice Institute
Charles Sturt University, Australia

CONTRIBUTORS

Edwina Adams BAppSc, MAppSc, PhD
The Education For Practice Institute
Charles Sturt University, Australia

Rola Ajjawi BAppSc(Physiotherapy) Hons, PhD
Medical Education Institute
University of Dundee, Scotland
Adjunct Senior Lecturer, The Education For Practice Institute, Charles Sturt
University, Australia

Hugh Barr MPhil PhD
Emeritus Professor, University of Westminster, UK
President, The UK Centre for the Advancement of Interprofessional Education

Peter Hani Tawfik Cosman BA, MB,BS, PhD, FRACS
School of Medicine
The University of Western Sydney, Australia

Anaise Cottrell BIntStud, LLB(Hons), GDLP
School of Medicine
Flinders University, Australia

Julia Coyle MManipPhys., PhD
School of Community Health
Charles Sturt University, Australia

Alma Dender PhD Candidate, DipEd, B.Sc. (Occupational Therapy)
School of Occupational Therapy and Social Work
Curtin University of Technology, Australia

Marcia Devlin BA, DipEd, Grad Dip Appld Psych, MEd, PhD
Open Universities Australia

Elaine Duffy RN, RM, DipAppSc(CHN),BAppSc(AdvNsg),MN, PhD, FRCNA
School of Nursing and Midwifery
Griffith University, Australia
Adjunct Professor, Charles Sturt University, Australia

CONTRIBUTORS

Dawn Forman PhD MBA PG Dip Research PG Dip Executive Coaching MDCR
TDCR
Curtin Health Innovation Research Institute
Faculty of Health Sciences
Curtin University of Technology, Australia

Kirsty Foster PhD
Sydney Medical School
The University of Sydney, Australia

Susan Furness Dip Hlth Sc Nursing, Dip Amb Para, Grad Dip Emerg Health,
MHSc
La Trobe Rural Health School
La Trobe University, Australia

Janet Gerzina RT
Specialist Magnetic Radiation Imaging
Royal Prince Alfred Medical Centre, Australia

Tania Gerzina PhD
Faculty of Dentistry
The University of Sydney, Australia
Adjunct Associate Professor, The Education For Practice Institute, Charles Sturt
University, Australia

Nigel Gribble MBA, B.Sc. (Occupational Therapy) (Hons)
School of Occupational Therapy and Social Work
Curtin University of Technology, Australia

Joy Higgs AM BSc MHPEd PhD
The Education For Practice Institute
The Research Institute For Professional Practice, Learning & Education
Charles Sturt University, Australia

Belinda Kenny BAppSc(SpPath)PhD
Speech Pathology
The University of Sydney, Australia

Mike Keppell PhD
Australian Digital Futures Institute
University of Southern Queensland, Australia

Andrew Kilgour PhD candidate
Faculty of Health Sciences
The University of Sydney, Australia

Helen Larkin BApp Sc (OT),MAppSc, Grad Dip Health Admin, Grad Cert Higher
Education
School of Health and Social Development, Faculty of Health
Deakin University, Australia

Tracy Levett-Jones RN PhD
The School of Nursing and Midwifery
The University of Newcastle, Australia

Melinda J. Lewis BAppSc (MRA) MHlthScEd (Syd)
Faculty of Nursing & Midwifery & Sydney e-learning
The University of Sydney, Australia

Michelle Lincoln PhD
Faculty of Health Sciences
The University of Sydney, Australia

Iris Lindemann BSc, BNutDiet, MEd, APD
School of Medicine
Flinders University, Australia

Stephen Loftus PhD
The Education For Practice Institute
Charles Sturt University, Australia

Patricia Logan PhD
The School of Biomedical Sciences
Charles Sturt University, Australia

Claire Macrae BMSc (Hons), PGCE
Medical Education Institute
University of Dundee, Scotland

Sue McAllister PhD
School of Medicine
Flinders University, Australia

Patricia McCabe BAppSc(SpPath), PhD
Speech Pathology
The University of Sydney, Australia

Anthony McKenzie BA, DipEd, MSc(Hons)
The Education For Practice Institute
Charles Sturt University, Australia

CONTRIBUTORS

Graham Munro MHSM, BHSc, CCP
School of Biomedical Sciences
Charles Sturt University, Australia

Peter O'Meara BHA, MPP, PhD
La Trobe Rural Health School
La Trobe University, Australia

Narelle Patton BAppSc(Phty), MHSc, PhD Candidate
School of Community Health
Charles Sturt University, Australia

David Prideaux Dip T (Prim), BA (Hons), MEd, PhD
School of Medicine
Flinders University, Australia

Wayne (Colin) Rigby RN, BSW, MHSc(PHC)
Clinical Leader Rehab
Mental Health
Murrumbidgee Central, Australia

Chris Roberts MBChB MRCGP MMedSci PhD
Charles Perkins Centre
The University of Sydney, Australia

Gary D. Rogers MBBS, MGPPsych, PhD
School of Medicine and Health Institute for the Development of Education and
Scholarship (Health IDEAS)
Griffith University, Australia

Doreen Rorrison PhD
School of Teacher Education
Charles Sturt University, Australia

Susie Schofield BSc (Hons), PGCE, MSc, PhD
Medical Education Institute
University of Dundee, Scotland

Maree Donna Simpson BPharm BSc (Hons) PhD
School of Biomedical Sciences
Charles Sturt University, Australia

Megan Smith BAppSc (Phty), PhD
Faculty of Science
Charles Sturt University, Australia

Olanrewaju Sorinola PhD Candidate
Faculty of Medicine
University of Warwick, UK

Teresa Swirski PhD
The Education For Practice Institute
Charles Sturt University, Australia

Jill Thistlethwaite PhD
School of Medicine
University of Queensland, Australia

Mary-Helen Ward BA, MA(Hons), MPhil
Sydney e-learning
The University of Sydney, Australia

Sandra West RN BSc, PhD
Faculty of Nursing and Midwifery
The University of Sydney, Australia